Anaesthesia for Patients with Endocrine Disease

Anaesthesia for Patients with Endocrine Disease

Edited by

MFM James

Department of Anaesthesia, University of Cape Town, South Africa
Groote Schuur Hospital, Cape Town, South Africa

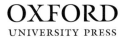

OXFORD
UNIVERSITY PRESS

UNIVERSITY PRESS

Great Clarendon Street, Oxford OX2 6DP

Oxford University Press is a department of the University of Oxford.
It furthers the University's objective of excellence in research, scholarship,
and education by publishing worldwide in

Oxford New York

Auckland Cape Town Dar es Salaam Hong Kong Karachi
Kuala Lumpur Madrid Melbourne Mexico City Nairobi
New Delhi Shanghai Taipei Toronto

With offices in

Argentina Austria Brazil Chile Czech Republic France Greece
Guatemala Hungary Italy Japan Poland Portugal Singapore
South Korea Switzerland Thailand Turkey Ukraine Vietnam

Oxford is a registered trade mark of Oxford University Press
in the UK and in certain other countries

Published in the United States
by Oxford University Press Inc., New York

© Oxford University Press, 2010

The moral rights of the authors have been asserted
Database right Oxford University Press (maker)

First published 2010

British Library Cataloguing in Publication Data
Data available

Library of Congress Cataloging-in-Publication Data
Anaesthesia for patients with endocrine disease / edited by M. F. M. James.
      p. ; cm.
  Includes bibliographical references and index.
  ISBN 978-0-19-957025-6 (alk. paper)
  1. Endocrine glands—Surgery—Complications. 2. Anesthesia. I. James,
Michael F. M. [DNLM: 1. Anesthesia—methods. 2. Endocrine System Diseases—surgery.
3. Endocrine System Diseases—complications. 4. Endocrine System
Diseases—physiopathology. WK 148 A532 2010]
  RD599.A53 2010
  617.9'6744—dc22

                                                           2010011179

Typeset in Minion by Glyph International, Bangalore, India
Printed in Great Britain by the MPG Books Group, Bodmin and King's Lynn

ISBN 978–0–19–957025–6

10 9 8 7 6 5 4 3 2 1

Preface

Apart from diabetes mellitus, endocrine diseases requiring surgical treatment are relatively uncommon. However, when they occur, they frequently present major clinical anaesthetic problems that require extensive knowledge of the pathophysiology of the underlying condition and considerable anaesthetic expertise. The purpose of this book is to provide the practising specialist in anaesthesia with a ready reference for the underlying pathophysiological problems presented by each of the endocrine conditions and to offer guidance as to optimal anaesthetic care. Inevitably, given the relative infrequency of endocrine problems, many of the recommendations presented in this book are based on accumulated knowledge and experience rather than firm evidence. The authors contributing to this publication have substantial experience in the field, and have applied their practical knowledge as well as their understanding of the literature to the development of sound clinical recommendations.

The book covers a range of endocrine diseases, commencing with an overview of the function of the endocrine system followed by detailed discussions of each area. A number of endocrine conditions, particularly those affecting reproductive physiology, will not be dealt with as these present no special anaesthetic problems.

Diabetes mellitus is the most common endocrine challenge presented to anaesthetists, and extensive coverage has been given to this particular problem by one of the leading experts in the field, dealing with the various approaches to the anaesthetic management of these patients. Secreting endocrine tumours provide major anaesthetic challenges and these have been dealt with in a systematic fashion. Section authors have provided a detailed description of the pathophysiology of the diseases of their particular organ system together with recommendations for clinical practice that are evidence based as far as is possible. There is a concluding section to each chapter consisting of around two pages summarizing the major features of the disease process and outlining a suggested anaesthetic approach. A section on endocrine emergencies has been included, covering the spectrum of urgent conditions in the endocrine field that the clinical anaesthetist may encounter. The concept is that these sections will provide a 'ready reference' for the anaesthetist faced with a rare but challenging problem. In addition, we have presented recent evidence on the use of endocrine substances as pharmacological agents and a chapter on surgery for endocrine conditions to give the clinician an understanding of the surgical approaches and considerations.

We trust that this book will provide a valuable resource for the practical clinical management of these intriguing and challenging clinical problems.

Contents

Contributors

John GT Augoustides
Associate Professor, Cardiovascular and
Thoracic Anesthesiology and Critical
Care, Department of Anesthesiology and
Critical Care, University of Pennsylvania
School of Medicine, USA

Anis S Baraka
Professor of Anesthesiology, American
University of Beirut, Beirut, Lebanon

Insung Chung
Senior Resident in Cardiac Anesthesiology
and Critical Care, Department of
Anesthesiology and Critical Care,
University of Pennsylvania School of
Medicine, Philadelphia, PA, USA

Joel Dave
Department of Medicine, University of
Cape Town, Faculty of Health Sciences,
Cape Town, South Africa

PA Farling
Royal Victoria Hospital, Belfast, UK

MFM James
Department of Anaesthesia, University of
Cape Town, and Groote Schuur Hospital,
Cape Town, South Africa

Tom R Kurzawinski
Consultant Endocrine and Pancreatic
Surgeon, Centre for Endocrine Surgery,
University College London Hospitals,
Royal Free Hospital, and Great Ormond
Street Hospital for Children, London, UK

Naomi Levitt
Department of Medicine, University of
Cape Town Faculty of Health Sciences,
Cape Town, South Africa

Jeffrey J Pasternak
Assistant Professor of Anesthesiology,
Mayo Clinic College of Medicine,
Rochester, MN, USA

Prakash Patel
Senior Resident in Cardiac Anesthesiology
and Critical Care, Department of
Anesthesiology and Critical Care,
University of Pennsylvania School of
Medicine, Philadelphia, PA, USA

Philipp Riss
Section of Endocrine Surgery, Division of
General Surgery, Department of Surgery,
Medical University Vienna, Vienna,
Austria

Ian Ross
Department of Medicine, University of
Cape Town Faculty of Health Sciences,
Cape Town, South Africa

WJ Russell
Department of Anaesthesia, Royal
Adelaide Hospital, Adelaide, Australia

Eva Schaden
Department of Anaesthesia, General
Intensive Care, and Pain Management,
Medical University Vienna, Vienna,
Austria

John W Sear
Nuffield Department of Anaesthetics,
University of Oxford, UK

JA Silversides
Specialty Registrar in Anaesthesia and
Intensive Care Medicine,
Royal Victoria Hospital,
Belfast, UK

Christian K Spiss
Department of Anaesthesia, General
Intensive Care, and Pain Management,
Medical University Vienna, Vienna,
Austria

Abbreviations and Acronyms

5-HIAA	5-hydroxy-indole acetic acid		GH	growth hormone
ACC	adrenocortical carcinoma		GHRH	GH-releasing hormone
ACCM	American College of Critical Care Medicine		GIP	glucose-dependent insulinotrophic polypepetide, gastric inhibitory peptide
ACE	angiotensin-converting enzyme		GLP-1	glucagon-like peptide 1
ACTH	adrenocorticotrophic hormone		GnRH	gonadotrophin-releasing hormone
ADA	American Diabetes Association		HbA1C	glycated haemoglobin
ADH	antidiuretic hormone		hCG	human chorionic gonadotrophin
ALP	alkaline phosphatase		HHS	hyperglycaemic hyperosmolar state
APUD	amine precursor uptake and decarboxylation		HPA	hypothalamic–pituitary–adrenal
ARB	angiotensin receptor blocker		HPLC	high-pressure liquid chromatography
ARDS	adult respiratory distress syndrome		HRE	hormone-response element
ATP	adenosine triphosphate		iCa	ionized calcium
ATPase	adenosine triphosphatase		ICP	intra-cranial pressure
AUC	area under the curve		ICRH	insulin counter-regulatory hormone
AVP	arginine vasopressin		ICU	intensive care unit
BMI	body mass index		IGF	insulin-like growth factor
BP	binding protein		IL	interleukin
CAD	coronary artery disease		ILGF	insulin-like growth factor
cAMP	cyclic adenosine-3',5'-monophosphate		IP$_3$	inositoltriphosphate
CaR	calcium-sensing receptor		kDa	kilodalton(s)
CBG	cortisol-binding globulin		LA	laparoscopic adrenelectomy
CI	confidence interval		LAR	long-acting release
CIRCI	critical-illness-related corticosteroid insufficiency		LH	luteinizing hormone
CoA	coenzyme A		LMA	laryngeal mask airway
COMT	catechol-O-methyl transferase		MAO	monoamine oxidase
CPB	cardiopulmonary bypass		MEN	multiple endocrine neoplasia
CRH	corticotrophin-releasing hormone		MIBG	meta-iodo-benzylguanethidine
CT	computed tomography		MRI	magnetic resonance imaging
DDAVP	1-desamino-8-ᴅ-arginine vasopressin		NE	noradrenaline
DHPG	dihydroxyphenylglycol		NET	neuroendocrine tumour
DI	diabetes insipidus		NNT	number needed to treat
DKA	diabetic ketoacidosis		NR	nuclear receptor
DPP-IV	peptidase dipeptidyl peptidase IV		ODF	osteoclast differentiating factor
FFA	free fatty acid		OR	odds ratio
FSH	follicle-stimulating hormone		PA	primary aldosteronism
GFR	glomerular filtration rate		PEEP	positive end-expiratory pressure
			PFK	phosphofructokinase

PHPT	primary hyperparathyroidism	RXR	retinoid-X-receptor
PNET	pancreatic neuroendocrine tumour	SHBG	sex-hormone-binding globulin
PNMT	phenylethanolamine-*N*-methyl transferase	SIADH	syndrome of inappropriate antidiuretic hormone secretion
POMC	pro-opiomelanocortin	SSTR	somatostatin receptor
PONV	post-operative nausea and vomiting	STATs	signal transducers and activators of transcription
PPAR	peroxisome proliferator-activated receptor	T_3	tri-iodothyronine
PTH	parathyroid hormone	T_4	thyroxine
PZI	insulin zinc suspension	TNF-α	tumour necrosis factor α
RFA	radiofrequency ablation	TRPC	transient receptor potential operated type C channels
RHPT	renal hyperparathyroidism		
RLN	recurrent laryngeal nerve	TSH	thyroid-stimulating hormone
rT_3	reverse tri-iodothyronine	VMA	vanillylmandelic acid

Chapter 1

Basic endocrine concepts in health and critical illness

Naomi Levitt, Ian Ross, and Joel Dave

The endocrine and nervous systems are primarily responsible for the flow of information between different cells and tissues and, by so doing, regulate many functions of the body. The disciplines of cellular and molecular biology have enabled a much greater appreciation of the intricacies of the endocrine system than was available prior to the last few decades, but the basic principles which underpin its function remain unchanged.

In this chapter we provide a brief overview of the physiology of the endocrine system, the endocrine response to stress, and endocrine dysfunctions associated with critical illness.

Endocrine signals

Hormones have classically been defined as chemical substances released by specific cells in endocrine glands which enter the bloodstream and act on receptors on distant target tissues to regulate some function. In addition, certain organs not traditionally viewed as endocrine glands, such as the heart and kidneys, have the potential to synthesize and release hormones. Hormones may also act in a number of ways other than the traditional view of their action, i.e. following their release and transport into the circulation. Selected hormones can act on a receptor on the surface of the same endocrine cell (autocrine), act on a receptor within the same endocrine cell (intracrine), remain within the cell membrane of the same cell and act on a receptor on a juxtaposed cell (juxtacrine), or act on a receptor on a neighbouring non-endocrine cell (paracrine).[1] Certain hormones may act in more than one way. For example, insulin may have an autocrine action (i.e. it is able to inhibit its own release by pancreatic β-cells) in addition to the more distant effects following binding to insulin receptors on target tissues.[2] Insulin-like growth factor-1(IGF-1) has both endocrine and paracrine effects by virtue of its actions after release into the circulation from the liver in response to growth hormone (GH) and its control of cellular proliferation in multiple tissues after its local release (e.g. in bone).[3]

Structure and synthesis of hormones

Most hormones are derived from larger molecules such as proteins or lipids and therefore can be grouped as large proteins, glycoproteins, peptides or peptide derivatives,

Table 1.1 Basic structures of hormones with examples

Derivation	Examples
Large proteins	Insulin
	Parathyroid hormone (PTH)
Glycoproteins	Luteinizing hormone (LH)
	Thyroid-stimulating hormone (TSH)
	Follicle-stimulating hormone (FSH)
	Human chorionic gonadotrophin (hCG)
Peptides or peptide derivatives	Gonadotrophin-releasing hormone (GnRH)
	Thyrotrophin-releasing hormone (TRH)
	Somatostatin
	Vasopressin
Amino acid derivatives	Thyroid hormone (T_4, T_3)
	Catecholamines
Lipids	Steroid hormones
	Vitamin D
	Eicosanoids

or lipids (Table 1.1).[4,5] Some hormone families share a common structure and exhibit a degree of cross-reactivity at their receptors. Examples of hormones demonstrating cross-reactivity are the insulin–IGF family and the parathyroid hormone (PTH)–PTH-related peptide (PTHrP) family.[6] Although members of the glycoprotein hormone family (luteinizing hormone (LH), follicle-stimulating hormone (FSH), thyroid-stimulating hormone (TSH), and human chorionic gonadotrophin (hCG)) share a common α-subunit, the distinct β-subunit confers a specific function on each of these hormones.

The peptide hormones are synthesized following a series of steps which include transcription, post-transcriptional processing, and translation, whereas most of the lipid-containing hormones are synthesized by the modification of cholesterol (see Chapter 7 for steroid hormone synthetic pathways). Many of the hormones are derived from the synthesis of larger inactive precursor polypeptides (e.g. adrenocorticotrophic hormone (ACTH) from proopiomelanocortin (POMC), insulin from pro-insulin, and glucagon from pro-glucagon), which require cleavage by proteases for their activation.[7] A pro-sequence in these inactive hormones is recognized by the cell as a secretory signal, which is the precursor to the release and secretion of an active hormone. During translocation through various intra-cytoplasmic organelles (Golgi apparatus and endoplasmic reticulum), some hormones (e.g. TSH, FSH, and LH) undergo post-translational modification including: glycosylation and phosphorylation. Some hormones are critically dependent on specific enzymes for synthesis. For example, thyroid peroxidase coordinates the iodination of tyrosine residues in thyroglobulin to produce thyroid hormone (Chapter 4) and tyrosine hydroxylase catalyses the formation of L-dihydroxyphenylalanine (L-dopa) from tyrosine, which is the initial step in the synthesis of catecholamines (Chapter 8).

Secretion and transport of hormones

Polypeptide hormones are classically released via vesicle-mediated secretion.[5,7] These secretory vesicles reside below the plasma membrane and release pre-formed hormone when a specific signal (releasing factor, neural signal, or other) stimulates fusion of the vesicles with the plasma membrane. Some non-polypeptide hormones, such as catecholamines, are also secreted in this way. In contrast, steroid hormones are released into the circulation immediately after synthesis, but it is uncertain whether this takes place by simple diffusion or is mediated by specific transporters.

Following secretion into the circulation most hormones are transported bound to serum-binding proteins. For example, thyroxine (T_4) and tri-iodothyronine (T_3)) are bound to thyroxine-binding globulin, albumin, and thyroxine-binding pre-albumin,[8] androgens and oestrogen bind to sex-hormone-binding globulin (SHBG), and cortisol binds to cortisol-binding globulin (CBG).[1,7] The liver is the site of synthesis of many of the carrier proteins and their concentrations are affected by a number of conditions such as cirrhosis, obesity, and severe illness. These carrier proteins ensure a constant reservoir of hormone by preventing or limiting degradation. Binding proteins may restrict access of hormone to certain sites and help modulate the unbound 'free' fraction of the hormone. Physiologically, this is important as it is the 'free' fraction that is mostly available for biological action.[9]

Action of hormones

The 'free' fraction of a hormone exerts a biological action by binding to a specific receptor on a target tissue. In the case of polypeptide hormones, the receptor is located on the membrane of the target cell, whereas for lipid-derived hormones, the receptor is located intracellularly and in the nucleus.[5,10,11] Each membrane receptor (Figure 1.1) activates a specific intracellular signalling molecule. These receptor-signalling molecule combinations can be divided into four major groups:

- **G-protein coupled receptors** These receptors have seven transmembrane domains, an α-subunit, a β-subunit, and a γ-subunit. Ligand binding induces the dissociation of the α-subunit from the $\beta\gamma$-subunit which then mediates signal transduction via adenylate cyclase activation (Gsα stimulates and Giα inhibits) of cyclic adenosine-3',5'-monophosphate (cAMP) and protein kinase A or phospholipase C (Gqα), and activation of diacylglycerol and inositol triphosphate (IP$_3$). IP$_3$ activates ryanodine receptors on the endoplasmic reticulum to stimulate the release of calcium. Most polypeptide hormones act via these G-protein-coupled receptors to increase production of adenylate cyclase (LH, FSH, TSH, catecholamines, PTH, ACTH) or phospholipase C (TSH, PTH).

- **Tyrosine kinase receptors** These receptors have a single transmembrane domain, an extracellular ligand-binding domain, and an intracellular tyrosine kinase catalytic domain. Ligand binding induces dimerization of the receptor which then induces autophosphorylation of the intracellular tyrosine kinase catalytic domain. This domain

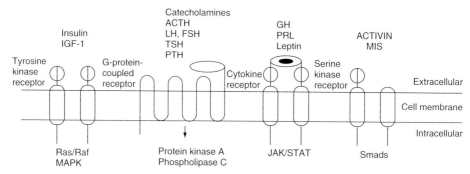

Fig. 1.1 Hormone receptors and subcellular signalling molecules. From left: tyrosine kinase receptors with a single transmembrane domain. G-protein-coupled receptors have seven transmembrane domains, and α-, β-, and γ-subunits. Cytokine receptors resemble tyrosine kinase receptors, but lack inherent tyrosine kinase activity. Serine kinase receptors have type I and type II subunits.

undergoes a conformational change and is then capable of phosphorylating other downstream proteins. Insulin and various growth factors use this type of receptor.

- **Cytokine receptors** These receptors resemble tyrosine kinase receptors, but do not have inherent tyrosine kinase activity. Rather, ligand binding activates a tyrosine kinase from the Janus family (JAK1–3, TYK2). The cytokine receptor–JAK complex then recruits signalling molecules, including signal transducers and activators of transcription (STATs). Once activated, the STATs bind to specific sequences in the promoter region of cytokine-responsive genes. GH, prolactin, and leptin bind to this receptor.

- **Serine kinase receptors** These receptors have type I and type II subunits and signal through the activation of Smads (fusion of terms for *Caenorhabditis elegans* sma + mammalian mad).[5] Activins and Müllerian-inhibiting substance use these receptors.

Hormones derived from lipids (e.g. cortisol, sex steroids, and aldosterone as well as thyroid hormones) gain access to intracellular nuclear receptors (Figure 1.2) by passive diffusion across the cell membrane or through active transport by a membrane transport protein. Once inside the cell, the hormone is transported to the nucleus where it binds with high affinity to the carboxy-terminal domain (ligand-binding domain) of its nuclear receptor (NR). Nuclear receptors can be grouped into two major subtypes: the steroid receptor family (e.g. glucocorticoid receptor, mineralocorticoid receptor, androgen receptor) and the thyroid receptor family (e.g. thyroid hormone receptor, oestrogen receptor, vitamin D receptor, retinoic acid receptor).[5,10,11] There are also many 'orphan receptors' for which the ligand is unknown. The central DNA-binding domain of the nuclear receptor mediates binding to a hormone-response element (HRE), usually situated upstream of the promoter region of a specific gene. Both the ligand-binding domain and the DNA-binding domain mediate dimerization with the same NR or the retinoid-X-receptor (RXR) prior to binding to the HRE. Once bound to the HRE the

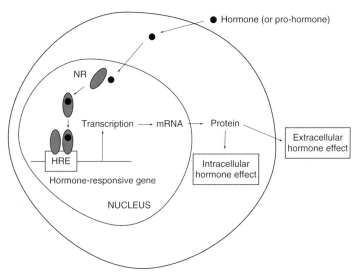

Fig. 1.2 Nuclear-stimulating hormones gain access to intracellular nuclear receptors by passive diffusion across the cell membrane or through active transport by a membrane transport protein. Once bound to the relevant receptors, these hormones mediate gene activation, producing a cellular response. Adapted from Kronenberg H, Melmed S, Larsen P, Polonsky K (2003). Principles of endocrinology. In: Larsen P, Kronenberg H, Melmed S, Polonsky K (eds), *Williams Textbook of Endocrinology*, 10th edn. WB Saunders, Philadelphia, PA. © Elsevier (2003) with permission.

H–NR complex mediates gene activation; repression of transcription or negative regulation of transcription may occur.

Regulation of hormones

Maintenance of circulating hormone concentrations within a required range which permits normal physiological function is ensured by regulating the rate of production, delivery to target tissues, clearance, and degradation. Production is the most highly regulated of these processes and control is exerted at multiple levels. Most peptide hormones have a short half-life, usually a few minutes (e.g. insulin and ACTH). However, the glycosylated glycoproteins, such as hCG, are more stable and have a half-life of hours.

Positive feedback control of hormonal synthesis and release is poorly understood. However, the negative feedback mechanisms which regulate most of the important hypothalamic–pituitary axes and certain additional hormonal systems are better known.[1] In addition, a great deal of cross-talk exists across the traditional hormonal axes. A few examples of negative feedback control are as follows: thyroid hormones inhibit the release of TRH and TSH, cortisol inhibits the release of corticotrophin-releasing hormone (CRH) and ACTH (Chapter 7), gonadal steroids inhibit the release of GnRH, LH, and FSH, calcium inhibits the release of PTH (Chapter 5), and glucose inhibits the release of insulin.[1,4]

Hormonal systems are also regulated by various environmental factors, such as seasonal changes, sleep, nutritional changes, day–night cycle, systemic illness, and stress, facilitating appropriate adaptation to the environment. Most pituitary hormones exhibit a circadian rhythm ensuring a peak of hormone at times when there is greatest demand, as illustrated by the peak secretion of ACTH and cortisol which occurs early in the morning. This rhythm is repeated every 24 hours, but may be influenced by alterations in the sleep–wake cycle. Several pituitary hormones (e.g. FSH and LH) are released in a pulsatile fashion throughout the day in response to altered GnRH frequency. Specific central nervous system input and inherent properties of certain endocrine cells dictate to what extent the pulsatility may be influenced.

The role of endocrinology in the stress response

Critical illness is characterized by profound dysregulation of the endocrine system which appears to occur in a biphasic manner, i.e. an early acute phase and a later prolonged phase.[12] It is important that the anaesthetist has some knowledge of the physiology of the endocrine response to stress and its disorders, which they may encounter in perioperative and critically ill patients. These may occur in all hypothalamic–anterior pituitary– end-organ axes, not exclusively in the hypothalamic–pituitary–adrenal (HPA) axis, and may manifest with, *inter alia*, stress hyperglycaemia.

The endocrine system is an essential part of the body's response when exposed to stressors which threaten dynamic equilibrium or homeostasis. Once activated, the stress system induces behavioural and physical changes in order to enhance the chances of survival. The behavioural adaptation includes increased alertness and arousal, improved cognition and attention span, analgesia, and inhibition of appetite and reproduction. The physical changes are primarily orchestrated to promote adequate redirection of energy. Initially the redirection of blood flow conveys oxygen and nutrients to the heart, brain, lungs, and skeletal muscle, and away from the gut, liver, and kidneys, thereby facilitating recovery and healing. However, activation of the adaptive processes of the stress response depends on the stressor exceeding a threshold of severity or duration or both, whilst the possible outcomes are threefold: a perfect match with restoration of homeostasis, an inadequate response, or an exaggerated response, the last two of which may result in a diminished chance of survival.[13,14]

The neuroendocrine effectors of the stress response are found in the hypothalamus, brainstem, peripheral limbs of the HPA axis, the efferent sympathetic adrenomedullary system, and the parasympathetic system (Figure 1.3). The major peripheral effectors are glucocorticoids, adrenaline, and noradrenaline, while the respective central effectors include CRH and arginine vasopressin (AVP) released from the hypothalamus. Some of the total pool of noradrenaline is produced in the brainstem. The central components of the stress system have multiple interactions; for example, CRH and noradrenergic neurons of the central stress system function synergistically. The central and peripheral components of the autonomic nervous system play critical roles in the stress response. The resultant haemodynamic and metabolic changes found during the stress response

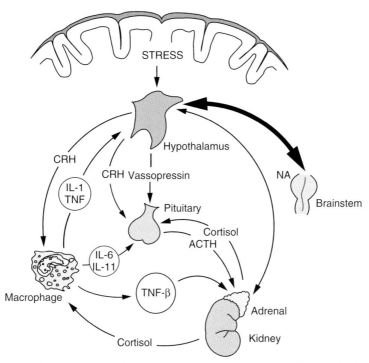

Fig. 1.3 Hormonal components of the stress response: CRH, corticotrophin releasing hormone; IL, interleukin; TNF, tumour necrosis factor; ACTH, adrenocorticotrophic hormone; NE, noradrenaline. Adapted from Marik PE (2009). Critical illness-related corticosteroid insufficiency. *Chest*, **135**, 181–93, with permission.

are: redirection of blood flow, an increased heart rate and cardiac output, and an increased rate of metabolism, with hyperglycaemia and increased biolysis through inhibition of insulin secretion and stimulation of hormone-sensitive lipase.

Hypothalamic–pituitary–adrenal axis

CRH is the most important regulator of ACTH release, but it acts in synergy with AVP to exert control on the pituitary–adrenal axis. Under non-stressful conditions, the release of CRH and AVP occurs in a circadian pulsatile fashion, with the greatest amplitude found in the early hours of the morning. Acute stress results in a marked increase of periventricular nuclei CRH and AVP pulsatile release into the portal circulation of the pituitary gland and subsequent stimulation of peptides derived from POMC. These include ACTH, the opioid peptide β-endorphin, and α-melanocyte-stimulating hormone. ACTH then stimulates the synthesis of cortisol from the adrenal cortex. Depending on the magnitude of the stressor, additional factors, such as various cytokines (tumour necrosis factor α (TNF-α) and interleukins 6 and 1(IL-6 and IL-1)), angiotensin II, and lipid mediators of inflammation, may be secreted into the circulation in order to enhance the HPA stress response. IL-6 is the major immune stimulator of the HPA axis. Cortisol regulates the secretion of CRH, AVP, and ACTH through its well-known negative feedback actions in the hypothalamus to inhibit the synthesis and secretion of CRH and AVP, and in the anterior pituitary gland where corticotrophs become less responsive to CRH and AVP. The net result of this negative feedback is that it places a limit on tissue exposure to cortisol, curtailing an excessive metabolic, cardiovascular, and immune response in times of stress.

If the stress response is short lived, it will induce very few adverse consequences. On the other hand, prolonged stress will result in higher levels of CRH and glucocorticoid secretion. Examples of conditions associated with increased HPA activity include chronic stress, anorexia nervosa, malnutrition, panic disorder, alcohol withdrawal, increased visceral adiposity, reduced lean body mass, and reduced osteoblastic activity, similar to the phenotype of Cushing's syndrome. Insulin resistance *per se* may be a manifestation of the prolonged stress response as gluconeogenesis is increased.[13-15] The degree to which an individual responds to a given stress may be determined by genetic polymorphisms of CRH and AVP, and their receptors and regulators. It is believed that an individual's vulnerability to stress is accounted for by multiple genes.

Critical illness adrenal insufficiency

The endocrine changes in critical illness are summarized in Table 1.2. In the early stages of critical illness, cortisol levels increase through a rise in CRF and ACTH secretion, but the diurnal rhythm is lost. Concurrently, cortisol-binding globulin (CBG), which binds 90% of cortisol, declines by as much as 50%, resulting in a significantly greater portion of free cortisol than in health. Cortisol is a particularly important stress hormone because of its stimulation of gluconeogenesis, inhibition of glucose uptake in the adipose tissue, and lipolysis. It also has a permissive effect on catecholamines and glucagon essential for normal cardiovascular reactivity, cardiac contractility, vascular tone, and blood pressure.

Adrenal insufficiency is becoming increasingly recognized among critically ill patients. The reported incidence of critical-illness-related corticosteroid insufficiency (CIRCI) varies widely, from zero to 77%, because of differences in the criteria used for diagnosis, as well as in the patient groups included. An incidence as high as 65% has been found in patients with septic shock and up to 20% in medical intensive care unit (ICU) patients.[16,17] CIRCI can be defined as inadequate corticosteroid activity for the severity for the patient's illness and differs from Addison's disease or chronic adrenal insufficiency. A small number of patients with apparent CIRCI may actually have structural damage to the adrenal glands caused by haemorrhage, infarction, or blunt trauma, which may result in permanent adrenocortical dysfunction. However, in the vast majority of cases, critically ill patients develop reversible dysfunction of the HPA axis. This is manifested by a decreased production of cortisol and/or ACTH and may be associated with tissue resistance to cortisol because of abnormalities of the glucocorticoid receptor. A variety of factors have been suggested to play a role in the pathogenesis of CIRCI. For example, TNF-α impairs both ACTH secretion and action on the adrenal glands, yet TNF-α and IL-1 reduce glucocorticoid receptor transcription and expression. A fall in cortisol production may also be caused by a lack of high-density lipoprotein (HDL), which is the major

Table 1.2 Overview of the neuroendocrine changes in critical illness

	Hormone	Acute phase	Prolonged phase
1.	Growth hormone–IGF-1 axis		
	Pulsatile GH release	↑	↓
	IGF-1	↓	↓↓
	IGFBP-3	↓	↓↓
2.	Thyroid axis		
	Pulsatile TRH release	↑≡	↓
	T_4	↑≡	↓
	T_3	↓	↓↓
	rT3	↑	↑≡
3.	Gonadal axis		
	Pulsatile LH release	↑≡	↓
	Testosterone/oestradiol	↓	↓↓
4.	Adrenal axis		
	Corticotrophin	↑	↓
	Cortisol	↑↑	↑≡↓
	CBG	↑	≡
5.	Lactotrophic axis		
	Pulsatile PRL release	↑	↓

↑, increase in circulating levels; ↓, decrease in circulating levels; ≡, return to normal circulating levels.

Adapted from Langouche L, Van den Berghe G (2006). The dynamic neuroendocrine response to critical illness. *Endocrinology and Metabolism Clinics of North America* **35** 777–91.

substrate required for cortisol synthesis. The most significant result of corticosteroid insufficiency in critically ill patients, frequently affecting outcome, is an excessive systemic inflammatory response with overproduction of pro-inflammatory mediators such as NF-κβ.

CIRCI should be considered in all patients admitted to the ICU requiring vasopressor support. The following specific features may also suggest the presence of CIRCI: hypotension resistant to fluids, eosinophilia, and mild hypoglycaemia. A number of non-specific features may also be observed, such as unexplained fever, unexplained mental changes, anaemia, and, in particular, a hyperdynamic circulation (see also Chapter 10). In contradistinction to chronic adrenal insufficiency (Addison's disease), hyponatraemia and hyperkalaemia are uncommon.

As controversy surrounds the diagnosis of CIRCI, an international task force of the American College of Critical Care Medicine was established to examine the evidence for the diagnostic criteria. An increment of less than 248 nmol/L of cortisol following a 250 μg ACTH stimulation test or a random plasma cortisol of less than 276 nmol/L was considered to be compatible with CIRCI, based on available evidence to be the most robust diagnostic criteria.[18]

Hydrocortisone should be considered in the management strategy of patients with septic shock, particularly those who respond inadequately to fluid resuscitation vasopressor agents. If CIRCI is suspected, hydrocortisone doses of 200–300 mg per day should be administered for at least 7 days up to a maximum of 14 days, followed by a gradual wean. The management of septic shock with steroids is controversial, as the benefits in mortality are not clear. On the other hand, glucocorticoids resulted in shorter duration of ventilation and reduced mortality in five randomized studies of patients with adult respiratory distress syndrome (ARDS). Nevertheless, it should be considered that adverse effects of steroids may occur, particularly myopathy and super-infection.[18]

The thyroid axis

Stress also has a major impact on the thyroid axis, and therefore changes in thyroid function are commonly encountered in patients with critical illness. It is important for the practising anaesthetist to be cognisant of these changes, as failure to recognize the sick euthyroid syndrome may result in erroneous and potentially hazardous administration of therapy.

It is widely appreciated that thyroid hormone has ubiquitous actions on growth, normal physiological functions, and metabolism. The hypothalamic TRH controls the release of TSH, which in turn stimulates the thyroid gland release of thyroxine (T_4). Conversion of the pro-hormone T_4 to the metabolically active hormone tri-iodothyronine (T_3) occurs in the periphery. T_3 may undergo conversion to the inactive metabolite reverse T_3 (rT_3). This conversion occurs at a very low level in health (Chapter 4).

Within 2 hours of the onset of acute stress, circulating levels of T_3 decline and those of rT_3 increase, accompanied by a short-lived rise in T_4 and TSH levels. An altered feedback mechanism is indicated by the finding that TSH levels return to normal when the T_3 levels remain low and the normal nocturnal TSH surge is lost. This is known as the low T_3 syndrome, and the extent of fall in T_3 is a function of the severity of the stress or illness. When the stress or critical illness is prolonged and severe, low levels of both T_4 and T_3 may be noted, together with inappropriately normal TSH concentrations. In some individuals T_3 may be extremely low or even undetectable. Reduced TRH gene expression and an impaired ability to secrete TSH may partly explain this condition. Moreover, peripheral metabolism of T_4 to T_3 is compromised as type 1 deiodinase is reduced while the action of type 3 deiodinase is increased, resulting in enhanced conversion of T_4 to inactive rT_3. It is reasonable to assume that tissue concentrations of T_4 and T_3 are also low, resulting in upregulation of thyroid hormone receptors. The recognition that low levels of T_3 frequently coexist with critical illness poses the question as to whether these changes are adaptive or protective in response to a hypercatabolic state. Administration of T_4 in these circumstances has not been associated with any clinical benefit, although the lack of endogenous conversion to T_3 may have contributed to the lack of success. However, the fact that administration of T_3 has failed to demonstrate any benefit in prolonged critical illness supports the notion that these changes in the thyroid axis are protective.[12,19]

The growth hormone axis

Growth hormone (GH), whch is secreted by the pituitary somatotrophin cells, exerts its indirect effects on growth, for example, via IGF-1, whose effect is in turn controlled by a number of binding proteins, the IGF binding proteins (IGF-BPs). Stress has a major effect on the growth axis, acting at multiple levels. Acutely, there is an increase in GH secretion caused by a rise in its pulse frequency as well as high peak and trough levels resulting from enhanced stimulation of the GH gene by a rapid rise in circulating glucocorticoids. The high levels of the circulating cytokines IL-6 and TNF-α induce a degree of peripheral GH resistance, corroborated by the finding that IGF-I levels are frequently reduced. Consequently anabolism, mediated primarily by IGF-1 (teleologically not required when survival is threatened), is inhibited whilst the non IGF-1-mediated GH effects on metabolism, such as stimulation of lipolysis, are enhanced.

In contrast, prolonged stress leads to the reduction of GH secretion through inhibition of its pulsatile secretion and low levels of both IGF-1 and its most important GH-dependent carrier protein, IGF-BP3. Hypothalamic dysfunction with defective secretion or action of GH secretogogues is thought to be responsible for these findings, which may play a part in the wasting that occurs with prolonged stress. In extreme emotional deprivation, GH is also inhibited by prolonged excess levels of glucocorticoids, and these individuals may manifest with profound short stature.[12,13,20]

The gonadal axis

Pulsatile hypothalamic GnRH release is necessary for the stimulation of LH and FSH from the pituitary gonadotrophs. In men, at the gonadal level, LH stimulates the synthesis and secretion of androgens which, in concert with FSH, induces spermatogenesis. In women, LH causes ovarian androgen production and FSH is responsible for the aromatization of androgens to oestrogen. In turn, these sex steroids exert a negative feedback action on both GnRH at the level of the hypothalamus and the pituitary gland, inhibiting FSH and LH.

The stress response mediated by an increase in glucocorticoids inhibits all levels of the reproductive axis. CRH suppresses GnRH through a paracrine effect at the level of the hypothalamus, and glucocorticoids not only inhibit GnRH, but also inhibit the pituitary gonadotrophic cells and the gonads, and render the targets of the sex steroids resistant to their actions. Cytokines produced during inflammatory stress also suppress reproductive function at the hypothalamic and gonadal levels in tandem with glucocorticoids. In acute illness there is a fall in testosterone levels and a rise in LH, but prolonged critical illness suppresses LH concentrations, resulting in low levels of testosterone in men and oestradiol in women. Elite athletes of both sexes often display elevated levels of cortisol and reduced gonadal function.[12,13]

Prolactin levels are high following acute stress, and its secretion is blunted during prolonged critical illness. There is uncertainty as to whether the suppressed prolactin levels contribute to increased susceptibility to infection during the prolonged phase of critical illness.[12]

Stress hyperglycaemia

There is profound alteration in glucose metabolism during stress.[21–23] The development of stress hyperglycaemia occurs as a consequence of activation of counter-regulatory hormones, such as glucagon, catecholamines, and cortisol. These result in enhanced gluconeogenesis and subsequent increased hepatic glucose output into the circulation. Simultaneously, cytokines (e.g. IL-1 and IL-6) promote insulin resistance. The liver is thought to be the major site of insulin resistance in this context, and the enhanced hepatic glucose output is the major contributor to the hyperglycaemia observed. Interestingly, overall glucose uptake in insulin-independent tissues (e.g. red blood cells, wounds, and brain) is increased during critical illness, but this is offset because insulin-stimulated glucose intake by muscle and heart is reduced. Hyperglycaemia has a number of deleterious effects, including increasing the generation of free oxygen radicals with resultant oxidative stress and altered vascular reactivity, formation of micro-thrombi and altered organ perfusion, reducing chemotaxis and phagocytosis, and thus compromising immune function, and impairment of fluid balance, and as a consequence a worse outcome of morbidity and mortality can be expected.

Hyperglycaemia is a frequent feature in patients with acute or critical illness. This hyperglycaemia may occur naturally in those with a prior diagnosis of diabetes, in which case the degree of hyperglycaemia may be worse than might be expected for their usual degree of glycaemic control, or it may reflect pre-existing undiagnosed diabetes or stress hyperglycaemia, defined as transient hyperglycaemia with return to normal glucose tolerance after discharge. The relative contributions of these two conditions to the number of patients not known to be diabetic who have hyperglycaemia in the acute setting will be dependent on the background prevalence of diabetes in the population. Thus in a country or population with low diabetes prevalence, the majority of cases are likely to turn out to be stress hyperglycaemia, while the reverse will hold if the background prevalence and numbers of undiagnosed cases of diabetes are high.

In the acute setting it may be difficult to differentiate between the two conditions. Theoretically, an elevated glycated haemoglobin (HBA1c) which reflects glycaemic control over a 2–3 month period would be of assistance, but there is considerable debate currently as to whether this test can be used as a diagnostic test for diabetes. Moreover, even if HBA1c is accepted as a diagnostic test with a cut-off of >6.5%, there may be additional factors which may affect the validity of its measurement during critical illness; for example, changes of red cell turnover, such as major blood loss or blood transfusions, will lead to spurious HbA1C results, and haemoglobin traits, such as HbS, HbC, HbF, and HbE, will interfere with some A1C assay methods.[24]

The initial enthusiasm for the use of intensive insulin therapy in critically ill patients in the ICU[23] has been tempered by recent studies demonstrating that it actually increases the risk of hypoglycaemia significantly, without mortality benefit.[22,25–27] Therefore this form of therapy may not be currently justified, but if used, it must be done cautiously to ensure that hypoglycaemia is prevented. Moderate glycaemic control, aiming at glucose concentrations between 6 and 10 mmol/L may be more appropriate than tight glucose control with a target range of 4.5–6 mmol/L.

References

1. Kronenberg H, Melmed S, Larsen P, Polonsky K (2003). Principles of endocrinology. In: Larsen P, Kronenberg H, Melmed S, Polonsky K (eds), *Williams Textbook of Endocrinology*, 10th edn. WB Saunders, Philadelphia, PA.
2. Cheatham B, Kahn CR (1995). Insulin action and the insulin signaling network. *Endocrine Reviews*, **16**, 117–42.
3. Jones JI, Clemmons DR (1995). Insulin-like growth factors and their binding proteins: biological actions. *Endocrine Reviews*, **16**, 3–34.
4. Baxter J, Ribeiro R, Webb P (2004). Introduction to endocrinology. In: Greenspan F, Gardner D (eds), *Basic and Clinical Endocrinology*, 7th edn. McGraw-Hill, New York.
5. Jameson JL (2005). Principles of endocrinology. In: Kasper DL, Braunwald E, Fauci AS, Hauser S, Longo D, Jameson JL (eds), *Harrison's Principles of Internal Medicine*, 16th edn. McGraw-Hill, New York.
6. Strewler GJ (2000). The physiology of parathyroid hormone-related protein. *New England Journal of Medicine*, **342**, 177–85.
7. Lingappa V, Mellon S (2004). Hormone synthesis and release. In: Greenspan F, Gardner D (eds), *Basic and Clinical Endocrinology*, 7th edn. McGraw-Hill, New York.
8. Mendel CM, Weisiger RA, Jones AL, Cavalieri RR (1987). Thyroid hormone-binding proteins in plasma facilitate uniform distribution of thyroxine within tissues: a perfused rat liver study. *Endocrinology*, **120**, 1742–9.
9. Mendel CM (1989). The free hormone hypothesis: a physiologically based mathematical model. *Endocrine Reviews*, **10**, 232–74.
10. Lazar M (2003). Mechanism of action of hormones that act on nuclear receptors. In: Larsen P, Kronenberg H, Melmed S, Polonsky K (eds), *Williams Textbook of Endocrinology*, 10th edn. WB Saunders, Philadelphia, PA.
11. Gardner D, Nissenson R (2004). Mechanisms of hormone action. In: Greenspan F, Gardner D (eds), *Basic and Clinical Endocrinology*, 7th edn. McGraw-Hill, New York.
12. Langouche L, Van den Berghe G (2006). The dynamic neuroendocrine response to critical illness. *Endocrinology and Metabolism Clinics of North America*, **35**, 777–91.
13. Charmandari E, Tsigos C, Chrousos G (2005). Endocrinology of the stress response. *Annual Review of Physiology*, **67**, 259–84.
14. Chrousos GP (2007). Organization and integration of the endocrine system. *Sleep Medicine Clinics*, **2**, 125–45.
15. Chrousos GP (2009). Stress and disorders of the stress system. *Nature Reviews. Endocrinology*, **5**, 374–81.
16. Marik PE (2007). Mechanisms and clinical consequences of critical illness associated adrenal insufficiency. *Current Opinion in Critical Care*, **13**, 363–9.
17. Annane D, Maxime V, Ibrahim F, Alvarez JC, Abe E, Boudou P (2006). Diagnosis of adrenal insufficiency in severe sepsis and septic shock. *American Journal of Respiratory and Critical Care Medicine*, **174**, 1319–26.
18. Marik PE, Pastores SM, Annane D, *et al.* (2008). Recommendations for the diagnosis and management of corticosteroid insufficiency in critically ill adult patients: consensus statements from

an international task force by the American College of Critical Care Medicine. *Critical Care Medicine*, **36**, 1937–49.

19. Mebis L, Debaveye Y, Visser TJ, Van den Berghe G (2006). Changes within the thyroid axis during the course of critical illness. *Endocrinology and Metabolism Clinics of North America*, **35**, 807–21.

20. Mesotten D, Van den Berghe G (2006). Changes within the growth hormone/insulin-like growth factor I/IGF binding protein axis during critical illness. *Endocrinology and Metabolism Clinics of North America*, **35**, 793–805.

21. Annetta MG, Ciancia M, Soave M, Proietti R (2006). Diabetic and nondiabetic hyperglycemia in the ICU. *Current Anaesthesia and Critical Care*, **17**, 385–90.

22. Dungan KM, Braithwaite SS, Preiser JC (2009). Stress hyperglycaemia. *Lancet*, **373**, 1798–1807.

23. Vanhorebeek I, Van den Berghe G (2009). Diabetes of injury: novel insights. *Endocrinology and Metabolism Clinics of North America*, **35**, 859–72.

24. Nathan DM, Balkau B, Bonora E, *et al.* (2009). International Expert Committee report on the role of the A1C assay in the diagnosis of diabetes. *Diabetes Care*, **32**, 1327–34.

25. Finfer S, Chittock DR, Su SY, *et al.* (2009). Intensive versus conventional glucose control in critically ill patients. *New England Journal of Medicine*, **360**, 1283–97.

26. Preiser JC (2009). NICE-SUGAR: the end of a sweet dream? *Critical Care*, **13**, 143.

27. Van den Berghe G, Schetz M, Vlasselaers D, *et al.* (2009). Clinical review: intensive insulin therapy in critically ill patients: NICE-SUGAR or Leuven blood glucose target? *Journal of Clinical Endocrinology and Metabolism*, **94**, 3163–70.

Chapter 2

The pituitary gland

Jeffrey J Pasternak

Introduction

The pituitary gland, also known as the 'master gland', is under the control of the hypoth-alamus and secretes a variety of substances which either have direct effects on tissues or control the regulation of other endocrine substances. The normal functions of a plethora of biological processes and organs depend on the pituitary gland. Consequently, the dys-function of even a subset of normal pituitary functions can have broad-ranging manifes-tations in the organism as a whole.

This chapter will address normal pituitary anatomy and physiology, pathophysiology, and issues pertaining to the pre-operative care of patients with disorders affecting the pituitary gland. Surgery for pituitary tumours will then be reviewed. Cushing's disease will be addressed in Chapter 6.

Anatomical relationships and physiology of the pituitary gland

The cross-sectional diameter of the normal pituitary gland is approximately 8–10 mm. It is located within the sella turcica, a region encompassing a mere 600 mm^3 of space within the sphenoid bone inferior to the hypothalamus (Figure 2.1). Lateral to the pitui-tary gland is the cavernous sinus which contains a plexus of veins and the carotid artery, in addition to the oculomotor (III), trochlear (IV), abducens (VI), and ophthalmic (V$_1$), and maxillary (V$_2$) branches of the trigeminal nerve. The distance between the carotid artery and the pituitary gland is 2–7 mm in an adult. The stalk of the pituitary gland extends superiorly, through an orifice in the diaphragm sella, to join the hypothalamus and comes in close proximity to the optic chiasm.

The basic structure of the pituitary gland strongly reflects upon its ontogeny. The gland consists of two major regions—the anterior region, or adenohypophysis, and the posterior region, or neurohypophysis. The adenohypophysis arises from ectodermal tissue derived from Rathke's pouch, a depression in the roof of the developing mouth. The neurohypo-physis develops as a direct extension of neural mesodermal tissue. As a result, the anterior and posterior portions of the pituitary gland are structurally and functionally different.

The adenohypophysis consists of both secretory and non-secretory cells (i.e. null cells). Each secretory cell synthesizes, stores, and secretes a hormone in response to hormones secreted by the hypothalamus (Table 2.1). The most common cell type is the

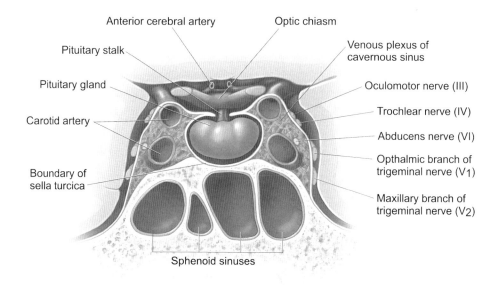

Fig. 2.1 Coronal section of the sella turcica demonstrating the anatomical relationship between the pituitary gland and the cranial nerves, carotid arteries, and cavernous and sphenoid sinuses. Copyrighted and used with permission of Mayo Foundation for Medical Education and Research, all rights reserved.

Table 2.1 Hypothalamic hormones and adrenohypophyseal responses

Hypothalamic hormone	Pituitary cell target	Pituitary response	Overall effect
Corticotrophin-releasing hormone (CRH)	Corticotrophs	Increased production of adrenocorticotrophic hormone (ACTH)	Increased production of cortisol by the adrenal gland
Thyrotrophin-releasing hormone (TRH)	Thyrotrophs	Increased production of thyroid-stimulating hormone	Increased production of T3 and T4 by the thyroid gland
Gonadotrophin-releasing hormone (GnRH)	Gonadotrophs	Increased production of follicle-stimulating hormone (FSH) and luteinizing hormone (LH)	Regulates oestrogen, progesterone, testosterone, and inhibin production by gonads
Growth-hormone-releasing hormone (GHRH)	Somatotrophs	Increased production of growth hormone	Increased production of insulin-like growth factor
Somatostatin	Somatotrophs	Decreased production of growth hormone	Decreased production of insulin-like growth factor
Prolactin-releasing factor	Lactotrophs	Increased production of prolactin	Lactation
Dopamine	Lactotrophs	Decreased production of prolactin	Inhibition of lactation

somatotroph, which secretes growth hormone (GH). Approximately 50% of the cells of the normal anterior pituitary gland are somatotrophs. Other cell types include cortico-trophs (which secrete adrenocorticotrophic hormone (ACTH)), lactotrophs (which secrete prolactin), and gonadotrophs (of which there are two subgroups, one secreting follicle-stimulating hormone (FSH) and the other secreting luteinizing hormone (LH)). The least common cell types found in the anterior pituitary gland, each accounting for less than 5% of the cells, are the thyrotrophs (which secrete thyroid-stimulating hormone (TSH)) and the null cells, which are non-secretory.

Hypothalamic hormones are released into a capillary bed supplied by afferent arterioles (Figure 2.2). These hypothalamic capillaries give rise to tributaries of portal vessels which then form a second capillary bed within the adenohypophysis. Hypothalamic hormones are released into the adenohypophysis proper where they stimulate or inhibit the

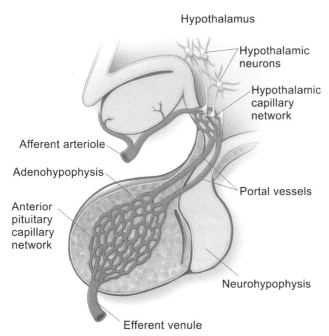

Fig. 2.2 Physiology of the adenohypophysis. Afferent arterioles enter the hypothalamus where hypothalamic neurons secrete hormone into the circulation. Blood then leaves the hypothalamus via portal vessels and enters the adenohypophysis (i.e. anterior pituitary gland) where the hypothalamic hormones enter a second capillary network and act upon adenohypophyseal cells, thus regulating the secretion of hormones. Hormones produced by the adenohypophysis enter the capillary network and hence the systemic circulation by the efferent venule. The advantage of a portal system is that it allows low volumes of hypothalamic hormones to be secreted since their concentration will be much higher in the portal vessels than in the systemic circulation. This also allows rapid regulation of hormone secretion by the adenohypophysis. Copyrighted and used with permission of Mayo Foundation for Medical Education and Research, all rights reserved.

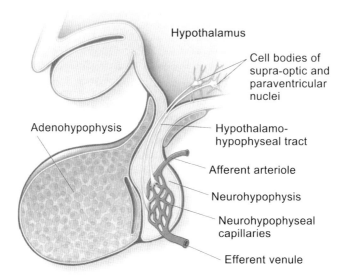

Fig. 2.3 Physiology of the neurohypophysis. The axons of neurons located in the supra-optic and paraventricular nuclei of the hypothalamus extend via the hypothalamo-hypophysial tract to the neurohypophysis. When stimulated, these neurons secrete either oxytocin or vasopressin into the capillary network of the neurohypophysis. Copyrighted and used with permission of Mayo Foundation for Medical Education and Research, all rights reserved.

secretion of hormones by the cells of the adenohypophysis. The hormones produced by the adenohypophysis are released into the capillary network and enter the systemic circulation. The advantage of such a portal system allows strict control of adenohypophyseal hormone secretion, as small amounts of hypothalamic hormones need be produced since the concentrations of hypothalamic hormone within the portal vessels supplying the adenohypophysis greatly exceed those found in the systemic circulation.

The neurohypophysis consists mostly of unmyelinated axons in addition to fenestrated capillaries and glial cells. The cell bodies of these neuronal axons are located in the supra-optic and paraventricular nuclei of the hypothalamus (Figure 2.3). These neurons synthesize, store, and secrete either oxytocin or vasopressin, along with the carrier protein neurophysin, into the capillary network of the neurohypophysis.

Tumours of the pituitary gland

Symptomatic tumours of the pituitary gland are rare, with an estimate annual incidence of 2 per 100,000 per year. However, pituitary tumours are reported in 14% of autopsies and as an incidental finding in 23% of radiological studies performed for unrelated reasons.[1] Pituitary tumours are the most common reason for primary pituitary gland dysfunction in adults. Resection of pituitary adenomas represents approximately 20% of all intracranial neurosurgical procedures.[2] Given the diverse functions of the pituitary gland, diseases affecting this structure can have far-reaching systemic implications. In caring for patients with pituitary gland diseases in the peri-operative period, the clinician must be aware of these implications.

A very wide array of tumour pathologies can affect the pituitary gland. The majority of pituitary tumours are adenomas, which comprise about 85% of all pituitary tumours.[3] Approximately 55% of adenomas are manifested by the hypersecretion of one, or rarely more than one, hormone. The remaining 45% of adenomas produce clinical signs and symptoms due to compression of either normal gland (resulting in decreased hormone production) or structures adjacent to the sella turcica. Other tumour types include craniopharyngiomas (3.2%), meningiomas (1%), tumours which have metastasized to the pituitary gland (0.6%), and primary pituitary carcinoma (0.1%). Although very rare, even astrocytomas, sarcomas, haemangiomas, and hamartomas, have been known to affect the pituitary gland.

Pituitary adenomas are typically composed of a single cell type derived from the adenohypophysis. A pituitary adenoma, along with parathyroid hyperplasia and islet cell tumours of the pancreas (typically insulinomas), is found in patients with multiple endocrine neoplasia type 1 (MEN 1, Wermer's syndrome). Tumours derived from cell types which secrete a specific hormone will typically manifest with clinical signs reflecting inappropriate excess hormone production. Rarely, some tumours secrete multiple hormones, the most common combination being GH and prolactin. Signs and symptoms of excessive hormone production usually allow the offending adenoma to come to attention earlier, when the tumour is much smaller, than those derived from non-secreting cell lines where signs and symptoms result from increasing tumour size and compression of surrounding structures. Therefore pituitary tumours were classically divided based on the diameter at the time of diagnosis into micro-adenomas (<1 cm) and macro-adenomas (>1 cm). Most clinically diagnosed micro-adenomas are hormone-secreting tumours, and most macro-adenomas are non-secreting tumours. However, this relationship between tumour size at the time of diagnosis and tumour type does not always hold true. Therefore a more current classification system for pituitary tumours is based on excessive hormone production such that tumours are classified as either functional (i.e. hormone secreting) or non-functional.

In addition to endocrine manifestations, pituitary tumours can cause signs and symptoms from compression of surrounding structures commensurate with the tumour volume breaching the confines of the sella turcica. Typically, these tumours are derived from either non-secreting cells (i.e. null cells) or a cell type which may not produce overt clinical hormonal disturbances such as cells which produce either FSH or LH, especially in males. Extension superiorly can result in compression of the optic chiasm (Figure 2.4). Contained within the optic chiasm are afferent neurons from the medial retina. As the tumour grows from the inferiorly located sella turcica, chiasmic compression progresses superiorly such that disruption of axons from the inferior retina are typically affected first, resulting in a bitemporal superior quadrantanopia in which there is loss of the

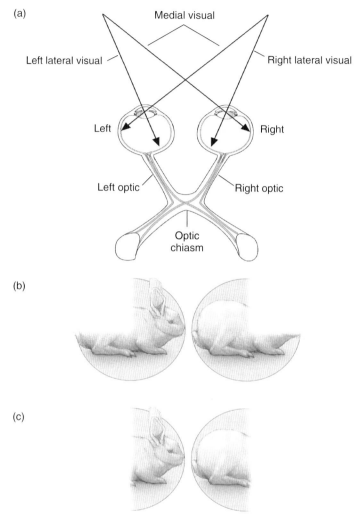

Fig. 2.4 Visual fields. (a) Light from the left and right lateral (or temporal) visual fields strikes the left and right medial regions of the retina, respectively. Afferent neurons originating from the medial regions of the retina cross in the optic chiasm. Injury to the optic chiasm results in dysfunction of these neurons and thus loss of the lateral visual fields. Early in the course of enlargement of the contents of the sella turcia, axons located within the inferior portion of the optic chiasm are compressed. These axons carry information from the inferiomedial bilateral retinas and visual information from the superiolateral visual fields resulting in loss of the superiolateral quadrants of the visual field (i.e. bitemporal superior quadrantanopia). Later, as all axons within the optic chiasm become compressed, full loss of the lateral visual fields occurs (i.e. bitemporal hemianopia). (b) Bitemporal superior quadrantanopia. (c) Bitemporal hemianopia. Copyrighted and used with permission of Mayo Foundation for Medical Education and Research, all rights reserved.

superior lateral visual fields. Later, complete inhibition of these pathways results in loss of the lateral visual fields (i.e. bitemporal hemianopia). Further superior extension can result in obstruction of cerebrospinal fluid flow, typically by impingement upon the third ventricle, resulting in obstructive hydrocephalus. Likewise, lateral extension leads to invasion of the cavernous sinus and can result in dysfunction of the cranial nerves that traverse the cavernous sinus or compression of the carotid artery.[4]

Growth hormone excess

GH is a 191 amino acid polypeptide which is normally secreted by the somatotrophs of the anterior pituitary. Secretion is under hypothalamic control via at least two hormones, GH-releasing hormone (GHRH) and somatostatin, which stimulate and inhibit GH production, respectively. GH exerts its effect via interaction with a specific GH receptor and target cells. Systemic actions of GH are quite diverse (Figure 2.5). GH directly stimulates chondrocyte proliferation, muscle sarcomere hyperplasia, bone mineralization,

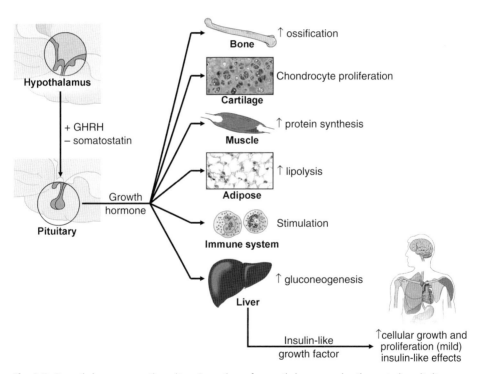

Fig. 2.5 Growth hormone action sites. Secretion of growth hormone by the anterior pituitary gland is regulated by the hypothalamus. Hypothalamic secretion of growth-hormone-releasing hormone (GHRH) and somatostatin serve to stimulate and inhibit, respectively, the secretion of growth hormone. Growth hormone receptors are quite diverse. In the liver, growth hormone stimulates the secretion of somatomedin C, which is also known as insulin-like growth factor. Copyrighted and used with permission of Mayo Foundation for Medical Education and Research, all rights reserved.

and protein synthesis, and thus stimulates the growth of all internal organs except the brain. Proliferation of chondrocytes and subsequent mineralization of the epiphyseal growth plates in children and adolescents results in growth of long bones. GH also directly reduces hepatic glucose uptake, upregulates hepatic gluconeogenesis, and directly stimulates hepatic production of insulin-like growth factor 1 (ILGF-1), formerly known as somatomedin C. However, ILGF-1 is also produced in the target tissues of GH such that it acts in an endocrine and paracrine manner. ILGF-1 is one of the most potent stimulators of cell growth and proliferation, affecting almost all cells of the body.

The clinical manifestations of GH excess depend on the ossification state of epiphyseal plates in bones. Specifically, GH excess results in gigantism if the epiphyseal chondrocytes are still active and acromegaly when the epiphyseal cartilage has ossified. Although they are classified as different disorders, gigantism and acromegaly are manifestations of the same disorder and share most of the same characteristics. Further, if gigantism is not controlled, with the passage of adolescence patients with gigantism continue to develop similar characteristic to those with acromegaly.

The estimated incidence of acromegaly is 3–4 cases per million per year.[5] Gigantism is quite rare, with about 100 cases reported to date.[6] Approximately 95% of patients with GH excess (i.e. acromegaly or gigantism) harbour a growth-hormone-secreting pituitary adenoma. The remaining 5% of cases are due to production of GH at extra-pituitary sites, such as: intramesenteric islet cell tumours, non-Hodgkin's lymphoma, or hypothalamic tumours, or from residual ectopic pituitary remnants in surrounding structures such as the nasal cavity and sphenoid sinus.[7] GH excess can also be associated with a variety of genetic aberrations such as MEN 1, McCune–Albright syndrome, and the Carney complex.

The clinical manifestations of GH excess are widespread in view of the ubiquitousness of GH receptors on most cell types. Bone and soft tissue changes associated with acromegaly include growth of hands and feet such that patients may initially notice an increase in ring, glove, or shoe size. Patients with acromegaly develop characteristic coarse facial features due to excessive bone hypertrophy and prognathism. Airway manifestations include a thick tongue and hypertrophy of the tonsils, epiglottis, and larynx. This makes the presence of obstructive sleep apnoea common in this population and also leads to difficulty with mask fit and visualization of the larynx for tracheal intubation. Difficult direct laryngoscopy is three times more common in patients with acromegaly than in patients with other types of pituitary tumour.[8] Further factors which can complicate airway management include an increased incidence of vocal cord dysfunction secondary to stretching of the recurrent laryngeal nerve from soft tissue enlargement and impaired mobility of the crico-arytenoid joints. Sleep apnoea occurs in up to 70% of patients with acromegaly and is due to both anatomical airway changes and centrally mediated depression of respiratory drive.[9]

The cardiovascular system is often affected by GH excess. Cardiovascular issues account for most deaths from untreated acromegaly. Hypertension is observed in half of patients; the cause is probably multifactorial. The development of cardiac hypertrophy is probably due to a combination of GH-induced sarcomeric hypertrophy and a response to increased afterload secondary to hypertension. Left ventricular hypertrophy can be observed even in normotensive acromegalic patients. Classic cardiac findings include diastolic dysfunction with preserved systolic function at rest; however, left ventricular ejection fraction may not increase appropriately with stress.[10,11] Patients also typically exhibit arrhythmias and electrocardiographic abnormalities.[12] Coronary arterial insufficiency is related to increased oxygen demand by the hypertrophied ventricle and a reduction of diastolic blood flow due to diastolic myocardial dysfunction.

Peripheral neuropathies are common in patients with acromegaly: carpal tunnel syndrome occurs in up to 64% and 80% have abnormal nerve conduction studies.[13] The aetiology is probably multifactorial, and clinical symptoms may result from a combination of oedema of the nerve proper and demyelination.[14] The origins of this oedema and demyelination remain obscure.

Other endocrine and metabolic disturbances are found in acromegalics. Because of GH-enhanced hepatic gluconeogenesis, glucose intolerance or diabetes mellitus can occur despite hyperinsulinaemia. About 30% of patients with acromegaly also have coexisting hyperprolactinaemia, since somatotrophic and mammotrophic cells of the pituitary gland are thought to arise from the same stem cell. Finally, with larger tumours, patients may develop signs and symptoms of compression or invasion of neighbouring structures, such as headache or visual changes (i.e. bitemporal hemianopia or superior quadrantanopia), or, rarely, symptoms of increased intracranial pressure (ICP) due to cerebrospinal fluid flow obstruction.

Diagnosis of acromegaly is based on history and physical finding as well as on diagnostic tests. Normal adult serum GH concentrations are typically less than 5 ng/ml. However, because of normal variation in GH secretion, a single GH concentration is often inadequate to make the diagnosis of acromegaly. Because GH production decreases with carbohydrate intake, an oral glucose tolerance test will cause a decrease in serum GH concentration to less than 1 ng/ml within 1–2 hours in patients with normal pituitary function. Nadir concentrations greater than 1 ng/ml are suggestive of acromegaly. Of note, attempted diagnosis using an oral glucose tolerance test can be unreliable in patients with diabetes mellitus, those with hepatic or renal disease, or those receiving oestrogen therapy.[15] Currently, the cut-off for the diagnosis of acromegaly following an oral glucose tolerance test is debated. Some suggest a serum growth hormone cut-off of 0.4 ng/ml to reduce the number of false positives that are identified with the current 1 ng/ml cut-off.[16] Since serum concentrations of ILGF-1, a product of GH action on cells, vary less than those of GH, this makes serum ILGF-1 concentration a possible alternative to GH concentrations for the biochemical diagnosis of acromegaly. However, variability in the current clinical assay and lack of agreement of normal reference ranges for ILGF-1 at the time of publication of this chapter have not allowed accurate chemical diagnosis of acromegaly depending solely on serum ILGF-1 concentrations.[16] Magnetic resonance imaging (MRI) of the pituitary gland often demonstrates the presence of an adenoma.

Surgical resection of well-circumscribed non-invasive adenomas is the mainstay treatment. Cure rates can be as high as 91% for micro-adenomas but is reduced with larger, more invasive tumours.[17] Medical therapy with dopamine agonists (i.e. bromocriptine and carbogerline), somatostatin analogues such as octreotide, and newer GH receptor antagonists such as pegvisomant, as well as radiation therapy, are available for patients who are not surgical candidates or who fail surgical treatment.[16]

Management of anaesthesia for patients with GH excess

Given the diverse organ system involvement of acromegaly and gigantism, peri-operative management of these patients prior to surgery should start with a comprehensive history and physical examination with appropriate testing. A thorough evaluation of the airway should be conducted. Hypertrophy of the mandible and other facial bones makes mask ventilation difficult. This is further complicated by probable airway obstruction from a large tongue, epiglottis, and glottic structures. Mandibular hypertrophy may lead to an increased distance from the lips to the vocal cords. Despite an apparently adequate inter-incisor distance, Mallampati score, and thyromental distance, direct laryngoscopy may still prove difficult because of involvement of the epiglottis and glottis, structures not typically assessed on a pre-operative examination of the airway. The presence of hoarseness or stridor may indicate significant laryngeal or recurrent laryngeal nerve involvement, suggesting that a smaller-diameter tracheal tube may be required. Given these findings, the safest means of placing a tracheal tube is probably by awake fibreoptic intubation during spontaneous ventilation. If tracheal intubation is planned after the induction of anaesthesia, the clinician should consider maintaining spontaneous ventilation. This will avoid the need to mask ventilate with positive pressure, given the likelihood of a poor mask fit or airway obstruction due to enlarged airway structures. Further, a larger laryngoscope blade, other back-up airway equipment, and back-up personnel should be readily available. In patients with acromegaly and gigantism, special attention should be paid to the possible need to deliver larger than normal tidal volumes from the anaesthesia ventilator.

Particular attention should be paid to the cardiovascular system. Assessment of pre-operative control of hypertension may help guide intra- and post-operative blood pressure management. Since electrocardiographic changes and arrhythmias are common, a baseline 12-lead electrocardiogram may prove helpful to detect new-onset changes. Exercise capacity and a history of congestive heart failure should be assessed. In those with congestive heart failure or reduced exercise tolerance, a pre-operative echocardiogram may help to assess the degree of myocardial involvement. Further, a stress test may identify either classic coronary disease or poor oxygen delivery to the myocardium due to small vessel disease which is commonly found in acromegalics. If diastolic dysfunction is present, maintenance of sinus rhythm and the avoidance of hypovolaemia, tachycardia, and bradycardia will help optimize cardiac function. Intra-operative invasive monitoring should be guided by the nature of the surgery and the degree of cardiovascular involvement by acromegaly. Assessment of alterations in blood pressure and cardiac function should continue into the post-operative period.

Given the high incidence of peripheral neuropathies and abnormal nerve conduction in patients with acromegaly, care should be taken to avoid positioning the extremities in a manner that may impact already altered peripheral nerve function. For example, the patient's elbows should remain extended to minimize tension of the ulnar nerve at the elbow. Extension of the hands should also be avoided as this could potentially stretch the ulnar and median nerves. Theoretical concerns of inadequate arterial blood flow and inadequate collateral circulation for the hand were once factors for avoiding radial arterial cannulation. However, subsequent research determined that the radial artery is not contained within the space enclosed by the transverse carpal ligament and carpal bones, and no increased risk of ischaemic complications was identified in a case series of acromegalic patients having radial artery cannulation.[18]

Pre-operative panhypopituitarism may be present with larger adenomas. Patients with panhypopituitarism should receive pre-operative corticosteroids; assessment of thyroid function may also be prudent. Abnormalities in serum calcium and glucose concentration may indicate the presence of MEN 1 and may require treatment in the peri-operative period. Hyperglycaemia may exist because of the actions of GH on hepatic gluconeogenesis and may require peri-operative monitoring and treatment.

Pre- and post-operative assessment for cranial nerve deficits should be conducted. Evidence of elevated ICP, such as the presence of papilloedema, alterations in mental status, or significant hypertension or alterations in heart rate, should be assessed. Patients with pre-operative intracranial hypertension may benefit from treatment prior to surgery. Hypercarbia and hypoxaemia should also be avoided since cerebral vasodilatation, which would ensue, may further exacerbate intracranial hypertension.

As patients with acromegaly and gigantism may have a larger than normal body girth or may be excessively tall, special consideration should be made to assure that the operating table will be sufficiently large to accommodate their atypical body habitus safely.

Given the high incidence of obstructive sleep apnoea, special considerations should be made to manage airway obstruction post-operatively. These patients will require monitoring for hypoxia and apnoea. In those with airway obstruction, continuous positive-pressure ventilation is likely not to be an available option following trans-sphenoidal pituitary surgery, given that elevations of pressure within the airway, and thus the sphenoid sinus, may cause disruption of the surgical site. Other than the use of an orally inserted airway device and adjustment of head position, there are limited non-invasive options available to manage airway obstruction post-operatively. In severe cases, patients may require replacement of the tracheal tube post-operatively and ventilatory assistance until the effects of general anaesthesia have sufficiently dissipated.

Hyperprolactinaemia

Prolactin is a 199 amino acid polypeptide produced by the mammotrophic cells of the adenohypophysis. Although the hypothalamus produces releasing factors which upregulate prolactin secretion, prolactin production is predominantly controlled via hypothalamic dopamine. Dopamine binds to the dopamine D_2 receptor on lactotrophs and results in a suppression of prolactin production.[19] Pregnancy, oestrogen (i.e. in menstruating women), sleep, and exercise cause an increase in serum prolactin concentrations. Prolactin concentrations can also be elevated in renal failure[20] and hypothyroidism[21] owing to reduced clearance. Various pituitary pathologies can lead to an increased serum prolactin concentration; however, a prolactin-producing mammotrophic adenoma is probably the most common pituitary cause. The presence of a non-prolactin-secreting pituitary mass which compresses the stalk and blocks hypothalamic dopamine from reaching the normal mammotrophic cells can also cause an increase in pituitary prolactin production. Factors that lead to hypothalamic dysfunction, such as the presence of eosinophilic granulomas, gliomas, histiocytosis X, or sarcoidosis, can attenuate hypothalamic dopamine secretion and increased prolactin production by a normal pituitary gland. Drugs that decrease dopamine synthesis or function as dopamine receptor antagonists, such as α-methyldopa and phenothiazines, can also cause hyperprolactinaemia.[22,23]

Prolactin receptors are present on a variety of cell types, including breast, liver, prostate, gonads, prostate, lung, myocardium, brain, and lymphocytes. Although prolactin has many important effects in other animals, its effects in humans are limited. Given the diverse differences in the physiological roles of prolactin between lower animals and humans, research on the mechanism of action of prolactin in humans is difficult because of the paucity of useful animal models. Prolactin plays no significant role in breast development in humans; however, it is vital for milk production, which occurs as oestrogen and progesterone concentrations fall after pregnancy while the blood concentration of prolactin remains elevated. Prolactin also modulates reproduction and affects accessory reproductive organs in human males and females. The specific mechanisms of this interaction have not been elucidated, although direct suppression of gonadotrophin-stimulating hormone production by hyperprolactinaemia is believed to play a major role in causing reproductive system dysfunction in both men and women.

Signs of hyperprolactinaemia are more concrete in women and include galactorrhoea, amenorrhoea, and infertility; loss of libido and osteopenia may also be noted. In men, signs and symptoms of hyperprolactinaemia are usually very non-specific, such as decreased libido, impotence due to oligospermia, and erectile dysfunction. Galactorrhoea may also occur in men, but may not be as evident as in women given the smaller amount of breast tissue in men. Therefore prolactin-secreting adenomas have a propensity to be larger in men at the time of diagnosis.[24]

The evaluation of a patient with signs and symptoms of increased prolactin production begins with obtaining a serum prolactin concentration. Normal serum prolactin concentrations are 3–20 ng/ml in women and 3–15 ng/ml in men. Causes other than a pituitary secreting adenoma (i.e. hypothyroidism, renal failure, medications such as antipsychotics, and pituitary stalk compression due to a non-prolactin-secreting tumour) will typically not result in serum prolactin concentrations greater than 150 ng/ml. Therefore a serum prolactin concentration above 150 ng/ml is highly predictive of a prolactin-secreting adenoma. Initial therapy of a prolactinoma involves treatment with a dopamine agonist such as bromocriptine, carbergoline, or pergolide. If pharmacological manage-ment does not produce a decrease in tumour size and control the signs and symptoms of hyperprolactinaemia, or if the patient is unable to tolerate the side-effects associated with medical therapy, surgical treatment is indicated.

Management of anaesthesia in patients with hyperprolactinaemia

The presence of hyperprolactinaemia warrants no specific anaesthetic or peri-operative concerns. However, in patients presenting for surgery, the clinician should not only be aware of consequences of tumour mass and local invasion (i.e. increased ICP, cranial nerve deficits, or intra-operative bleeding due to the close proximity of the sagittal sinus and carotid artery to the pituitary gland), but consider adverse effects related to the drugs used for the medical management of hyperprolactinaemia. Patients with medically controlled hyperprolactinaemia may present for surgery unrelated to their endocrinopathy. Also, patients who have failed medical management may still be using a dopamine agonist or may suffer from longer-term complications of these agents. Common side-effects of dopamine agonists (i.e. bromocriptine, carbergoline, pergoline) include nausea and ortho-static hypotension,[25] both of which can be exacerbated by general anaesthesia. Long-term use of higher-dose carbergolide and pergolide have both been associated with the develop-ment of cardiac valvular lesions.[26–30] Since these valvulopathies resemble those associated with carcinoid syndrome,[26,27,31] and both carbergoline and pergoline, unlike bromocrip-tine, possess serotonin receptor agonist properties, it is believed that the cardiac manifesta-tions associated with the use of carbergoline and pergoline are due to a serotonin-mediated mechanism. Therefore the presence of a murmur or evidence of heart failure should alert the clinician to suspect valvular disease in patients taking these medications.

Pituitary hyperthyroidism (see also Chapter 4)

TSH-secreting tumours are rare, with an overall prevalence of 0.5–2.8% in patients with pituitary tumours.[32,33] TSH-secreting tumours can also co-secrete other hormones such as GH, prolactin, or ACTH; therefore signs and symptoms of acromegaly, hyperpro-lactinaemia, or Cushing's disease may coexist. TSH-secreting tumours are usually large and locally invasive at the time of diagnosis; however, distant metastases are rare. Patients with a TSH-secreting adenoma can present with symptoms of both tumour size (i.e. visual changes, headache, or cranial nerve palsies) and thyroid hormone overproduc-tion (i.e. palpitations, nervousness, heat intolerance, tremor, or arrhythmias). In many circumstances, symptoms of thyroid hormone overproduction occur first and patients undergo treatment for Graves' disease. It is only later, when tumour growth causes signs and symptoms, that a TSH-secreting adenoma is identified. At the time of diagnosis, approximately 60% are locally invasive.[34] A patient presenting with elevated serum concentrations of thyroid hormones (i.e. tri-iodothyronine (T_3) and thyroxine (T_4)) and an elevated or inappropriately normal serum TSH should undergo MRI of the head in search of a pituitary tumour.

Surgical resection is usually the first-line treatment for TSH-secreting pituitary adenomas. However, the percentage of patients who have remission (i.e. absence of tumour upon imaging and biochemical evidence of hypo- or euthyroidism) is at most 50%.[35] Radiation and medical management with antithyroid agents, somatostatin analogues, and β-adrenergic antagonist agents are usually reserved for patients who were not cured with, or are not candidates for, surgery.[36]

Management of anaesthesia in patients with pituitary hyperthyroidism

Unless vision is acutely threatened, tumour resection should commence after the patient is rendered physiologically euthyroid. A somatostatin analogue, such as octreotide, should be considered as a first-line agent in patients with TSH-secreting adenomas prior to surgery. Octreotide is known to reduce TSH production by an adenoma.[37] In adults, octreotide can be initiated at 50 μg injected subcutaneously twice daily and can be increased, as tolerated, to 500 μg three times daily. Control of tachycardia and a reduction of clinical symptoms of hyperthyroidism serve as a useful endpoint for pre-operative optimization. Use of β-antagonist agents, in addition to octreotide, may be helpful in reducing symptoms of hyperthyroidism and the conversion of T_4 to T_3.

As many patients with pituitary hyperthyroidism may have initially been treated for primary hyperthyroidism or Graves' disease with radioactive-iodine-based thyroid ablation or surgical thyroidectomy, some patients may be clinically hypothyroid when they present for pituitary adenoma resection and require thyroid hormone replacement. Hypothyroid patients should continue to receive thyroid hormone supplementation in the peri-operative period.

Intra-operative management is based on an awareness of the impact of the existing endocrinopathy (i.e. hyperthyroidism, hypothyroidism) on clinical management as discussed in Chapter 4. The potential for the intra-operative precipitation of thyroid storm is possible, but unlikely. Invasive arterial blood pressure monitoring may be helpful to avoid extremes of blood pressure or blood pressure lability in non-euthyroid patients. Adequate large-bore intravenous access is necessary, given the high likelihood of tumour invasiveness at the time of diagnosis and the potential for significant, and possibly rapid, bleeding owing to the close proximity of the carotid arteries and venous plexus of the cavernous sinus to invasive tumours.

Gonadotrophin-secreting pituitary tumours

Pituitary gonadotrophs secrete either FSH or LH, and the complex secretory patterns of these hormones represent complex interactions between the hypothalamus, pituitary gland, and peripheral target organs (i.e. ovaries or testes). Dysregulation of the hypothalamic–pituitary–gonadal axis can occur from a wide variety of causes, including genetic disorders, physical or emotional stress, and gonadal or pituitary disorders. Gonadotrophin-secreting pituitary adenomas are common, accounting for a quarter of all pituitary adenomas.[3] Gonadotrophin-secreting tumours potentially may manifest as disorders pertaining to sexual function and reproduction. However, these tumours overwhelmingly present as macro-adenomas with symptoms related to mass effect, and thus peri-operative anaesthetic management will be similar to that of non-secreting pituitary tumours.

Non-secreting pituitary tumours

A wide variety of tumour pathologies, which do not result in overt hormonal hypersecretion, can affect the pituitary gland. In fact, approximately half of pituitary pathologies requiring surgical biopsy or treatment are not associated with hormonal hypersecretion.[3] The majority of non-functioning pituitary tumours are adenomas consisting of either chromophobe (i.e. non-staining, non-hormone-producing 'null cells') or gonadotrophin-secreting cells without overt endocrinological manifestations. Other common masses include craniopharyngiomas, cysts, and meningiomas. Most non-functioning pituitary masses become symptomatic because of their growth and compression of surrounding structures, and they are often larger than their hormone-secreting counterparts at the time of diagnosis. Common signs and symptoms include headache, visual changes, cranial nerve deficits, and hypopituitarism. Headaches are often bifrontal or bitemporal and are due to direct pressure on surrounding structures, such as the diaphragm sella, or to obstruction of cerebrospinal fluid resulting in increased ICP. Papilloedema, nausea, and vomiting may occur. With compression of the optic chiasm, visual changes can occur and will often manifest as loss of visual fields. Bitemporal hemianopia is the classic finding, and occurs because of compression of the afferent axons originating in the medial portion of the retina, which is responsible for the lateral visual fields (see Figure 2.4). Complete loss of the lateral visual fields is usually a later finding because upward extension of the growing pituitary mass will typically result in dysfunction of the more inferior axons within the chiasm, resulting in the loss of the superior lateral visual field quadrants (i.e. bitemporal superior quadrantinopia) earlier in the course of tumour growth. Cranial nerve dysfunction is often due to infiltration of the sagittal sinus, which contains cranial nerves III, IV, V, and VI. The most common symptom of cranial nerve compression is diplopia due to dysfunction of the extra-ocular muscles.

Management of anaesthesia in patients with non-secreting pituitary tumours

Since non-functioning pituitary masses are usually large at the time of diagnosis, the likelihood of invasion of surrounding structure, and the existence of both increased ICP and hypopituitarism, is greater than for adenomas which secrete GH, ACTH, or prolactin. Pituitary imaging (e.g. with MRI) should be evaluated for the presence of tumour invasion of surrounding structures. Lateral or superior invasion, resulting in breech of the sagittal sinus or past the diaphragm sella, respectively, increases the likelihood of intra-operative bleeding, given the location of the sagittal sinus venous plexus, the carotid artery, and the circle of Willis. If there is tumour invasion of these regions, one should consider having blood products readily available as well as large-bore intravenous and arterial access.

Pre-operative elevated ICP may be evidenced by the presence of altered mental status, nausea, vomiting, headache, and ventriculomegaly, and may indicate superior extension of the mass. In those with increased ICP, pre-operative sedation, if used at all, should be carefully administered since these patients may be sensitive to sedative drugs, and drug-induced hypoventilation can further exacerbate intracranial hypertension due to hypercarbia-induced cerebral vasodilatation. Anaesthesia induction agents should be titrated to avoid hypotension, thus reducing cerebral perfusion pressure. Ketamine and high-dose volatile anaesthetics should be avoided, given their adverse effect on ICP. Hypotension should be treated aggressively.

Given that hypopituitarism is common in this group of patients, peri-operative corticosteroid supplementation should be considered unless contraindicated. Thyroid function should be assessed and severe hypothyroidism, although unlikely, should be treated. Diabetes insipidus (DI) may also be present and should alert the clinician to the probable presence of hypovolaemia and electrolyte abnormalities. Blood glucose may increase with the administration of corticosteroids.[38] Blood glucose concentrations should be monitored and hyperglycaemia should be treated with insulin. These should be evaluated pre-operatively, and frequently intra-operatively, and abnormalities should be corrected. If present, cranial nerve deficits, especially those related to ocular movement and mastication, should be documented since new deficits or exacerbation of pre-existing deficits post-operatively could indicate surgical trauma or haematoma formation.

Hypopituitarism

Pituitary failure, or hypopituitarism, refers to impaired synthesis of one or more hormones produced by the pituitary gland. The most common causes of hypopituitarism are pituitary tumours or a history of traumatic head injury, pituitary surgery, or head irradiation. Other causes include infections (e.g. meningitis, encephalitis), inherited disorders (e.g. Prader–Willi syndrome, Kallmann's syndrome, Lawrence–Moon–Biedl syndrome, or hormone or hormone receptor mutations), inflammatory diseases (e.g. sarcoidosis, Wegener's granulomatosis, hypophysitis, or histiocytosis X), and vascular disorders (e.g. sickle cell disease, Sheehan's syndrome, apoplexy, and aneurysms of the circle of Willis which can compress the hypothalamic–pituitary axis). Pituitary failure can occur acutely or may be chronic. Common causes of acute pituitary failure include pituitary apoplexy (haemorrhagic infarction of a pituitary adenoma), Sheehan's syndrome (ischaemic pituitary infarction usually associated with obstetric haemorrhage), traumatic head injury, or following pituitary surgery. Acute causes of pituitary failure can lead to chronic hypopituitarism. Pituitary tumours can lead to pituitary failure by (i) causing compression of the pituitary gland proper, (ii) causing compression of the pituitary stalk or portal vessels such that hypothalamic releasing factors cannot reach target cells of the pituitary, (iii) leading to reduced pituitary gland tissue following surgical resection or radiation, or (iv) causing acute or chronic pituitary apoplexy (i.e. haemorrhagic infarction and necrosis of a pituitary tumour).

Table 2.2 Clinical features of hypopituitarism

Growth hormone deficiency
Reduced exercise tolerance
Fatigue
Decrease in muscle mass
Increase in central body fat
Hyperlipidaemia
Short stature (if deficiency begins in childhood)
Adrenocorticotrophic hormone deficiency
Fatigue
Weightless
Hypoglycaemia
Dilutional hyponatraemia
Severe hypotension*
Gonadotrophin deficiency
Amenorrhoea
Infertility
Decreased libido
Loss of body hair
Decreased muscle mass
Thyroid-stimulatinghormone deficiency
Fatigue
Cold intolerance
Weight gain
Bradycardia

*Occurs if adrenocortictrophic hormone deficiency is acute (as in pituitary apoplexy)

Signs and symptoms of hypopituitarism are often non-specific and depend on the deficient hormone(s) and the degree of deficiency (Table 2.2). In acute pituitary failure, as can occur with acute pituitary apoplexy, acute adrenal insufficiency (see Chapters 7 and 9) may develop, given that the serum half-lives of ACTH and cortisol are very short (approximately 10 min and 70–120 min, respectively). Symptoms of acute adrenal insufficiency include nausea, dilutional hyponatraemia, and profound hypotension or shock. Treatment with corticosteroids can be life-saving in this setting. In chronic and progressive pituitary failure, GH deficiency usually occurs prior to deficiency of other hormones, and deficiency of either ACTH or TSH usually occurs late in the course. Prolactin deficiency is exceedingly rare. In fact, given the disparity in the control of hormonal secretion between prolactin and other adenohypophyseal hormones (i.e. control of prolactin secretion depends predominantly on tonic inhibition from hypothalamic dopamine, whereas control of other hormones depends of stimulation of hypothalamic releasing factors), patients with hypopituitarism often have hyperprolactinaemia. In many cases, reduced antidiuretic hormone (ADH) production can also occur, leading to DI. Diagnosis of hypopituitarism is based on serum hormone concentrations, the hormonal response to the administration of stimulating agents (i.e. corticotrophin, GH-releasing hormone, thyrotrophin-releasing hormone), and imaging. Treatment involves rectifying the cause, if possible, and hormonal supplementation as appropriate.

Management of anaesthesia in patients with hypopituitarism

Patients with acute pituitary failure due to apoplexy may present for emergency surgical decompression to prevent vision loss. Given that glucocorticoids are essential to maintain vasomotor tone,[39,40] and since the half-lives of both ACTH and cortisol are short, failure of the HPA axis occurs quickly following apoplexy and is usually associated with hypotension, which can be profound. Support of airway, breathing, and circulation is the first priority. Patients may be resistant to the effects of vasopressors and, because of generalized loss of vasomotor tone, may be relatively hypovolaemic, requiring intravascular volume expansion preferably with a colloid. The early supplementation of glucocorticoids can be of great value in the management of severe hypotension. An initial dose of 100 mg of intravenous hydrocortisone (or equivalent) should be considered, with 50 mg intravenously every 6 hours for the first hospital day. Although rare, DI may occur in the setting of pituitary apoplexy, and the administration of vasopressin for haemodynamic support may not only increase blood pressure but will also serve to supplement ADH deficiency.[41] Large-bore intravenous access is required, and arterial access will be helpful for haemodynamic management. Supplementation of other hormones is usually not required acutely since the half-life of T_4 is 6.8 days and the manifestations of GH and gonadotrophin deficiency are usually not immediately life-threatening.

Patients with chronic hypopituitarism often present for surgery unrelated to their pituitary gland disorder. In patients with a normally functioning hypothalamic–hypophyseal–adrenal axis, serum cortisol concentrations increase in response to the physiological stress of surgery and often remain elevated for up to 24 hours following minor to moderate surgery, but can remain elevated for up to 3 days follow major surgery, such as cardiac surgery.[42] Therefore patients with hypopituitarism should receive their scheduled dose of corticosteroid replacement on the morning of surgery, and additional corticosteroids should be administered to compensate for the increased corticosteroid requirement facilitated by the stress of surgery or critical illness. Dosing of additional corticosteroids will depend on the severity of the physiological stress. For minor surgery, such as herniorrhaphy, replacement with 25 mg of hydrocortisone (or equivalent) at induction of anaesthesia may be sufficient. For moderate or major surgery or critical illness, patients should receive 25–100 mg parenteral hydrocortisone (or equivalent) with induction of anaesthesia, and subsequent scheduled corticosteroid supplementation thereafter (see Chapter 7).

In patients with concurrent DI, supplementation of ADH should continue in the perioperative period. Supplementation with intranasal, parenteral, or oral desmopressin (i.e. DDAVP) or parenteral vasopressin are all options for management. Assessment of thyroid function should be considered, especially if symptoms of hypothyroidism exist, with subsequent administration of thyroid hormone supplements if necessary.

Posterior pituitary gland

Unlike the anterior pituitary gland, which consists of cells that respond to hormone secreted by the hypothalamus, the posterior pituitary gland consists of neural tissue—the distal axons of peptidergic neurons with cell bodies located primarily in the paired paraventricular and supra-optic nuclei of the hypothalamus. These neurons synthesize either oxytocin or vasopressin, along with their carrier proteins (the neurophysins), within the hypothalamus. These octapeptides are then transported within the axons and stored in secretory granules within the posterior pituitary gland. Upon stimulation, the secretory granules are released, and the hormones enter the systemic circulation via capillaries within the posterior pituitary gland (see Figure 2.3).

Arginine vasopressin, also known as ADH, is secreted by the posterior pituitary primarily in response to changes in serum osmolality. Osmoreceptors are believed to exist within the organum vasculosum of the lamina terminalis, a structure located anterior to the hypothalamus and perfused by fenestrated capillaries, and thus located outside the blood–brain barrier. Increases in serum osmolality (normal serum osmolality is approximately 285 mOsm/kg body water) stimulate secretion of ADH stored in neuronal secretory granules within the posterior pituitary gland. Serum osmolality is normally very tightly controlled. Small changes in serum osmolality will cause rapid changes in the output of ADH by the posterior pituitary gland (Figure 2.6). As serum osmolality decreases, ADH output rapidly decreases and, given the short serum half-life of ADH (approximately 15 minutes), serum ADH concentration falls rapidly.

ADH release is also affected by changes in blood pressure and volume. Mediated by afferents from arterial baroreceptors located in the aortic arch and carotid sinus and low-pressure baroreceptors in the atria and pulmonary venous system, decreases in blood volume, reflected by changes in arterial and venous blood pressure, stimulate ADH release (Figure 2.6). Of note, modulation of ADH release is much more sensitive to changes in serum osmolality than to changes in blood volume and pressure, since very little change in ADH release occurs when blood volume and pressure decrease by up to 10%. However, severe hypotension and hypovolaemia are strong triggers for ADH release, as noted by the exponential increase in ADH release when in blood pressure and volume decrease by more than 10%. This phenomenon is believed to be related to sympathetic reflexes. With mild hypovolaemia, sympathetic reflexes prevent significant decreases in arterial blood pressure. It is when this compensatory mechanism is exhausted that exponential increases in ADH release occur.[43,44]

The physiological effects of ADH are mediated via specific vasopressin receptors: V_1 receptors are located predominantly on vascular smooth muscle and mediate ADH-induced vasoconstriction,[45] and V_2 receptors are located on the cells of the renal collecting duct. ADH-induced increases in the permeability of these cells to water cause an

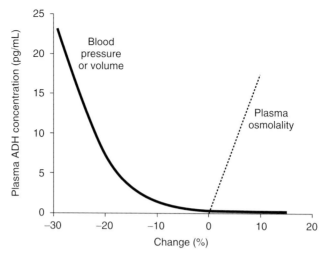

Fig. 2.6 Comparative sensitivity of antidiuretic hormone (ADH) secretion in response to increases in plasma osmolality versus decreases in blood volume or blood pressure in human subjects. Note that ADH secretion is much more sensitive to small changes in blood osmolality than to changes in volume or pressure. Also, exponential increases in ADH output occur with moderate to severe decreases in blood pressure or volume. Adapted from Robertson GL (1986). Posterior pituitary. In: Felig P, Baxter J, Frohman LA (eds), *Endocrinology and Metabolism*, pp. 338–86. McGraw Hill, New York. Reproduced with permission from The McGraw Hill Companies.

increase in water re-absorption from the urine, thus increasing urine osmolality and decreasing urine output.

Syndrome of inappropriate antidiuretic hormone secretion

The syndrome of inappropriate antidiuretic hormone secretion (SIADH) occurs when plasma concentrations of ADH are inappropriately elevated when, from a physiological standpoint, secretion of ADH by the posterior pituitary gland should be suppressed. The hallmark finding in SIADH is hypo-osmolality. SIADH is the most common cause of euvolaemic hypo-osmolality and is found in 20–40% of patients with hypo-osmolality.[46,47] Serum osmolality can be estimated based on the three major solutes in plasma:

$$\text{plasma osmolality (mOsm/kg body water)} = 2[\text{Na}] \text{ (mmol/L)}$$
$$+ [\text{glucose}] \text{ (mg/dl)}/18$$
$$+ \text{BUN (mg/dl)}/2.8$$

where BUN is blood urea nitrogen. Alternatively, it can be directly determine by measuring the freezing point depression or the vapour pressure of plasma. Given that sodium is the primary cationic osmolar agent in plasma, hypo-osmolality is often manifested as hyponatraemia. There are many causes of SIADH, but it is generally due to inappropriate secretion of ADH by the pituitary gland, extra-pituitary production of ADH, or potentiation of the renal effects of ADH, which result in the impaired excretion of water by the kidney. The clinical criteria required to diagnose SIADH, developed by Bartter and Schwartz,[48] are as follows:

- decreased osmolality of the extracellular fluid space (plasma osmolality <275 mOsm/kg water) after the exclusion of pseudo-hyponatraemia and hyperglycaemia
- inappropriately high urine osmolality (>100 mOsm/kg water) with normal renal function
- clinical euvolaemia as defined by the absence of signs or symptoms of hypovolaemia (i.e. tachycardia, orthostatic hypotension, decreased skin turgor) or hypervolaemia (i.e. generalized oedema or ascites)
- elevated urine sodium excretion with a normal salt and water intake
- absence of other causes (i.e. hypercortisolism, hypothyroidism, diuretic use).

Patients with mild hypo-osmolality and hyponatraemia may be asymptomatic. As sodium continues to decrease, patients may complain of nausea, headache, lethargy, and confusion. Stupor, seizures, and coma do not usually occur until sodium acutely falls below 120 mmol/L. In patients with chronic hyponatraemia, adaptive mechanisms tend to minimize symptoms despite a very low serum sodium concentration.

Treatment begins by treating the cause of SIADH, if possible (i.e. limit drugs that may cause ADH-mediated hypo-osmolality (Table 2.3)). Patients with symptomatic hyponatraemia and hypo-osmolality, especially if acute, should be treated urgently. Sodium replacement with hypertonic saline (3%) should be considered, with the aim of increasing serum sodium concentration by no more than 0.5 mmol/L/h in patients with mild neurological symptoms and no more than 1–2 mmol/L/h in patients with severe symptoms.[49,50] An initial infusion rate of hypertonic saline can be estimated using the following equation:

$$\text{volume of 3\% NaCl/h} = \text{body weight (kg)} \times \text{expected change in serum sodium (mmol/L/h)}.$$

For example, in a person weighing 70 kg, an infusion of 70 ml/h of 3% NaCl will increase serum sodium by approximately 1 mEq/L/h). Treatment with hypertonic saline should be terminated when (i) symptoms are abolished, (ii) a safe serum sodium level is achieved (120–125 mmol/L), or (iii) a total magnitude of correction of 20mEq/L is obtained. Correcting serum sodium concentration too rapidly is associated with the development of central pontine myelinolysis.[51]

In asymptomatic patients, fluid management usually begins by limiting water intake and enhancing water excretion. Standard first-line therapy is water restriction in mild cases and may require days before a significant improvement is observed. In mildly symptomatic patients or those in whom water restriction fails, administration of a loop diuretic, such as furosemide, will reduce the ability of the kidney to excrete concentrated urine and, when combined with sodium replacement (i.e. high-sodium diet, sodium chloride tablets), can enhance free water excretion. Currently, the use of vasopressin

Table 2.3 Causes of antidiuretic hormone dysregulation

Causes of SIADH	Causes of diabetes insipidus
Tumours	Central
Bronchogenic carcinoma, mesothelioma	Traumatic brain injury
Non-pulmonary cancers	Anoxic brain injury
Central nervous system disorders	Surgical hypophysectomy
Mass lesions	Pituitary tumours (especially craniopharyngeoma, suprasellar germinoma, pinealoma, and primary pituitary carcinoma)
Inflammatory diseases (meningitis, encephalitis, multiple sclerosis	
Degenerative diseases (Guillain–Barré)	Primary central nervous system lymphoma
Subarachnoid haemorrhage	Leukaemic involvement of the hypothalamus
Head trauma	Genetic disorders associated with defective vasopressin production
Hydrocephalus	
Pituitary disorders (pituitary stalk transection, hypophysectomy)	Meningitis, encephalitis
	Tuberculosis
Drugs	Syphilis
Stimulation of ADH release (nicotine, tricylic antidepressants, phenothiazines	Granulomatous disease (Wegener's granulomatosis, histiocytosis X, sarcoidosis)
Potentiation of ADH in the kidney (DDAVP, oxytocin)	Pregnancy (increased metabolism of ADH)
Angiotensin-converting enzyme inhibitors	Brain death
Serotonin re-uptake inhibitors	Nephrogenic
Vincristine and cyclophosphamide	Congenital (i.e. mutation of ADH receptor)
Non-malignant pulmonary diseases	Polycystic kidney disease
Infections (tuberculosis, pneumonia)	Renal infarcts
Chronic obstructive pulmonary disease	Sickle-cell disease
Acute respiratory failure	Drugs
Positive-pressure ventilation	Lithium carbonate
Other	Demeclocycline
Prolonged strenuous exercise	
Aquired immunodeficiency syndrome	

receptor antagonist drugs, such as contivaptan or satavaptan, is being investigated for the long-term treatment of SIADH.[52,53]

Diabetes insipidus

Diabetes insipidus (DI) is the physiological condition where an excessive volume of hypotonic (and tasteless, i.e. insipid) urine is inappropriately produced. There are two physiological conditions which can cause DI: (i) failure of the posterior pituitary to secrete adequate amounts of ADH (central DI) or (ii) failure of the kidney to respond appropriately to ADH (nephrogenic DI). The causes of DI are diverse (see Table 2.3). DI is a common complication of pituitary surgery or traumatic head injury. The diagnosis of DI is made in the setting of increased urine output with a specific gravity of less than 1.010 or a urine osmolality of less than 300 mOsm/kg water despite serum hypertonicity (serum osmolality greater than 295 mOsm/kg water). One must first rule out the use of diuretic agents. Central and nephrogenic DI can be distinguished by either a reduction in urine output following the administration of 5 U subcutaneous vasopressin or a low serum vasopressin concentration. In those with nephrogenic DI, serum ADH concentrations are usually greater than 5 pg/ml after dehydration and there is no response in urine production to the administration of exogenous ADH.

The aims of treatment in patients with DI are to correct the water deficit and stop ongoing water loss. In severely hypovolaemic patients, expansion of the intravascular compartment is a priority and may be accomplished with intravenous 0.9% NaCl. This affords the ability to replace the intravascular volume component, increasing organ perfusion and avoiding rapid correction of serum sodium concentration. In patients with mild to moderate volume depletion, the total body free-water deficit can be calculated as follows:

$$\text{free-water deficit (L)} = (\text{plasma } [Na^+] - 140)/140 \times \text{total body water (L)}.$$

Oral free-water replacement is preferred, if possible. If intravenous replacement is selected, care must be taken to avoid rapid correction of hypernatraemia. In those with DI existing for more than 24 hours or in whom the duration is unknown, the free-water deficit should be corrected over 48–72 hours and plasma sodium concentration should not decrease by more than 1 mmol/L every 2 hours. The slow rate of correction is necessary because in the setting of chronic DI with hypernatraemia, the brain is able compensate for the serum hypertonicity by generating compounds which increase intracellular osmolality, thus minimizing cellular shrinkage. Rapid correction of the free-water deficit can cause water to enter the relatively hypertonic intracellular compartment in the brain, leading to the development of cerebral oedema. Use of 0.45% NaCl or lactated Ringer's solution, with 500 mL and 100 mL of free water per litre of solution, respectively, are both reasonable options

Stopping water loss in patients with central DI is accomplished by either using the oral hypoglycaemic agent chlorpropamide, which potentiates the effect of ADH in the kidney, or replacing ADH with either an intravenous vasopressin infusion or administering 1-desamino-8-D-arginine vasopressin (DDAVP), the synthetic analogue of ADH. DDAVP can be administered intranasally (5–10 μg every 12–24 hours), intramuscularly or intravenously (1–2 μg every 12 hours), or orally (0.1–0.8 mg/day in divided doses).

No specific treatment exists for nephrogenic DI. Salt restriction and thiazide diuretics may reduce urine output. Thiazide diuretics work in this setting by inhibiting sodium reabsorption in distal nephrons, resulting in natriuresis. This leads to hypovolaemia, decreased glomerular filtration, and subsequent sodium reabsorption, resulting in decreased urine output. Thiazide diuretics may also enhance water reabsorption in the collecting duct independent of the action of vasopressin.[54,55]

Surgical management of pituitary disorders

The pituitary gland may be approached via three different routes: transnasally, translabially, or via craniotomy. The translabial approach is usually reserved for children, since the smaller diameter of the nares limits the size of instrument which can be introduced into the surgical field. Craniotomy, usually via a lateral approach, is used for either large invasive tumours with significant suprasellar extension or situations where nearby pathology may complicate tumour resection (i.e. a nearby arterial aneurysm). The transnasal approach is the most commonly used technique. Pre-operative evaluation should assess the implications of any endocrinopathy (e.g. acromegaly, Cushing's disease, hypopituitarism) on anaesthetic management. Pre-existing neurological deficits (i.e. visual field and cranial nerve) should be documented, and tumour size and extension should be noted to stratify the risk of intra-operative bleeding (e.g. cavernous sinus or suprasellar involvement). Arterial and large-bore intravenous access, as well as available blood products, should be considered in patients at risk for significant intra-operative bleeding.

Following the induction of general anaesthesia, the surgical technique typically begins with the administration of a topical or submucosal local anaesthetic. Using an endoscope, a tunnel is then created in the nasal cavity to reach the sphenoid sinus, where the floor of the sella turcica is removed (Figure 2.7).

The tumour is resected with the use of an operating microscope, and if a cerebrospinal fluid leak is noted, thigh or abdominal fat may be harvested to seal the leak. Intra-operative complications include hypertension (if a vasoconstrictor is added to the submucosal anaesthetic)[56] and bleeding, which may be severe and fatal given the proximity of the pituitary gland to the cavernous sinus and carotid arteries (see Figure 2.1). Oral packing should be employed to minimize gastric accumulation of blood, which may increase the risk of nausea and vomiting post-operatively. Avoidance of patient movement will minimize the risk of injury to adjacent structures, especially the carotid artery. Some surgeons may request the placement of a lumbar cerebrospinal fluid drainage catheter. Injection of saline or air will transiently increase ICP and displace the sellar contents inferiorly. Likewise, drainage of cerebrospinal fluid will decrease ICP and superiorly displace a pituitary mass. If air is injected via a lumbar catheter, nitrous oxide should not be used given its effect on the volume of gases in closed spaces.

Most complications from pituitary surgery become evident post-operatively, and include nausea and vomiting, pain, cerebrospinal fluid leakage, disorders of ADH production, hypopituitarism, injury to neurological structures, bleeding, and infection. Neurological injury is quite rare following pituitary surgery; however, it is probably the most feared complication. In the immediate post-operative period, a cranial nerve examination is often performed to assess gross visual function and identify injury to the cranial nerves that pass through the cavernous sinus. Assessment of visual function (i.e. cranial

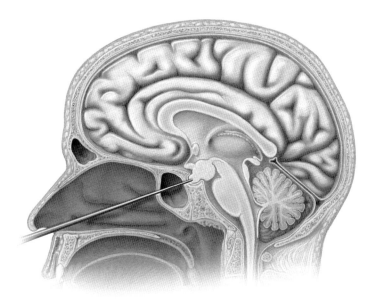

Fig. 2.7 The trans-sphenoidal route is the most common approach for the resection of pituitary tumours in adults. Instruments are advanced through the nasal cavity, usually with the aid of an operating microscope. The sphenoid sinus is entered, its roof is opened, and the pituitary gland is approached through the floor of the sella turcica. Copyrighted and used with permission of Mayo Foundation for Medical Education and Research, all rights reserved.

nerve II, especially the lateral visual fields), extra-ocular movements (i.e. cranial nerves III, IV, and VI), pupillary constriction (i.e. cranial nerve III), and facial sensation (i.e. the first and second branches of cranial nerve V) are typically employed. A gross neurological examination is often performed to rule out vascular injury or stroke. Post-operative nausea and vomiting are common, occurring in up to 40% of trans-sphenoidal surgery patients.[57]

Cerebrospinal fluid leakage into the sella is evident intra-operatively in over half (56%) of cases. Local treatment with a fat graft, with or without collagen sponges, titanium mesh, or fibrin glue, is generally effective as continued leakage post-operatively only occurs in 2.5% of cases.[58] Patients will often complain of rhinorrhoea; however, nasal discharge can also occur following a transnasal approach independent of a cerebrospinal fluid leak. The presence of β_2-transferrin, a glycoprotein found almost exclusively in cerebrospinal fluid, in the fluid strongly suggests cerebrospinal fluid leakage. Most leaks will respond to lumbar cerebrospinal fluid diversion where a lumbar drainage catheter is placed, enabling cerebrospinal fluid to exit via the catheter instead of through the dural defect, thus allowing the dural defect to close. Operative repair is reserved for patients who do not respond to lumbar diversion. Complications associated with prolonged cerebrospinal fluid leakage include meningitis and pneumocephalus. Thus detection and treatment of leaks should be accomplished prior to hospital discharge.

Disorders of ADH release are common following pituitary surgery. Specifically, DI and SIADH have been reported in up to 31% and 25% of cases, respectively.[59,60] A triphasic response in urine output is often described. This consists of an initial phase of increased urine output, thought to be due to the inability of axons in the hypothalamic–neurohypophyseal tract to propagate action potentials, which typically starts immediately post-operatively and generally lasts for 6 days. The second phase, usually lasting for about 5 days, consists of a decrease in urine output due to the unregulated release of stored ADH. The third phase, the recurrence of DI, occurs after the stored ADH is released. This third phase can eventually resolve or may become permanent. In reality, the classical triphasic response is rare, as most patients with a post-operative ADH release disorder exhibit either a monophasic pattern (DI or SIADH only) or a biphasic pattern (DI followed by SIADH with resolution). DI lasting for 3 months and 1 year following pituitary surgery occurs in 0.9% and 0.25% of patients, respectively.[59]

New-onset post-operative failure of at least one hypothalamic–pituitary–end-organ axis is reported in 7–21% of patients having pituitary surgery.[61,62] All patients who have had pituitary surgery should be screened for hypopituitarism prior to hospital discharge. Typically if patients are feeling well and morning serum cortisol on the day following surgery is greater than 10 µg/dL, patients are unlikely to develop new-onset anterior pituitary failure.[63,64] Few patients with pre-existing hypopituitarism will have recovered adequate pituitary function prior to hospital discharge and thus will require hormone replacement. In these patients, hormone supplementation can be reduced as tolerated in the months following surgery.

Summary

The proper function and regulation of the hypothalamic-pituitary axis is critical to a plethora of biological processes so that dysfunctional regulation of even a single hormone can have broad-reaching effects. The peri-operative care of patients with pituitary disease requires a broad understanding of not only the local anatomical relationships of the pituitary gland but also the impact and appropriate management of hormonal dysregulation.

Key clinical management points

Diagnosis

Tumours may cause anatomical and hormonal consequences.

Anatomical

- Raised ICP
  - Visual field changes
  - Compression of other cranial nerves, cavernous sinus, and carotid artery

Endocrine

- Hypopituitarism
- Growth hormone excess
  - Gigantism and acromegaly
- Hyperprolactinaemia—little anaesthetic implication
  - Consequences of therapy
- TSH excess
  - Hyperthyroidism
- Gonadotrophin excess—little anaesthetic implication

Diagnostic tests

Anatomical

- Standard cranial imaging
- Growth hormone excess
  - Clinical signs
  - Single GH estimations unreliable
  - Serum ILGF-1 concentration a possible alternative
- TSH secretion
  - Thyroid function tests and MRI

Growth hormone excess

Pre-operative preparation

Comprehensive history and physical essential

- Airway: thorough evaluation necessary
  - Enlarged tongue and jaw, swollen soft tissues, glottis abnormalities
  - Standard pre-anaesthetic airway examination may not be very reliable to predict airway difficulty

Key clinical management points (continued)

- CVS screening
  - Blood pressure and cardiac dysfunction
- Neurological deficits

Anaesthetic management

- Avoid sedative premedication
- Monitoring and equipment
  - Standard anaesthetic monitoring
  - Consider large operating table and high-capacity ventilator

Anaesthetic induction

- Without airway problems
  - Standard intravenous induction, neuromuscular blockade, and endotracheal intubation
- Suspected airway difficulty
  - Awake fibreoptic intubation
  - Gas induction and attempted airway inspection
  - Intubation with a flexible armoured tube of appropriate size

Anaesthetic maintenance

- Standard neurosurgical technique for pituitary surgery
- Lumbar drain and possible injection of air or saline to deliver gland

Post-operative care

- Ensure adequate airway function following extubation
- Monitor blood glucose
- Cerebrospinal fluid leak possible

Hypopituitarism

Diagnosis

- Serum hormone concentrations
- Response to stimulating agents

Anaesthesia

- Anticipate haemodynamic unresponsiveness, hypovolaemia
- Hydrocortisone 100 mg on induction, 50 mg 6 hourly on day of surgery

Key clinical management points (continued)

Pituitary tumours

Anaesthesia

- Standard neurosurgical anaesthesia
- Vasoconstrictor to nasal mucosa
- Throat pack to avoid gastric accumulation of blood
- Consider effects of lumbar injection (air/saline)

Post-operative care

- Nausea, vomiting, cerebrospinal fluid leak common
- ADH disorders common
  - DI or SIADH

References

1 Ezzat S, Asa SL, Couldwell WT, Barr CE, *et al.* (2004). The prevalence of pituitary adenomas: a systematic review. *Cancer*, **101**, 613–19.

2 Laws ER, Jane JA, Sulton LD (2004). Surgery for primary brain tumors in US academic training centers. Presented at: Congress of Neurological Surgeons Annual Meeting, San Francisco, CA.

3 Saeger W, Ludecke DK, Buchfelder M, Fahlbusch R, Quabbe HJ, Petersenn S (2007). Pathohistological classification of pituitary tumors: 10 years of experience with the German Pituitary Tumor Registry. *European Journal of Endocrinology*, **156**, 203–16.

4 Yaghmai R, Olan WJ, O'Malley S, Bank WO (1996). Nonhemorrhagic pituitary macroadenoma producing reversible internal carotid artery occlusion: case report. *Neurosurgery*, **38**, 1245–8.

5 Etxabe J, Gaztambide S, Latorre P, Vazquez JA (1993). Acromegaly: an epidemiological study. *Journal of Endocrinological Investigation*, **16**, 181–7.

6 Sotos JF (1996). Section III other hormonal causes. *Clinical Pediatrics*, **35**, 637–48.

7 Lloyd RV, Chandler WF, Kovacs K, Ryan N (1986). Ectopic pituitary adenomas with normal anterior pituitary glands. *American Journal of Surgical Pathology*, **10**, 546–52.

8 Nemergut EC, Zuo Z (2006). Airway management in patients with pituitary disease: a review of 746 patients. *Journal of Neurosurgical Anesthesiology*, **18**, 73–7.

9 Fatti LM, Scacchi M, Pincelli AI, Lavezzi E, Cavagnini F (2001). Prevalence and pathogenesis of sleep apnea and lung disease in acromegaly. *Pituitary*, **4**, 259–62.

10 Lopez-Velasco R, Escobar-Morreale HF, Vega B, *et al.* (1997). Cardiac involvement in acromegaly: specific myocardiopathy or consequence of systemic hypertension? *Journal of Clinical Endocrinology and Metabolism*, **82**, 1047–53.

11 Fazio S, Cittadini A, Cuocolo A, *et al.* (1994). Impaired cardiac performance is a distinct feature of uncomplicated acromegaly. *Journal of Clinical Endocrinology and Metabolism*, **79**, 441–6.

12 Kahaly G, Olshausen KV, Mohr-Kahaly S, *et al.* (1992). Arrhythmia profile in acromegaly. *European Heart Journal*, **13**, 51–6.

13 Baum H, Ludecke DK, Herrmann HD (1986). Carpal tunnel syndrome and acromegaly. *Acta Neurochirurgica*, **83**, 54–5.

14 Jenkins PJ, Sohaib SA, Akker S, *et al.* (2000). The pathology of median neuropathy in acromegaly. *Annals of Internal Medicine*, **133**, 197–201.

15 Melmed S (2006). Medical progress: acromegaly. *New England Journal of Medicine*, **355**, 2558–73.

16 Ben-Shlomo A, Melmed S (2008). Acromegaly. *Endocrinology and Metabolism Clinics of North America*, **37**, 101–22.

17 Swearingen B, Barker FG, 2nd, Katznelson L, *et al.* (1998). Long-term mortality after transsphenoidal surgery and adjunctive therapy for acromegaly. *Journal of Clinical Endocrinology and Metabolism*, **83**, 3419–26.

18 Losasso T, Dietz NM, Muzzi DA (1990). Acromegaly and radial artery cannulation. *Anesthesia and Analgesia*, 71, 204.

19 Horseman ND, Zhao W, Montecino-Rodriguez E, *et al.* (1997). Defective mammopoiesis, but normal hematopoiesis, in mice with a targeted disruption of the prolactin gene. *EMBO Journal*, **16**, 6926–35.

20 Travaglini P, Moriondo P, Togni E, *et al.* (1989). Effect of oral zinc administration on prolactin and thymulin circulating levels in patients with chronic renal failure. *Journal of Clinical Endocrinology and Metabolism*, **68**, 186–90.

21 Kleinberg DL, Noel GL, Frantz AG (1977). Galactorrhea: a study of 235 cases, including 48 with pituitary tumors. *New England Journal of Medicine*, **296**, 589–600.

22 Baldini M, Cornelli U, Molinari M, Cantalamessa L (1988). Effect of methyldopa on prolactin serum concentration. Comparison between normal and sustained-release formulations. *European Journal of Clinical Pharmacology*, **34**, 513–15.

23 Rubin RT, Hays SE (1980). The prolactin secretory response to neuroleptic drugs: mechanisms, applications and limitations. *Psychoneuroendocrinology*, **5**, 121–37.

24 Danila DC, Klibanski A (2001). Prolactin secreting pituitary tumors in men. *Endocrinologist*, **11**,105–11.

25 Lahlou S, Demenge P (1991). Contribution of spinal dopamine receptors to the hypotensive action of bromocriptine in rats. *Journal of Cardiovascular Pharmacology*, **18**, 317–25.

26 Pritchett AM, Morrison JF, Edwards WD, Schaff HV, Connolly HM, Espinosa RE (2002). Valvular heart disease in patients taking pergolide. *Mayo Clinic Proceedings*, **77**, 1280–6.

27 Lanier WL (2003). Additional insights into pergolide-associated valvular heart disease. *Mayo Clinic Proceedings*, **78**, 684–6.

28 Zanettini R, Antonini A, Gatto G, Gentile R, Tesei S, Pezzoli G (2007). Valvular heart disease and the use of dopamine agonists for Parkinson's disease. *New England Journal of Medicine*, **356**, 39–46.

29 Schade R, Andersohn F, Suissa S, Haverkamp W, Garbe E (2007). Dopamine agonists and the risk of cardiac-valve regurgitation. *New England Journal of Medicine*, **356**, 29–38.

30 Corvol JC, Anzouan-Kacou JB, Fauveau E, *et al.* (2007). Heart valve regurgitation, pergolide use, and Parkinson disease: an observational study and meta-analysis. *Archives of Neurology*, 64(12),1721–6

31 Horvath J, Fross RD, Kleiner-Fisman G, *et al.* (2004). Severe multivalvular heart disease: a new complication of the ergot derivative dopamine agonists. *Movement Disorders*, **19**, 656–62.

32 Beck-Peccoz P, Brucker-Davis F, Persani L, Smallridge RC, Weintraub BD (1996). Thyrotropin-secreting pituitary tumors. *Endocrine Reviews*, **17**, 610–38.

33 Mindermann T, Wilson CB (1993). Thyrotropin-producing pituitary adenomas. *Journal of Neurosurgery*, **79**, 521–7.

34 Brucker-Davis F, Oldfield EH, Skarulis MC, Doppman JL, Weintraub BD (1999). Thyrotropin-secreting pituitary tumors: diagnostic criteria, thyroid hormone sensitivity, and treatment outcome in 25 patients followed at the National Institutes of Health. *Journal of Clinical Endocrinology and Metabolism*, **84**, 476–86.

35 Clarke MJ, Erickson D, Castro MR, Atkinson JL (2008). Thyroid-stimulating hormone pituitary adenomas. *Journal of Neurosurgery*, **109**,17–22.

36 Fukuda T, Yokoyama N, Tamai M, *et al.* (1998). Thyrotropin secreting pituitary adenoma effectively treated with octreotide. *Internal Medicine (Tokyo, Japan)*, **37**, 1027–30.

37 Chanson P, Weintraub BD, Harris AG (1993). Octreotide therapy for thyroid-stimulating hormone-secreting pituitary adenomas. A follow-up of 52 patients. *Annals of Internal Medicine*, **119**, 236–40.

38 Pasternak JJ, McGregor DG, Lanier WL (2004). Effect of single-dose dexamethasone on blood glucose concentration in patients undergoing craniotomy. *Journal of Neurosurgical Anesthesiology*, **16**, 122–5.

39 Grunfeld JP, Eloy L (1987). Glucocorticoids modulate vascular reactivity in the rat. *Hypertension*, **10**, 608–18.

40 Saruta T, Suzuki H, Handa M, Igarashi Y, Kondo K, Senba S (1986). Multiple factors contribute to the pathogenesis of hypertension in Cushing's syndrome. *Journal of Clinical Endocrinology and Metabolism*, **62**, 275–9.

41 Rolih CA, Ober KP (1993). Pituitary apoplexy. *Endocrinology and Metabolism Clinics of North America*, **22**, 291–302.

42 Chernow B, Alexander HR, Smallridge RC, *et al.* (1987). Hormonal responses to graded surgical stress. *Archives of Internal Medicine*, **147**, 1273–8.

43 Thrasher TN (1994). Baroreceptor regulation of vasopressin and renin secretion: low-pressure versus high-pressure receptors. *Frontiers in Neuroendocrinology*, **15**, 157–96.

44 Robertson GL (1976). The regulation of vasopressin function in health and disease. *Recent Progress in Hormone Research*, **33**, 333–85.

45 Wakatsuki T, Nakaya Y, Inoue I (1992). Vasopressin modulates K(+)-channel activities of cultured smooth muscle cells from porcine coronary artery. *American Journal of Physiology*, **263**, H491–6.

46 Anderson RJ, Chung HM, Kluge R, Schrier RW (1985). Hyponatremia: a prospective analysis of its epidemiology and the pathogenetic role of vasopressin. *Annals of Internal Medicine*, **102**, 164–8.

47 Gross PA, Pehrisch H, Rascher W, Schomig A, Hackenthal E, Ritz E (1987). Pathogenesis of clinical hyponatremia: observations of vasopressin and fluid intake in 100 hyponatremic medical patients. *European Journal of Clinical Investigation*, **17**, 123–9.

48 Bartter FC, Schwartz WB (1967). The syndrome of inappropriate secretion of antidiuretic hormone. *American Journal of Medicine*, **42**, 790–806.

49 Ayus JC, Krothapalli RK, Arieff AI (1987). Treatment of symptomatic hyponatremia and its relation to brain damage. A prospective study. *New England Journal of Medicine*, **317**, 1190–5.

50 Sterns RH, Cappuccio JD, Silver SM, Cohen EP (1994). Neurologic sequelae after treatment of severe hyponatremia: a multicenter perspective. *Journal of the American Society of Nephrology*, **4**, 1522–30.

51 Sterns RH, Riggs JE, Schochet SS, Jr. (1986). Osmotic demyelination syndrome following correction of hyponatremia. *New England Journal of Medicine*, **314**, 1535–42.

52 Decaux G (2001). Long-term treatment of patients with inappropriate secretion of antidiuretic hormone by the vasopressin receptor antagonist conivaptan, urea, or furosemide. *American Journal of Medicine*, **110**, 582–4.

53 Soupart A, Gross P, Legros JJ, *et al.* (2006). Successful long-term treatment of hyponatremia in syndrome of inappropriate antidiuretic hormone secretion with satavaptan (SR121463B), an orally active nonpeptide vasopressin V_2-receptor antagonist. *Clinical Journal of the American Society of Nephrology*, 1(6), 1154–60.

54 Gronbeck L, Marples D, Nielsen S, Christensen S (1998). Mechanism of antidiuresis caused by bendroflumethiazide in conscious rats with diabetes insipidus. *British Journal of Pharmacology*, 123(4), 737–45.

55 Cesar KR, Magaldi AJ (1999). Thiazide induces water absorption in the inner medullary collecting duct of normal and Brattleboro rats. *American Journal of Physiology*, **277**, F756–60.

56 Pasternak JJ, Atkinson JL, Kasperbauer JL, Lanier WL (2004). Hemodynamic responses to epinephrine-containing local anesthetic injection and to emergence from general anesthesia in transsphenoidal hypophysectomy patients. *Journal of Neurosurgical Anesthesiology*, **16**, 189–95.

57 Manninen PH, Raman SK, Boyle K, el-Beheiry H (1999). Early postoperative complications following neurosurgical procedures. *Canadian Journal of Anaesthesia*, **46**, 7–14.

58 Esposito F, Dusick JR, Fatemi N, Kelly DF (2007). Graded repair of cranial base defects and cerebrospinal fluid leaks in transsphenoidal surgery. *Neurosurgery*, **60** (Suppl 2), 295–304.

59 Hensen J, Henig A, Fahlbusch R, Meyer M, Boehnert M, Buchfelder M (1999). Prevalence, predictors and patterns of postoperative polyuria and hyponatraemia in the immediate course after transsphenoidal surgery for pituitary adenomas. *Clinical Endocrinology*, **50**, 431–9.

60 Olson BR, Gumowski J, Rubino D, Oldfield EH (1997). Pathophysiology of hyponatremia after transsphenoidal pituitary surgery. *Journal of Neurosurgery*, **87**, 499–507.

61 Cappabianca P, Cavallo LM, Colao A, de Divitiis E (2002). Surgical complications associated with the endoscopic endonasal transsphenoidal approach for pituitary adenomas. *Journal of Neurosurgery*, **97**, 293–8.

62 Ciric I, Ragin A, Baumgartner C, Pierce D (1997). Complications of transsphenoidal surgery: results of a national survey, review of the literature, and personal experience. *Neurosurgery*, **40**, 225–36.

63 Jane JA, Jr., Thapar K, Kaptain GJ, Maartens N, Laws ER, Jr. (2002). Pituitary surgery: transsphenoidal approach. *Neurosurgery*, **51**, 435–42.

64 Vance ML (2003). Perioperative management of patients undergoing pituitary surgery. *Endocrinology and Metabolism Clinics of North America*, **32**, 355–65.

Chapter 3

Diabetes mellitus

Glucose control: what benefit, what cost in surgical patients?

John W Sear

Diabetes mellitus (DM) is the most common non-communicable disease worldwide. Currently there are about 150 million diabetics; DM affects 1–2% of the population of the UK, and about 10% of the population of the USA. There may also be an equal number of undiagnosed patients. Diabetes affects about 1 in 6 patients over the age of 65 years, and 1 in 4 over the age of 85 years; over 90% of patients are non-insulin dependent (type 2) diabetics.

The disease 'diabetes mellitus' has undergone a reclassification on the basis of the aetiology of the hyperglycaemia rather than therapy required. Therefore causes of hyperglycaemia include insulin deficiency, insulin resistance, excessive hepatic gluconeogenesis, or a combination of these. The American Diabetes Association (ADA) currently recognizes four types of diabetes mellitus:[1]

- type 1—due to β-cell destruction and insulin deficiency
- type 2—insulin resistance; also secretory defects ± resistance
- specific causes of DM: genetic defects of β-cell function, diseases of exocrine pancreas, endocrinopathies, drug or chemical induced DM, infections, genetic defects associated with diabetes
- gestational diabetes.

The development of diabetes is associated with a number of risk factors which, if treated, will improve control of hyperglycaemia and *importantly* will reduce morbidity and mortality.

The risk factors for diabetes mellitus are:

- age > 45 years
- obesity (body mass index (BMI) >27 kg/m^2)
- high-risk ethnic group (native American, African American, Hispanic, Asian)
- gestational DM
- impaired glucose tolerance test

- hypertension
- low high-density lipids or increased triglycerides

The ADA defines diabetes primarily on the basis of an A1C >6.5%. This may then be confirmed on the results of a fasting glucose >7.0 mmol/L, a random non-fasting glucose >11.1 mmol/L, or a blood glucose >11.1 mmol/L in a 2 hour sample after a 75 g glucose tolerance test. The normal value for fasting is 5.6 mmol/L; impaired glucose tolerance presents with a fasting glucose of 5.6–7.0 mmol/L, or a 2 hour post-prandial value >7.8 and <11.1 mmol/L.

Biochemistry of diabetes mellitus

The regulation of the blood glucose concentration is controlled by two key hormones, insulin and glucagon, although other hormones (steroids, epinephrine, and growth hormone) are also regulatory. Under normal circumstances, the blood glucose concentration is remarkably constant. Exercise results in lactate being cycled from muscle to the liver and then converted to glucose. In starvation, tissues become fat adapted, using free fatty acids and ketone bodies for energy. Amino acids are substrates for gluconeogenesis, and glucose is produced in the liver to prevent hypoglycaemia.

Insulin

Insulin is produced in the β-cells of the pancreas as the precursor pro-insulin. This is broken down by esterases to the active component insulin and C-peptide. The release of pro-insulin is stimulated by a rise in the blood glucose concentration, as well as by various gastrointestinal hormones including glucagon and gastric inhibitory peptide (GIP) (also known as glucose-dependent insulinotrophic peptide). Insulin promotes the removal of glucose from the blood through stimulation of the relocation of the insulin-sensitive GLUT-4 glucose transporter from the cytoplasm to the cell membrane, especially in adipose tissue and skeletal muscle. However, insulin is not essential for glucose uptake to occur.

Insulin also stimulates hepatic glucose uptake by induction of glucokinase, which is responsible for the phosphorylation of glucose to glucose-6-phosphate. This is an important step, as it maintains a low intracellular concentration of glucose and hence maintains the glucose gradient that facilitates continuous uptake of glucose from the blood. Insulin also stimulates glycogen synthesis (and in turn inhibits glycogenolysis) by a coordinated control mechanism (Figures 3.1 and 3.2).

In summary, the binding of insulin to its receptor leads to activation of the post-receptor pathway and phosphorylation of various effector proteins. These include the protein phosphoprotein phosphatase which dephosphorylates both glycogen synthase (thereby activating it and promoting glycogen synthesis) and phosphorylase kinase (rendering it inactive and thus preventing the activation of glycogen phosphorylase, the key enzyme of glycogenolysis). As a result of these actions, when insulin secretion is inhibited in the fasting state, hepatic glycogenolysis is stimulated and glucose is liberated into the blood.

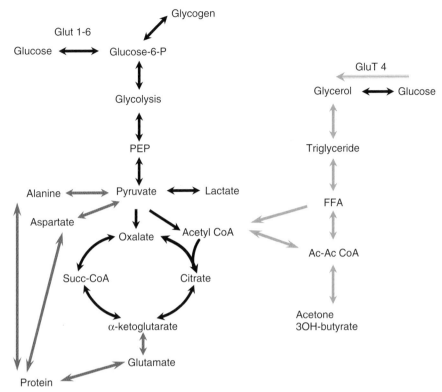

Fig. 3.1 Simplified diagram of the intermediary metabolism of carbohydrates, fats, and proteins; ➡, major carbohydrate pathways and citric acid cycle; ➡, interlinking energy pathways for protein; ➡, interlinking energy pathways for fat metabolism; GluT, glucose transporters; PEP, phosphoenolpyruvate; Ac-Ac CoA, aceto-acetyl co-enzyme A; FFA, free fatty acids.

Other actions of insulin are as follows.

♦ Control of glycolysis and gluconeogenesis—insulin stimulates the former and inhibits the latter by increased expression of the enzyme phosphofructokinase (PFK), pyruvate kinase, and the enzymes responsible for the synthesis of fructose-2,6-biphosphate, the key allosteric modifier of glycolysis.

♦ Stimulation of lipogenesis and inhibition of lipolysis.

♦ Stimulation of amino acid uptake into cells and incorporation into protein synthesis. This process is accompanied by intracellular potassium uptake.

The time-related actions of insulin are shown in Table 3.1.

Glucagon

This hormone is generated by the α-cells of the pancreas, and its secretion is decreased by an increase in the blood glucose concentration. In general, its effects are opposite to those

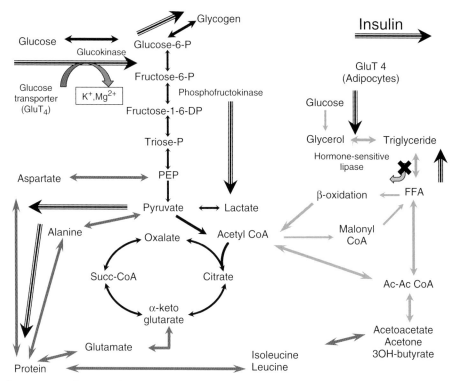

Fig. 3.2 Sites of action of insulin on intermediary metabolism: ➡, major carbohydrate pathways and citric acid cycle; ➡, interlinking energy pathways for protein; ➡, interlinking energy pathways for fat metabolism; GluT, glucose transporters; PEP, phosphoenolpyruvate; Ac-Ac CoA, aceto-acetyl co-enzyme A; FFA, free fatty acids; ✗, inhibited pathways. Note that insulin facilitates glucose entry into the cell, but is not essential other than for those tissues where glucose transporter 4 (GluT 4) is the major transporter (fat and muscle). Some insulin is essential for fat metabolism, and insulin is the only inhibitor of hormone-sensitive lipase.

Table 3.1 Time-related actions of insulin

Rapid
Intracellular transport of glucose, amino acids, K^+, and Mg^{2+}
Intermediate
Stimulation of protein synthesis
Inhibition of protein degradation
Glycogen synthesis
Inhibition of gluconeogenesis
Delayed
Increased lipogenesis

of insulin, i.e. stimulating hepatic but not muscle glycogenolysis through activation of glycogen phosphorylase, gluconeogenesis, lipolysis, and ketogenesis.

Classification of diabetes mellitus

Type 1 diabetes

Type 1 DM only accounts for 5–10% of all cases, and has an incidence of about 0.4% in the European and American populations. Most patients present as children, although about 33% are identified as adults. There are two different aetiologies—autoimmune and immune-mediated (type 1A) and idiopathic (type 1B)—with some patients showing various genetic markers and autoimmune antibodies against pancreatic cell islets, indicating an immunological basis to the disease. Diabetic keto-acidosis (DKA) is more common in type 1 than in type 2 diabetic patients.

In type 1 DM, there is an obligate need for insulin as there is usually an absolute insulin deficiency, although these patients normally have a lower insulin requirement than type 2 patients where there may be insulin resistance. Patients with type 1 DM are prone to developing ketosis and uncontrolled lipolysis.

Type 2 diabetes

Type 2 DM usually presents in older patients, but is increasingly being seen in certain younger patient groups (especially Native Americans, African Americans, and Hispanics). It accounts for about 90% of all diabetics (and has a prevalence of about 6.6% in the USA, equating to 15–20 million individuals). The incidence of type 2 DM has doubled over the last decade, and currently affects between 8–10% of all Americans!

Type 2 DM occurs because of a relative deficiency of insulin secretion to prevent hyperglycaemia, often because of peripheral resistance to its action. There may also be excess hepatic glucose release. It is associated with a significant risk of accompanying cardiovascular disease (see later in this chapter). Most type 2 diabetics produce adequate amounts of insulin to prevent ketosis occurring, but they are at risk of severe hyperglycaemia and hyperosmolar coma. Lipolysis is still controlled in type 2 DM, and hence disorders of lipid metabolism are rare.

The consequences of lack of insulin are shown in Table 3.2, and the clinical picture of types 1 and 2 DM is shown in Table 3.3 and illustrated in Figures 3.3 and 3.4.

Why is normoglycaemia the aim of therapy?

Pathophysiology of glucose control

The normal blood glucose concentration ranges from 4.0 to 11.0 mmol/L, with plasma concentrations tending to be about 10–15% greater than whole blood levels. Normoglycaemia has a number of important roles in the integrated physiology of the diabetic patient.

- It aids the maintenance of macrophage and neutrophil function.
- Insulin induces beneficial trophic changes on mucosal and skin barriers.

Table 3.2 Clinical picture of types 1 and 2 diabetes mellitus

	Type 1 DM	Type 2 DM
Typical age of onset	Children, young adults	Middle aged, elderly
Onset	Acute	Gradual
Habitus	Lean	Often obese
Weight loss	Usual	Infrequent
Ketone-prone	Usual	Usually not
PIC	Low or absent	Often normal, may be increased
Family history of DM	Less common	Common
HLA association	DR3, DR4, DQ2, DQ8	None

PIC, plasma insulin concentration.

Table 3.3 Summary of consequences of lack of insulin

Elevated fasting blood sugar
Increased gluconeogenesis
Decreased (but not absent) glucose utilization
Uncontrolled lipid metabolism
Glycerol metabolism to sugar
Ketoacidosis
Proteolysis
Gluconeogenesis
Ketone formation (ketogenic amino acids)
Diuresis and electrolyte losses
Water deficit, sodium, potassium, and magnesium deficits

- ◆ Normoglycaemia enhances red cell synthesis, decreases red cell haemolysis, and reduces the tendency to cholestasis.
- ◆ Normoglycaemia also reduces ventilation secondary to the direct anabolic effects of insulin on respiratory muscle function, and reduces the injurious effect on nerve axons seen with hyperglycaemia.

Hyperglycaemia

Hyperglycaemia occurs because of increased hepatic production of glucose, and to a lesser extent decreased removal of glucose from the blood. Acute and chronic hyperglycaemia increase the risk of ischaemic myocardial injury because of a reduction in coronary collateral blood flow. Furthermore, hyperglycaemia inhibits the development of coronary collateral blood vessels. At the cellular level, hyperglycaemia leads to decreased

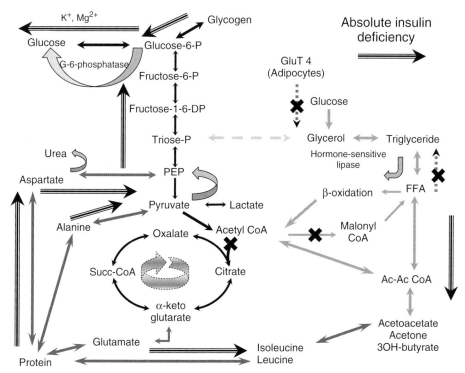

Fig. 3.3 The effects of absolute insulin deficiency (usually type 1 DM) on intermediary metabolism: ➡, major carbohydrate pathways and citric acid cycle; ➡, interlinking energy pathways for protein; ➡, interlinking energy pathways for fat metabolism; GluT, glucose transporters; PEP, phosphoenolpyruvate; Ac-Ac CoA, aceto-acetyl co-enzyme A; FFA, free fatty acids; ✖, inhibited pathways. Note that fat metabolism is markedly impaired, resulting in keto-acidosis. Relative impairment of the citric acid cycle in the liver leads to ketones becoming a major source of energy.

signal activation (as occurs with ischaemic and anaesthetic preconditioning), as well as K^+-ATP (adenosine triphosphate) channel activation. High blood glucose concentrations decrease microcirculatory dilatation, cause endothelial dysfunction, decrease coronary vasodilator reserve and coronary collateral blood flow, and are associated with the production of reactive oxygen species, enzyme and other protein glycosylation, and decreased nitric oxide (NO) production.

Glucose is normally filtered at the glomerulus and reabsorbed in the proximal convoluted tubule. However, when the renal threshold for glucose is exceeded (about 10 mmol/L), reabsorption is incomplete and glucose appears in the urine.

Glucose stimulates an osmotic diuresis which leads to increased water excretion and a rise in the plasma osmolality. In turn, the latter leads to stimulation of the thirst centre in the floor of the fourth ventricle. This combination of an osmotic dieresis (with fluid deficits of 5–6 litres, as well as Na^+, K^+, and Mg^{2+} deficiency) and thirst leads to the development of the 'classic symptoms' of diabetes, i.e. polyuria and polydypsia.

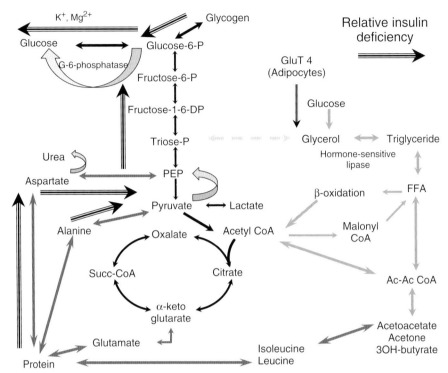

Fig. 3.4 The effects of relative insulin deficiency (only type 2 DM) on intermediary metabolism: ➡, major carbohydrate pathways and citric acid cycle; ➡, interlinking energy pathways for protein; ➡, interlinking energy pathways for fat metabolism; GluT, glucose transporters; PEP, phosphoenolpyruvate; Ac-Ac CoA, aceto-acetyl co-enzyme A; FFA, free fatty acids. Note that fat metabolism is usually preserved as minimal amounts of insulin are required for this pathway. Thus ketosis is uncommon, but severe hyperosmolar non-ketotic states may occur.

There are a number of long-term complications of hyperglycaemia, which can be classified into two separate groups with different aetiologies.

1. **Microvascular complications** These appear to be directly related to the increased blood glucose concentration, and lead to the complications of nephropathy, neuropathy, and retinopathy. In microvascular disease, there is narrowing of the lumen of small blood vessels because of the prolonged exposure to high glucose concentrations. This narrowing may be due to increased sorbitol formation (sorbitol is an alcohol derived from glucose through the action of aldose reductase). Sorbitol accumulates in the cells, leading to osmotic damage, alteration of the redox state of the cell, and reduction in the cellular myoinositol concentration. There may also be increased formation of advanced glycosylated products (e.g. plasma and tissue proteins). These products undergo cross-linking between molecules and accumulate in vessel walls and tissues, leading to structural and functional damage. Other possible

mechanisms of tissue damage include the generation of free radicals and the activation of tissue injury responses secondary to intracellular hyperglycaemia.

2. **Macrovascular complications** These are more closely related to insulin resistance, and present in the diabetic patient as exaggerated atherosclerosis. Although improved glucose control will lead to a decreased risk of the development of microvascular complications, there is only a 'trend' towards benefit for macrovascular issues.

Comorbidity and the surgical diabetic patient

Cardiovascular disease

Diabetic patients have an increased incidence of cardiovascular comorbidity, including arterial hypertension, coronary artery disease, peripheral vascular disease, and systolic and diastolic left ventricular dysfunction, leading to congestive cardiac failure. Cardiac pathologies are the main cause of death in diabetic patients.

If these patients are undergoing major non-cardiac surgery, they are at high risk of cardiovascular morbidity and mortality. The diabetic patient has an increased incidence of *silent* myocardial ischaemia, which may delay the diagnosis of overt coronary artery disease. The overall incidence of post-operative mortality and morbidity in these patients has recently been reported as 24% at a median follow-up time of 10 months.[2]

1. **Hypertension** Many diabetic patients are found to have coexisting hypertension at the time of diagnosis. In these patients, it seems that modest blood pressure control is more important than chronic tight glycaemia control. For example, the UK Prospective Diabetes Study[3] found that reduction of blood pressure in diabetic patients resulted in a decrease in cardiovascular and cerebrovascular events, while the Hypertension Optimal Treatment study[4] demonstrated that aggressive diastolic pressure reduction causes reduced cardiovascular mortality. The current aim of management of blood pressure in diabetics in the UK and USA is an arterial pressure below 130/80 mmHg; multiple drugs will often be needed to achieve this. Current drug treatments that afford the best outcomes include the combination of a thiazide plus either an ACE inhibitor or an angiotensin blocking drug. Many authorities consider ACE inhibitors to be the first-line treatment in younger non-black diabetic patients. In type 2 diabetic patients, hypertension may also be associated with the development of a progressive nephropathy, hyperinsulinaemia and insulin resistance, arterial vascular non-compliance, and chronic extravascular hypervolaemia (leading to syndrome X or insulin resistance syndrome).[5]

2. **Coronary artery disease (CAD)** DM increases the risk of CAD four to fivefold, and hence between 8% and 31% of type 2 diabetic patients have asymptomatic CAD. There is also a greater incidence of cardiac death after myocardial infarction than in the non-diabetic subject.[6] In the surgical patient, the presence of myocardial ischaemia or infarction should be suspected if unexplained confusion, hypotension, dysrhythmias, hypoxaemia, or non-specific ECG changes occur. Myocardial ischaemia or infarction may be clinically silent in the patient with DM if there is an associated

autonomic neuropathy. CAD in diabetic patients has been shown to be more extensive, to involve multiple vessels, and to be more progressive than in age-matched non-diabetic patients.

3. **Diabetic autonomic neuropathy** presents in its earliest stages as a lack of variation of the cardiac rate, with a tendency to higher than average resting heart rates. Other features include postural hypotension and intra-operative episodes of bradycardia and hypotension occurring unexpectedly without apparent precipitating causes. Cardiac neuropathy is present in 20–40% of all diabetics and is associated with a poor prognosis, but it is more common in type 1 than in type 2 DM (40% versus 17% incidence). Haemodynamic instability may occur in patients with autonomic neuropathy, especially during anaesthesia and surgery, with the risk being increased in patients with associated renal dysfunction. Another feature of the neuropathy is gastroparesis which is often unresponsive to kinetic agents.

4. **Left ventricular dysfunction** is found in diabetic patients at an incidence about four to five times that in the general population, and is often associated with hypertension and left ventricular hypertrophy, endothelial dysfunction, obesity, autonomic neuropathy, and metabolic complications secondary to hyperglycaemia and hyperlipidaemia. (Because of these various associated risk factors, many diabetic patients will receive other drug therapies including ACE inhibitors, low-dose aspirin, and lipid regulating drugs. All are beneficial in patients with the combination of diabetes and high cardiovascular risk.)

The high incidence of associated cardiovascular disease suggests that stress testing in diabetic patients presenting for major surgery should be routine where there is coexistence of diabetes and *any two* other factors (smoking, increased cholesterol or dyslipidaemia, hypertension, a family history of CAD, and males over 40 years of age). However, the role of peri-operative β-blockade in high-risk diabetic patients undergoing major noncardiac surgery has been questioned by the results of the DIPOM study.[7] Because of the high incidence of both latent and overt coronary artery disease, there is a good rationale for the pre-operative stress testing in many diabetic patients. Stress echocardiography has a high specificity and sensitivity, and is an effective tool for risk stratification in both diabetic and non-diabetic patients.[8–11] Myocardial stress scintigraphy is less effective as a risk predictor in these patients, with a lower diagnostic accuracy.[12] However, it is still useful.

Cerebrovascular disease

Diabetic patients have an increased incidence of cerebrovascular disease and stroke as a result of the accompanying increased frequency of hypertension, dyslipidaemia, accelerated atherosclerosis, and abnormal endothelial proliferation.

Renal disease

Diabetes mellitus is the leading cause of renal failure in the USA. Endstage renal disease occurs in about 30% of type 1 and up to 20% of type 2 diabetic patients. Prevention of further dysfunction is achieved by controlling hyperglycaemia and hypertension, avoiding nephrotoxic drugs or dyes, and maintaining adequate hydration, especially in the peri-operative period. No studies have shown the value of low-dose dopamine, mannitol, or diuretics as 'renal protective agents', but ACE inhibitors may decrease the long-term risk.

Diabetes and drug metabolism

There is some evidence that the disposition and metabolism of drugs and xenobiotics may be altered in patients with diabetes. DM is associated with suppression and induction of the expression of different isoforms of cytochrome P-450.

It is not only the effects of changes in pharmacokinetics that affect drug behaviour in diabetes; there is evidence that morphine analgesia is decreased in response to subcutaneous morphine in alloxanized mice.[13] Why? It is not due to decreased opiate receptor density or affinity, but rather diabetes causes glycosylation of proteins, leading to decreased drug binding and increases in the apparent volume of distribution of hydrophilic drugs such as morphine. This will lead to a decreased blood and effect-site drug concentration.

Glycosylated collagen

This presents as the 'stiff joint' syndrome and may also affect cervical mobility, leading to difficulty in endotracheal intubation.

Drug treatments for diabetes mellitus

Initially, many diabetic patients control their blood sugar by diet alone; some will need oral agents and insulin as the disease progresses, or during surgery or other stressful procedures. However, patients with type 1 DM require insulin at all times. The biochemical sequelae of insulin deficiency are shown in Figures 3.3 and 3.4.

Oral drugs

Sulphonylureas

Sulphonylureas act on the pancreas to increase β-cell sensitivity and thus augment insulin secretion (i.e. there is a need for residual β-cell activity) by binding to ATP-dependent K$^+$ channels. They may also have some long-term effects by increasing the numbers of insulin receptors on cell membranes. These drugs have a variable duration of action (usually less than 24 hours, but chlorpropamide has an effect for up to 72 hours). During long-term administration, these drugs may also show some extra-pancreatic actions, such as blockade of ischaemic preconditioning because of interference with K$^+$-ATP channel opening.

There are a number of different types of sulphonylureas:

- first generation—tolbutamide, chlorpropamide
- Second generation—these include glibenclamide, glyburide, glipizide, glimepiride.

Both first- and second-generation drugs should be withheld on the day of surgery. Although now less frequently prescribed, chlorpropamide should normally be stopped for 48 hours because of its longer half-life. These drugs can safely be combined with insulin therapy. It is rare for hypoglycaemia to be seen with these drugs, especially with the short-acting drugs (gliclazide and tolbutamide). Other long-acting drugs include glibenclamide (where there is a greater risk of hypoglycaemia) and glimepidine.

The major side-effect of sulphonylureas is hypoglycaemia, with minor episodes occurring in up to 20% of patients. The elderly are especially prone to these episodes, and use of longer-acting drugs, such as chlorpropamide and glibenclamide, is best avoided in these patients. The primary failure rate with sulphonylurea drugs is about 15%.

A few additional comments are relevant regarding the use of chlorpropamide. It is accompanied by more side-effects than other oral hypoglycaemic agents, and hence is no longer recommended (but there are still patients on this agent). Because chlorpropamide has a very prolonged duration of action, its use may be associated with the risk of hypoglycaemia. Other side-effects of chlorpropamide include facial flushing after drinking alcohol, enhanced ADH secretion, and very rarely hyponatraemia (which has also been reported after glimepiride and glipizide).

Other side-effects seen with the sulphonylureas include rare episodes of cholestatic jaundice, hypersensitivity reactions within the first 6–8 weeks of starting therapy, rare blood dyscrasias, and photosensitivity reactions (especially with chlorpropamide and glipizide).

Biguanides

Biguanides (e.g. metformin) act on the liver to decrease glucose output and on extra-hepatic sites to increase glucose utilization by shifting from an oxidative to an anaerobic metabolism and decreasing gluconeogenesis. Metformin only acts in the presence of some residual functioning β pancreatic islet cell activity, and it may also inhibit intestinal glucose absorption. Therefore it is the first-choice drug for overweight patients, where it may decrease obesity and lower mortality.

Metformin is associated with a lower risk of peri-operative hypoglycaemia than is the case with the sulphonylureas, but it should still be stopped for 24 hours pre-surgery, and its use should be avoided post-operatively in patients with renal or hepatic insufficiency. Other side-effects of metformin include gastrointestinal upsets, which are initially common and may persist in patients on high doses (>3 g per day). Like its predecessor phenformin, metformin can provoke lactic acidosis especially in patients with renal impairment. Compared with some of the other oral hypoglycaemics, metformin is less likely to be associated with hypoglycaemic episodes.

Metformin has other indications for use including as an unlicensed treatment for polycystic ovary syndrome, where it normalizes the menstrual cycle and improves hirsutism, as an adjunct in some diabetic patients to improve insulin sensitivity, and to achieve weight loss.

There are some contraindications to the use of metformin. It should be withdrawn if tissue hypoxia is likely (e.g. in patients with sepsis, respiratory failure, recent myocardial infarction, hepatic impairment), if iodine-containing X-ray contrast media are being used, and in the pregnant or breastfeeding patient. Lactic acidosis is most commonly seen in the elderly, in patients with renal or hepatic failure, and in patients undergoing major surgery.

In diabetic patients undergoing anaesthesia and surgery, it is recommended that the drug is suspended on the morning of surgery and not recommenced until renal function returns to normal.

Alpha-glucuronidase inhibitors (e.g. acarbose)

These drugs act to decrease gastrointestinal digestion and absorption of saccharides, and in turn glucose synthesis. They are useful in the reduction of post-prandial hyperglycaemia in type 1 DM, and can be used as an adjunct to metformin and sulphonylureas. Present evidence indicates no need to stop α-glucuronidase inhibitors pre-surgery. The side-effects of these inhibitors include increased incidence of flatulence and diarrhoea (in up to 50% of patients) resulting from the fermentation of unabsorbed carbohydrate in the large bowel. The incidence of these side-effects can be reduced by starting with low doses of the inhibitor.

Thiazolidinediones (e.g. pioglitazone, rosiglitazone)

The archetypal drug was troglitazone which was launched in the UK in 1997, but subsequently withdrawn because of concerns over a possible association with hepatotoxicity.

Generically, the glitazones act on extra-pancreatic sites to reduce peripheral insulin resistance, although their exact mechanism is not clear. The drugs bind to and activate one or more of the peroxisome proliferator-activated receptors (PPARs) which regulate gene expression in response to ligand binding. There are two types of PPAR: PPAR-γ is found mainly in adipose tissues, pancreatic β-cells, vascular endothelium, and macrophages, while PPAR-α is expressed in liver, heart, skeletal muscle, and vascular walls. Rosiglitazone (and troglitazone) act as a pure PPAR-γ agonist, while pioglitazone exerts some PPAR-α effects as well. This may explain the differences in the response of these drugs to lipids. The glitazones increase insulin sensitivity, increase insulin secretion, and act on the liver to inhibit gluconeogenesis.

The thiazolidinediones can be given either alone or in combination with metformin or a sulphonylurea. Inadequate drug response may indicate failure of intrinsic insulin release (a basic requirement for the effective action of the glitazones).

More recently (December 2007 and February 2008), advice on the cardiovascular safety of both rosiglitazone and pioglitazone has been offered in the UK. As a result, these drugs should not be used in patients with heart failure or a history of heart failure, as the incidence of heart failure is increased when one of these drugs is combined with insulin. Currently (August 2009), rosiglitazone is not recommended in patients with acute coronary syndrome, ischaemic heart disease, or peripheral arterial disease as it may cause a small but significant increase in the risk of cardiac ischaemia.

The glitazones act to reduce the levels of glycosylated haemoglobin, free fatty acids, and low-density lipid cholesterol, and may also improve lipaemic control. They also increase insulin-sensitive hepatic glucose uptake and inhibit gluconeogenesis.

Their use may be accompanied by a primary failure rate of about 25%.

Meglitinides (e.g. repaglinide, nateglinide)

These benzoic acid derivatives stimulate insulin secretion by binding to ATP-dependent K^+ channels in pancreatic cells. Both nateglinide and repaglinide have a rapid onset and short duration of action; therefore they should be given shortly before a meal. In the diabetic surgical patient, both the thiazolidinediones and meglitinides should be stopped on the day of surgery.

Most of the oral drugs mentioned so far bring about effective glycaemic control which decreases the microvascular but *not* the macrovascular complications of the disease.

New drugs

Three new classes of anti-diabetic agents have recently been reviewed.[14] Two of these are based on gastrointestinal hormones (the incretins and amylin) which have effects on blood glucose control. The other approach is the use of rimonabant, an antagonist of the endocannibinoid system, which acts through the CB1 receptor.

The 'incretin effect' The incretins are endogenous gut hormones which increase the secretion of insulin in response to oral glucose loads to levels that are greater than that seen when an intravenous glucose load is given to produce the same blood glucose concentration. The main incretins are glucose-dependent insulinotrophic polypepetide (GIP) and glucagon-like peptide 1 (GLP-1).

A GLP-1 effect persists in the patient with diabetes mellitus, with the hormone thought to be derived from enterendocrine L cells in the distal ileum and large intestine. Within a few minutes of food intake, GLP-1 concentrations in the blood increase three- to fivefold. The rapidity of response suggests that the secretion of GLP-1 is not simply the result of detection of food in the gastrointestinal tract, but that a fast endocrine or neutral mechanism may also be involved.

GLP-1 also reduces appetite, slows gastric emptying, reduces glucagon levels, enhances glucose-stimulated insulin secretion, and increases insulin biosynthesis. GLP-1 is rapidly biodegraded by the enzyme dipeptidyl peptidase IV (DPP-IV).

Two types of drug affect the incretin effect. The first type are naturally occurring peptide homologues of GLP-1 (exendin-4 or exenatide, and liraglutide). These are drugs which are resistant to breakdown by DPP-IV. Exenatide has a more rapid onset and duration of action of 6–12 hours, while liraglutide has a longer half-life (10–14 hours) and longer duration of effect. Exenatide is an incretin mimetic which increases insulin secretion, suppresses glucagon secretion, and slows gastric emptying. It is given by subcutaneous injection in type 2 DM patients, and can be used in combination with other treatments.

The second drug is sitagliptin, which acts as an inhibitor of DPP-IV and, in contrast to the other two compounds, does not affect gastric emptying. Sitagliptin has a half-life of about 12 hours, is well tolerated, and has no gastrointestinal symptoms. It is licensed for the treatment of type 2 DM patients when metformin or thioglitazone fail to give good glycaemic control.

Amylin

Amylin, another gastrointestinal hormone, is also produced by the pancreatic β-cells. In a similar manner to GLP-1, food intake stimulates amylin secretion. The glucose-decreasing effects of amylin seem to be independent of and additive to the effects of insulin.

Pramlintide is a synthetic amylin analogue which can be used as an adjunct to insulin therapy in both type 1 and type 2 DM. It has an onset time of about 20 minutes and a duration of action of 2–4 hours. As well as improving post-prandial glucose concentrations, pramlintide decreases glycated haemoglobin (HbA1C) levels and post-prandial triglyceride profiles. However, it has an important side-effect of nausea.

All of these classes of drugs have only recently been introduced into clinical practice, and currently there are few guidelines for the management of patients on these agents in the peri-operative period.[14] It is recommended that all three drugs are withheld on the day of surgery, but they can probably be taken on the day prior to surgery without any significant risk of hypoglycaemia whilst fasting.

Insulins

There are a number of different types of insulin based on their physiological profiles, and different sources (bovine, porcine, and human). Bovine insulin differs from the human insulin by three amino acids, and porcine insulin by one amino acid. When switching from an animal source to human insulin, a reduction of 10–20% of the overall daily dose is usually required to avoid episodes of hypoglycaemia. One useful classification is based on their duration of action.

Short-acting and ultra-short-acting insulins

Soluble insulin This is the archetypal insulin preparation. If it is used for maintenance regimens, it should given 15–30 minutes before meals. It has a rapid onset of action (30–60 minutes), with a peak effect at 2–4 hours and a duration of action up to 8 hours when given intravenously, intramuscularly, or subcutaneously. If given by the intravenous route, soluble insulin has a very short half-life (of about 5 minutes) and its effects dissipate within 30 minutes. However, its use is accompanied by a significant incidence of side-effects. These include local reactions and fat hypertrophy at the injection site. Very rarely it can cause hypersensitivity reactions including urticaria and rash. Overdose can cause hypoglycaemia.

Soluble insulin analogues Aspart, glulisine, and lispro are all recombinant human insulin analogues. All have a faster onset and shorter duration of action than soluble insulin, and can be given by subcutaneous infusion. When given intravenously, aspart and lispro are alternatives to soluble insulin for diabetic emergencies and at the time of surgery.

Thrice-daily regimens with soluble or similar insulin may be used for the introduction of insulin therapy, but long-term strategies will normally include:

- intermediate-acting insulin plus a short-acting insulin given together in the morning and evening

- intermediate- or long-acting insulin at bedtime and injections of short-acting insulin before each meal
- long-acting insulin in the morning plus short-acting insulin in the morning and evening
- long-acting insulin in the morning ± a short-acting insulin in the morning (see further below).

Intermediate and long-acting insulins

When given by subcutaneous injection, these preparations have a dynamic profile with an onset of 1–2 hours, maximum effect at 4–12 hours, and duration of 16–35 hours. They may be given twice daily in conjunction with short-acting (soluble) insulin *or* once daily, especially in elderly patients. Soluble insulin can often be mixed with other preparations in the same syringe (except with detemir and glargine insulin) with each formulation essentially retaining its own properties, although there may be a slight obtunding of the effect of the soluble insulin component if given with PZI (see below).

(a) Isophane is a mixture of insulin and protamine, and is of particular value in the initiation of twice-daily insulin regimens. It can be reliably mixed with soluble insulin, and is also prepared as 'ready-mixed' preparations (e.g. biphasic isophane insulin, biphasic insulin aspart, or biphasic insulin lispro).

(b) Insulin zinc suspension (PZI) is a mixture of 30% amorphous and 70% crystalline insulin, giving the insulin a more prolonged duration of action (24–46 hours). PZI is usually given once daily, but the formulation cannot be given by the intravenous route.

(c) Glargine and detemir are both human insulin analogues with prolonged durations of action. Glargine is given once daily, and detemir once or twice daily

- Intermediate insulin—isophane.
- Long-acting insulins—detemir, glargine, PZI.
- Biphasic insulins:
  - biphasic insulin aspart—30% aspart + 70% aspart protamine
  - biphasic insulin lispro—25% lispro + 75% lispro protamine
  - biphasic isophane insulin—30% soluble + 70% isophane.

As well as having a normoglycaemia action, insulin has a number of other non-metabolic effects which are advantageous to the surgical patient:

- maintenance of macrophage and neutrophil function
- insulin induces beneficial trophic changes on mucosal and skin barriers
- enhanced red cell synthesis and decreased haemolysis
- reduced cholestasis
- reduced ventilation secondary to direct anabolic effect of insulin on respiratory muscle function and less hyperglycaemic injury to axons
- less axon dysfunction and degeneration associated with hyperglycaemia and insulin deficiency.

Peri-operative handling of anti-glycaemic drugs

Patients on oral therapies (e.g. suphonylureas, biguanides, thiazolidinediones, or meglitinides) should have their drugs withheld prior to surgery. The patient who normally uses dietary control of their blood sugar concentration may require insulin therapy in the peri-operative period for glucose control.

There is no uniform approach for patients on different insulin regimens. Several different regimens have been suggested:

◆ withhold all insulin and start infusions of dextrose and insulin

◆ half or two-thirds of patient's usual intermediate-acting insulin subcutaneously

◆ combined insulin, glucose, and potassium

◆ separate insulin and glucose infusions

◆ insulin infusion and crystalloids

◆ conversion to use of subcutaneous insulin pumps

◆ use of an artificial pancreas.

Anaesthesia and the surgical diabetic patient

There is little consistency in the strategy used by anaesthetists to control glucose in the peri-operative period.[15]

Pre-operative assessment should include a full electrolyte, urea, and creatinine screen, blood count with white cell differential, chest radiograph, and electrocardiogram. Patients receiving other coincidental therapies should have them optimized before surgery. In the presence of uncontrolled diabetes, plasma and whole-body potassium levels may be decreased and therefore additional supplementation may be needed pre-surgery.

Strategies for control of blood glucose concentration in the peri-operative period are as follows:

◆ no hypoglycaemic agent, no glucose

◆ reduced hypoglycaemic dose with glucose

◆ combined insulin, glucose, potassium

◆ separate insulin and glucose infusions

◆ insulin infusion and crystalloids.

Elective surgery in non-insulin-dependent diabetics

Most patients will have sufficient endogenous insulin secretion to carry them through minor surgery (i.e. surgery not involving penetration of a body cavity or transection of a major limb bone) and avoid the need for transient insulin therapy. For major surgery, exogenous insulin will be needed to avoid the development of ketosis.

Elective surgery in insulin-dependent diabetics

The *laissez-faire* approach where there is no active management of the blood glucose concentration is inappropriate for most patients.[16]

Various approaches are adopted based on either regular administration of small doses of intravenous insulin or an infusion of insulin with the simultaneous infusion of 5% dextrose (with adjustment of the rates of infusion of the insulin and/or glucose based on frequent blood glucose estimations) or the glucose–insulin–potassium regimen.[17] Blood glucose estimations should be undertaken hourly until it is either well controlled or enteral feeding can be restarted.

If patients are already on a long-acting insulin preparation as part of their care, this can safely be given the evening before surgery to achieve basal normoglycaemia. Then half-hourly intravenous boluses of a rapid-acting insulin preparation (based on patient's weight, height, and existing blood glucose level) can be given to maintain the peri-operative plasma glucose level at 4–8 mmol/L.[18]

Hyperglycaemia is not the only physiological change that occurs during surgery in the diabetic patient. There is a well-characterized catabolic and sympathetic response to trauma—increased circulating catecholamines, growth hormone, glucagon, and cortisol, with an associated decrease in insulin levels promoting hepatic glycogenolysis and gluconeogenesis. The metabolic response may be *more pronounced* in diabetics undergoing surgery. For example, when type 2 diabetics were compared with non-diabetic patients undergoing colorectal surgery, the diabetic patients had higher plasma glucose concentrations, higher glucagon levels, and lower insulin levels post-surgery together with evidence of greater protein catabolism.[19]

Outcome measures and complications of treatment

Beyond the avoidance of hypoglycaemia, there is little reason to believe that any state other than euglycaemia (4.5–6.0 mmol/L) is best for the peri-operative patient. The benefits of glucose control and associated insulin therapy include decreased osmotic diuresis, enhanced innate immunity, improved endothelial function, and less impact on ischaemic tissues. These benefits occur through decreased lipolysis and less generation of free fatty acids (these act to exacerbate myocardial ischaemia and arrhythmias), inhibition of deleterious growth factors (e.g. AP-1, EGRG-1), enhanced production of nitric oxide synthase, and inhibition of pro-inflammatory mediators including cytokines, chemokines, acute phase proteins, and adhesion molecules. There is some evidence linking chronic hyperglycaemia and end-organ pathology in the long-term complications of diabetes.

Intra-operative control of glucose

There are few studies assessing whether intraoperative glycaemic control affects outcome in diabetic patients.

A retrospective study of over 6000 cardiac surgery patients showed that a high peak glucose concentration during bypass surgery was an independent risk factor for mortality and morbidity in both diabetic and non-diabetic patients.[20] Hyperglycaemia was a predictor of adverse outcome in other retrospective studies in cardiac surgery,[21,22] carotid endarterectomy,[23] and infra-inguinal arterial bypass surgery.[24]

In an attempt to assess the effects of different levels of hyperglycaemia, Malmstedt et al.[24] examined the intra-operative area under the curve (AUC) of glucose concentration versus time against major complications including death occurring in the first 90 days post-surgery. When the AUCs were divided into quartiles, the univariate odds ratio for the fourth versus the first quartile was 5.56 (1.27–24.49) for death, major amputation, or graft occlusion (adjusted ratio 13.35 (2.06–86.70)). Noordzij et al.[25] also showed that increased *pre-operative* glucose levels were associated with peri-operative mortality in patients undergoing non-cardiac non-vascular surgery. Using a cohort study based on a database of over 100 000 patients, they identified 989 cases where death occurred within 30 days of hospital stay and 1879 controls matched for age, sex, type of surgery, and calendar year. Patients were stratified into three groups (normal, random blood glucose <5.6 mmol/L; impaired = pre-diabetics, random blood glucose 5.6–11.1 mmol/L; diabetic, random blood glucose >11.1 mmol/L). About 18% of the deaths were cardiac in nature. Compared with the normoglycaemic patients, both the pre-diabetic and diabetic patients had a higher incidence of associated cardiovascular and all-cause deaths. Similar findings have been reported in studies on vascular surgical patients.[26,27]

Only one prospective intra-operative randomized control trial of intensive insulin therapy versus routine care in surgical patients is reported in the literature. Gandhi et al.[21] studied 400 cardiac surgery patients who received either intensive or conventional control intra-operatively, followed by intensive post-operative glycaemic control. While there was a significant difference in the mean intra-operative glucose concentrations, there were no differences in the incidence of a composite 30-day endpoint of death or major morbidity, with *more* deaths and strokes in the intra-operative intensive treatment group.

Other researchers have shown improved outcome in post-cardiac surgical patients where there was improved glycaemic control. Furnary et al.[28] found that improved control was associated with an absolute risk-adjusted decrease in mortality of 57% (a relative decrease of 50%). In two separate intensive care unit (ICU) studies (one retrospective and the other prospective), Krinsley[29,30] has shown an association between hyperglycaemia and mortality.

Although the influence of diabetes mellitus was not the primary aim of our case–control studies using the Oxford Record Linkage Study, we have found no association between diabetes and 30-day cardiac death in patients undergoing elective or emergency/urgent non-cardiac surgery.[31,32] More recently, Jeger et al.[33] examined long-term mortality after major cardiovascular surgery in a cohort study in patients with diabetes and coronary artery disease undergoing non-cardiac surgery. Mortality was only increased in patients treated with oral hypoglycaemics (odds ratio 3.3 (1.2–9.0)), suggesting a possible beneficial effect of insulin.

There is some evidence that a pre-operative shift of therapy from glibenclamide (a blocker of K^+-ATP channel opening) to insulin may be cardioprotective in diabetic patients undergoing coronary artery bypass surgery.[34] Further studies to support this finding are needed.

Tao *et al.*[35] studied a cohort of 107 non-cardiac patients to identify the predictors of post-operative complications in the diabetic patients.[35] The patients were chosen on the basis of either receiving insulin or oral hypoglycaemics drugs pre-admission or having been shown to have a fasting blood glucose >140 mg/dL on at least one occasion pre-operatively. All patients were followed up for 7 days post-operatively or until death, discharge, or re-operation. When univariate analyses were performed to identify preclinical risk factors that were predictive of peri-operative complications, only the Goldman Risk Index predicted both overall cardiac complications and myocardial infarction. The degree of glycaemic control did not improve the model. However, a number of risk factors were shown to be important for the development of long-term cardiac death and events. These unadjusted demographic, peri-operative, and post-operative variables included patient age, past history of myocardial infarction, peripheral vascular disease, Goldman Index class, duration of both DM and/or associated hypertension, and post-operative cardiac arrest or myocardial infarction. Again, peri-operative glucose control was not found to be important. After finally adjusting the odds ratio for confounders, a stepwise proportional hazards regression analysis showed that age, total comorbidity score, and total post-operative cardiac complications all predicted deaths. The duration of hypertension and total comorbidity score predicted cardiac deaths and events, while the history of stroke, Goldman Index, and total comorbidity score predicted vascular deaths and events. Thus the total comorbidity score was the only variable that predicted events of all types.[36]

Another study[27] has shifted interest away from diabetes mellitus *per se* to the risks associated with anaesthesia and surgery in the patient with new-onset hyperglycaemia. These 'pre-diabetic patients' have been shown to have an increased risk of peri-operative cardiac ischaemia (odds ratio 3.2) as well as showing impaired glucose regulation and an elevated level of HbA1A. A further paper[26] reports that these patients show increased troponin T levels post-surgery, and increased 30-day and long-term cardiac event rates. Clearly, the optimum management of these patients needs to be studied further.

There are no prospective data showing that intra-operative glycaemic control is associated with improved outcome. Hence there are still five key questions to be answered with respect to the care of diabetic patients undergoing surgery.

1. Is good glycaemic control relevant to all types of surgical patient? If tight glycaemic control is needed, what level of blood glucose should we aim for?

2. In the emergency case, does the duration of the presenting illness correlate with the need for tighter diabetic control?

3. Is the benefit of better outcome in diabetic patients due to infusing glucose, infusing insulin, or both?

4. Does early feeding help (as suggested by the work of Van den Berghe[49,50])?

5. Does insulin resistance increase the morbidity rate?

Another key issue is how and by whom should the glucose be managed during the peri-operative period?

Post-operative outcomes

Several studies and audits have looked at the outcome of anaesthesia and surgery in patients with diabetes mellitus. In one of the first, Treves (in 1898) states the following:

> Diabetes offers a serious bar to any kind of operation, and injuries involving open wounds, haemorrhage or damage to blood vessels are exceeding grave in subjects with the disease. A wound in the diabetic patient will probably not heal while the tissues appear to offer the most favourable soil for the development of putrefaction and pyogenic bacteria. The wound gapes, suppurates, and sloughs. Gangrene readily follows in injury in diabetics, and such patients show terrible proneness to the low form of erysipelas and cellulitis.

Many authors support this scenario, with Galloway and Shuman[37] reporting a mortality of 3.6% and morbidity of 17.2% in over 650 patients, Alieff[38] reporting a mortality of 13.2%, and Whelock and Marble[39] reporting a mortality of 3.7% among 2780 diabetic surgical patients. Other studies show the influence of diabetes mellitus on surrogate outcomes. Although Raby et al.[40] failed to show any association between diabetes and intra- and post-operative myocardial ischaemia, Hollenberg et al.,[41] using multivariate analysis, found that post-operative myocardial ischaemia occurred more frequently in treated diabetic patients. Based on further data from the same study, Browner et al.[42] found no association between diabetes and in-hospital and long-term mortality (odds ratio 2.1 (0.9–5.0)).

Recent data from Schmeltz et al.[43] report a mortality of 7.3% (compared with 3.3% in non-diabetic subjects) in over 600 patients undergoing cardiothoracic surgery. Krolikowska et al.[44] compared mortality in 274 consecutive diabetic patients and 282 non-diabetic patients matched for the same type of operation. Mortality in both the short term (within 21 days) and the long term (up to over 7 years) was higher in the diabetic patients (3.5% versus 0%, and 37.2% versus 15%, respectively. The major causes of death among the diabetic patients were diseases of the cardiovascular system (56.8% versus 18.6% in the non-diabetic subjects). Although diabetes per se was not a risk factor for post-operative mortality, a combination of variables (history of macroangiopathy, high-risk ASA class, urgent surgery, low-BMI quartile) had a significant effect on both short- and long-term mortality. This is in agreement with other studies.[6,45] Within a cohort of diabetic patients, Krolikowska et al.[44] found that those with type II diabetes had higher short- and long-term mortalities. However, these findings contrast with those of Axelrod et al.[46] who showed that, although there was a greater incidence of death and major cardiovascular events associated with diabetes in a study of 14 525 major vascular surgery patients, there was an association between insulin-dependent diabetics and adverse outcome (odds ratio 1.37 (1.13–1.64)) but not for those on oral therapies (odds ratio 1.07 (0.87–1.32)). This has not been confirmed by Hamdan et al.,[47] who found no increase in short-term major cardiovascular events (including death) in diabetic patients. However, there was a reduction in long-term survival.

A very recent retrospective observational study from Australia has identified a risk of death or cardiac events in diabetic patients as 12.2% at 30 days and 20% at 6 months after non-cardiac surgery.[48]

Effects of glycaemic control on outcome

There are few studies examining the effect of glycaemic control on patient outcome in the peri-operative period. In a study of patients randomized to intensive insulin (glucose 4.4–6.1 mmol/L) versus conventional therapy (glucose 10–11.1 mmol/L), Van den Berghe et al.[49] showed a reduction in mortality in critically ill ICU patients where the glucose was tightly controlled. In the former group, the aim was to maintain a blood glucose concentration between 80 and 110 mg/dL, while the aim of conventional therapy was to institute treatment if blood sugar rose above 215 mg/dL, and then to maintain the concentration between 80 and 200 mg/dL. The study was terminated early because of a significant reduction in ICU mortality in the intensive treatment group (4.6% versus 8.0%), as well as a significant reduction in in-hospital mortality, incidence of dialysis-dependent renal failure, number of transfusions, incidence of critical illness neuropathy, need for prolonged ventilation, and bloodstream infections. In a further prospective study of medical ICU critically ill patients, the same authors showed a similar reduction in morbidity, and a reduction in mortality in patients treated for 3 or more days.[50])

Furnary et al.[28] showed a similar benefit of improved glycaemic control in patients undergoing coronary artery bypass surgery. Krinsley[29,30] showed an association between hyperglycaemia and mortality. Similar findings have been reported when examining the effect of intra-operative glycaemic control on severe morbidity.[21,22]

A systematic review of 26 studies of of adult stroke patients showed that hyperglycaemia was associated with increased mortality and poorer functional recovery in survivors.[51] A similar association between hyperglycaemia and outcome was found in patients suffering myocardial infarction, where a raised blood glucose concentration was associated with an increased risk of the patient developing congestive cardiac failure and cardiogenic shock in patients *without* diabetes, and increased in-hospital mortality in patients both *with* and *without* diabetes.[52]

In April 2009, the results of the NICE-SUGAR study were published. This involved 6104 ICU patients randomized to either tight glucose control (4.5–6.0 mmol/L) or conventional treatment with blood glucose concentration maintained between 8.0 and 10.0 mmol/L. The main outcome measure was 90-day mortality which was *greater* in the tight-control group (27.5% versus 24.9%)! Deaths from cardiovascular causes were also more common in the tight-control group (41.6% versus 35.8%). There was a significant increase in the occurrence of hypoglycaemia, defined as blood sugar concentration <2.2 mmol/L (6.8% versus 0.5%).[53]

A new meta-analysis of the efficacy of tight glucose control in the ICU[54] came to the same conclusions (although it may have been biased by the inclusion of the NICE-SUGAR data), with a pooled relative risk for death of 0.93, and a relative risk ratio for hypoglycaemia of 6.0 associated with tight glucose control. These data cast doubt on the efficacy and safety of intensive insulin regimens in the post-operative period, but raise the important question of what blood sugar level the clinician should aim for in the post-operative surgical patient.

Key clinical management points

There are many different schemes for peri-operative care of the diabetic patient. This is a suggested approach, but others are equally acceptable.

Diagnosis

Suspect in patients with typical history of polyuria and polydypsia, patients with unusual septic presentations, and patients with extensive vascular pathology.

Diagnostic tests

- Glucose tolerance testing
- HbA1C will give an indication of control over the previous 2–3 months (life of the red cell)

General assessment

- Cardiovascular assessment, ischaemia risk, peripheral vascular lesions
  - ECG, possibly stress ECG for major surgery
  - Blood pressure control
- Assess renal function
- Peripheral neuropathy
  - Sensory deficits
  - Autonomic neuropathy
    - Valsalva manoeuvre, tilt table testing
- Joint mobility (glycosylated collagen)
  - Neck and jaw mobility, 'prayer sign'

Pre-operative preparation

All patients should be rendered normoglycaemic prior to surgery if possible (for emergency management see Chapter 9)

Type 1 diabetes mellitus

- Minor surgery
  - Omit morning insulin
  - Minimize starvation (glucose water up to 2 hours pre-operatively)
  - Early on list
- Major surgery
  - Convert to soluble insulin 24 hours pre-operatively *or*

Key clinical management points (continued)

- Give usual long-acting drug in the evening for basal insulin requirements
  - Measure blood sugar on morning of surgery
  - Titrate rapid-acting insulin
- Consider cardiac protective strategy
  - β-blockade, statins, aspirin

Type 2 diabetes mellitus

- Minor surgery—as for type 1
  - Omit oral hypoglycaemic agents on morning of surgery
- Major surgery—as for type 1
  - Convert to soluble insulin either pre-operatively or during surgery as indicated
  - Insulin may be needed in patients routinely controlled by diet alone

Autonomic instability

- Anticipate haemodynamic instability
- Consider H_2 antagonists and/or prokinetics with premedication

Anaesthetic management

- Minor surgery
  - Check starting blood sugar
  - Regional anaesthesia preferable
  - Monitor blood sugar hourly
  - Restart oral feeding and standard insulin therapy
- Major surgery
  - Insulin infusion starting at 1 unit per hour and adjusting to blood sugar; higher doses may be need in the obese, in cardiac and liver surgery, and in the uraemic patient
  - Monitor blood sugar hourly unless massive fluid shifts
- Consider airway protection if high risk of aspiration (severe autonomic dysfunction)
- Anticipate haemodynamic instability if autonomic instability present

Post-operative care

- Minor surgery in type 2 diabetes: restart oral therapy and feeding as soon as possible
- Ensure continued glucose control with insulin infusion until able to take orally
- Maintain adequate urine output

Further reading

Coursin DB, Connery LE, Ketzler JT (2004). Perioperative diabetic and hyperglycemic management issues. *Critical Care Medicine*, **32** (Suppl), s116–25.

Finney SJ, Zekveld C, Elia A, Evans TW (2003). Glucose control and mortality in critically ill patients. *Journal of the American Medical Association*, **290**, 2041–7.

Glister BC, Vigersky RA (2003). Perioperative management of type 1 diabetes mellitus. *Endocrinology and Metabolism Clinics of North America*, **32**, 411–36.

Gu W, Pagel PS, Warltier DC, Kersten JR (2003). Modifying cardiovascular risk in diabetes mellitus. *Anesthesiology*, **98**, 774–9.

Jacober SJ, Sowers JR (1999). A update on perioperative management of diabetes. *Archives of Internal Medicine*, **159**, 2405–11.

Roghi A, Palmieri B, Crivellaro W, Faletra F, Putini M (2001). Relationship of unrecognised myocardial infarction, diabetes mellitus and type of surgery to postoperative cardiac outcomes in vascular surgery. *European Journal of Vascular and Endovascular Surgery*, **21**, 9–16.

References

1. Garber AJ, Moghissi ES, Bransome ED, Jr, *et al.* (2004). American College of Endocrinology position statement on inpatient diabetes and metabolic control. *Endocrine Practice*, **10**, 77–82.

2. Juul AB, Wetterslev J, Kofoed-Enevoldsen A (2004). Long-term postoperative mortality in diabetic patients undergoing major non-cardiac surgery. *European Journal of Anaesthesiology*, **21**, 523–9.

3. UK Prospective Diabetes Study Group (1998). Tight blood pressure control and risk of macrovascular and microvascular complications in type 2 diabetes. *British Medical Journal*, **317**, 703–13.

4. Hansson L, Zanchetti A, Carruthers SG, *et al.* (1998). Effects of intensive blood-pressure lowering and low-dose aspirin in patients with hypertension: principal results of the Hypertension Optimal Treatment (HOT) randomised trial.. *Lancet*, **351**, 1755–62.

5. Alberti KG, Zimmet P, Shaw J (2006). Metabolic syndrome—a new world-wide definition. A consensus statement from the International Diabetes Federation. *Diabetic Medicine*, **23**, 469–80.

6. Rockman CB, Saltzberg SS, Maldonado TS, *et al.* (2005). The safety of carotid endarterectomy in diabetic patients: clinical predictors of adverse outcome. *Journal of Vascular Surgery*, **42**, 878–83.

7. Juul AB, Wetterslev J, Gluud C, *et al.* (2006). Effect of perioperative beta blockade in patients with diabetes undergoing major non-cardiac surgery: randomised placebo controlled, blinded multicentre trial. *British Medical Journal*, **332**, 1482.

8. Hennessy TG, Codd MB, Kane G, McCarthy C, McCann HA, Sugrue DD (1997). Evaluation of patients with diabetes mellitus for coronary artery disease using dobutamine stress echocardiography. *Coronary Artery Disease*, **8**, 171–4.

9. Cortigiani L, Bigi R, Sicari R, Landi P, Bovenzi F, Picano E (2006). Prognostic value of pharmacological stress echocardiography in diabetic and nondiabetic patients with known or suspected coronary artery disease. *Journal of the American College of Cardiology*, **47**, 605–10.

10. Elhendy A, Arruda AM, Mahoney DW, Pellikka PA (2001). Prognostic stratification of diabetic patients by exercise echocardiography. *Journal of the American College of Cardiology*, **37**, 1551–7.

11. Garrido IP, Peteiro J, Garcia-Lara J, *et al.* (2005). Prognostic value of exercise echocardiography in patients with diabetes mellitus and known or suspected coronary artery disease. *American Journal of Cardiology*, **96**, 9–12.

12. Kertai MD, Boersma E, Bax JJ, *et al.* (2003). A meta-analysis comparing the prognostic accuracy of six diagnostic tests for predicting perioperative cardiac risk in patients undergoing major vascular surgery. *Heart*, **89**, 1327–34.

13. Ginawi OT (1992). Morphine analgesia in normal and alloxanized mice. *Archives Internationales de Pharmacodynamie et de Thérapie*, **318**, 13–20.

14. Chen D, Lee SL, Peterfreund RA (2009). New therapeutic agents for diabetes mellitus: implications for anesthetic management. *Anesthesia and Analgesia*, **108**, 1803–10.

15. Eldridge AJ, Sear JW (1996). Peri-operative management of diabetic patients. Any changes for the better since 1985? *Anaesthesia*, **51**, 45–51.

16. Fletcher J, Langman MJS, Kellock TD (1965). Effect of surgery on blood-sugar levels in diabetes mellitus. *Lancet*, **286**, 52–4.

17. Robertshaw HJ, Hall GM (2006). Diabetes mellitus: anaesthetic management. *Anaesthesia*, **61**, 1187–90.

18. Holman RR, Turner RC (1985). A practical guide to basal and prandial insulin therapy. *Diabetic Medicine*, **2**, 45–53.

19. Schricker T, Gougeon R, Eberhart L, *et al.* (2005). Type 2 diabetes mellitus and the catabolic response to surgery. *Anesthesiology*, **102**, 320–6.

20. Doenst T, Wijeysundera D, Karkouti K, *et al.* (2005). Hyperglycemia during cardiopulmonary bypass is an independent risk factor for mortality in patients undergoing cardiac surgery. *Journal of Thoracic and Cardiovascular Surgery*, **130**, 1144.

21. Gandhi GY, Nuttall GA, Abel MD, *et al.* (2005). Intraoperative hyperglycemia and perioperative outcomes in cardiac surgery patients. *Mayo Clinic Proceedings*, **80**, 862–6.

22. Ouattara A, Lecomte P, Le MY, *et al.* (2005). Poor intraoperative blood glucose control is associated with a worsened hospital outcome after cardiac surgery in diabetic patients. *Anesthesiology*, **103**, 687–94.

23. McGirt MJ, Woodworth GF, Brooke BS, *et al.* (2006). Hyperglycemia independently increases the risk of perioperative stroke, myocardial infarction, and death after carotid endarterectomy. *Neurosurgery*, **58**, 1066–73.

24. Malmstedt J, Wahlberg E, Jorneskog G, Swedenborg J (2006). Influence of perioperative blood glucose levels on outcome after infrainguinal bypass surgery in patients with diabetes. *British Journal of Surgery*, **93**, 1360–7.

25. Noordzij PG, Boersma E, Schreiner F, *et al.* (2007). Increased preoperative glucose levels are associated with perioperative mortality in patients undergoing noncardiac, nonvascular surgery. *European Journal of Endocrinology*, **156**, 137–42.

26. Feringa HH, Vidakovic R, Karagiannis SE, *et al.* (2008). Impaired glucose regulation, elevated glycated haemoglobin and cardiac ischaemic events in vascular surgery patients. *Diabetic Medicine*, **25**, 314–19.

27. Dunkelgrun M, Schreiner F, Schockman DB, *et al.* (2008). Usefulness of preoperative oral glucose tolerance testing for perioperative risk stratification in patients scheduled for elective vascular surgery. *American Journal of Cardiology*, **101**, 526–9.

28. Furnary AP, Gao G, Grunkemeier GL, *et al.* (2003). Continuous insulin infusion reduces mortality in patients with diabetes undergoing coronary artery bypass grafting. *Journal of Thoracic and Cardiovascular Surgery*, **125**, 1007–21.

29. Krinsley JS (2003). Association between hyperglycemia and increased hospital mortality in a heterogeneous population of critically ill patients. *Mayo Clinic Proceedings*, **78**, 1471–8.

30. Krinsley JS (2004). Effect of an intensive glucose management protocol on the mortality of critically ill adult patients. *Mayo Clinic Proceedings*, **79**, 992–1000.

31. Howell SJ, Sear YM, Yeates D, Goldacre M, Sear JW, Foex P (1998). Risk factors for cardiovascular death after elective surgery under general anaesthesia. *British Journal of Anaesthesia*, **80**, 14–19.

32. Howell SJ, Sear JW, Sear YM, Yeates D, Goldacre M, Foex P (1999). Risk factors for cardiovascular death within 30 days after anaesthesia and urgent or emergency surgery: a nested case-control study. *British Journal of Anaesthesia*, **82**, 679–84.

33. Jeger RV, Seeberger MD, Keller U, Pfisterer ME, Filipovic M (2007). Oral hypoglycemics: increased postoperative mortality in coronary risk patients. *Cardiology*, **107**, 296–301.

34. Forlani S, Tomai F, De Paulis R, *et al.* (2004). Preoperative shift from glibenclamide to insulin is cardioprotective in diabetic patients undergoing coronary artery bypass surgery. *Journal of Cardiovascular Surgery*, **45**, 117–22.

35. Tao LS, Mackenzie CR, Charlson ME (2008). Predictors of postoperative complications in the patient with diabetes mellitus. *Journal of Diabetes and its Complications*, **22**, 24–8.

36. Charlson ME, Mackenzie CR, Gold JP, Ales KL, Topkins M, Shires GT (1991). Risk for postoperative congestive heart failure. *Surgery, Gynecology and Obstetrics*, **172**, 95–104.

37. Galloway JA, Shuman CR (1963). Diabetes and surgery. A study of 667 cases. *American Journal of Medicine*, 34, 177–91

38. Alieff A (1969). [Risks of surgical intervention in diabetics]. *Zentralblatt für Chirurgie*, **94**, 857–60.

39. Whelock FC, Marble A (1971). Surgery and diabetes. In: Marble A, White P, Bradley RF, Kroll LP (eds), *Joslin's Diabetes Mellitus*, Lea & Febiger, Philadelphia, PA.

40. Raby KE, Barry J, Creager MA, Cook EF, Weisberg MC, Goldman L (1992). Detection and significance of intraoperative and postoperative myocardial ischemia in peripheral vascular surgery. *Journal of the American Medical Association*, **268**, 222–7.

41. Hollenberg M, Mangano DT, Browner WS, London MJ, Tubau JF, Tateo IM (1992). Predictors of postoperative myocardial ischemia in patients undergoing noncardiac surgery. The Study of Perioperative Ischemia Research Group. *Journal of the American Medical Association*, **268**, 205–9.

42. Browner WS, Li J, Mangano DT (1992). In-hospital and long-term mortality in male veterans following noncardiac surgery. The Study of Perioperative Ischemia Research Group. *Journal of the American Medical Association*, **268**, 228–32.

43. Schmeltz LR, DeSantis AJ, Thiyagarajan V, *et al.* (2007). Reduction of surgical mortality and morbidity in diabetic patients undergoing cardiac surgery with a combined intravenous and subcutaneous insulin glucose management strategy. *Diabetes Care*, **30**, 823–8.

44. Krolikowska M, Kataja M, Poyhia R, Drzewoski J, Hynynen M (2009). Mortality in diabetic patients undergoing non-cardiac surgery: a 7-year follow-up study. *Acta Anaesthesiologica Scandinavica*, **53**, 749–58.

45. Aziz IN, Lee JT, Kopchok GE, Donayre CE, White RA, de Virgilio C (2003). Cardiac risk stratification in patients undergoing endoluminal graft repair of abdominal aortic aneurysm: a single-institution experience with 365 patients. *Journal of Vascular Surgery*, **38**, 56–60.

46. Axelrod DA, Upchurch GR, Jr, Demonner S, *et al.* (2002). Perioperative cardiovascular risk stratification of patients with diabetes who undergo elective major vascular surgery. *Journal of Vascular Surgery*, **35**, 894–901.

47. Hamdan AD, Saltzberg SS, Sheahan M, *et al.* (2002). Lack of association of diabetes with increased postoperative mortality and cardiac morbidity: results of 6565 major vascular operations. *Archives of Surgery*, **137**, 417–21.

48. Bolsin SN, Raineri F, Lo SK, Cattigan C, Arblaster R, Colson M (2009). Cardiac complications and mortality rates in diabetic patients following non-cardiac surgery in an Australian teaching hospital. *Anaesthesia and Intensive Care*, **37**, 561–7.

49. Van den Berghe G, Wouters P, Weekers F, *et al.* (2001). Intensive insulin therapy in the critically ill patient. *New England Journal of Medicine*, **345**, 1359–67.

50. Van den Berghe G, Wouters PJ, Bouillon R, *et al.* (2003). Outcome benefit of intensive insulin therapy in the critically ill: insulin dose versus glycemic control. *Critical Care Medicine*, 31(2), 359–66

51. Capes SE, Hunt D, Malmberg K, Pathak P, Gerstein HC (2001). Stress hyperglycemia and prognosis of stroke in nondiabetic and diabetic patients: a systematic overview. *Stroke*, **32**, 2426–32.

52. Capes SE, Hunt D, Malmberg K, Gerstein HC (2000). Stress hyperglycaemia and increased risk of death after myocardial infarction in patients with and without diabetes: a systematic overview. *Lancet*, **355**, 773–8.

53. Finfer S, Chittock DR, Su SY, *et al.* (2009). Intensive versus conventional glucose control in critically ill patients. *New England Journal of Medicine*, **360**, 1283–97.

54. Griesdale DE, de Souza RJ, van Dam RM, *et al.* (2009). Intensive insulin therapy and mortality among critically ill patients: a meta-analysis including NICE-SUGAR study data. *Canadian Medical Association Journal*, **180**, 821–7.

Chapter 4

The thyroid gland

MFM James and PA Farling

Anatomical disease of the thyroid gland is common, presenting as both benign thyroid enlargement and thyroid malignancy. Disorders of thyroid gland function—hyperthyroidism and hypothyroidism—are less frequent, but may present significant challenges to the anaesthetist in terms of clinical management in the peri-operative period. The anatomy, physiology, and anaesthetic complications of thyroid disease are reviewed in this chapter, with particular emphasis on hormonal disturbance.

Anatomy

The thyroid gland is a bilobular structure with the two lobes joined by a narrow isthmus which crosses the trachea at the level of the first and second cartilaginous rings. The term 'thyroid' derives from the Greek word for shield and properly refers to the thyroid cartilage, from which the gland derives its name. Developmentally, the gland is derived from two separate embryological structures. The thyroid gland itself arises from primitive cells in the ranks between the anterior and posterior rudiments of the tongue. The calcitonin-producing cells arise from neural crest tissue in the ultimobranchial bodies of the fourth pharyngeal pouch. Both groups of cells migrate caudally to form the definitive thyroid gland in front of the trachea. The migration of the pharyngeal thyroid bud forms the thyroglossal duct from the base of the tongue, which gradually regresses but may leave residual thyroid tissue in its wake. In around 15% of the population, a pyramidal lobe arises from the thyroid isthmus along this developmental track. The two lobes develop on each side of the trachea, displacing the carotid sheath laterally, with the right lobe generally larger than the left (Figure 4.1).

The gland is very vascular and receives its arterial supply via the superior and inferior thyroid arteries on each side, and these vessels may form an extensive arteriolar network around the gland (Figure 4.1). Occasionally, an additional artery arises from the median unpaired thyroid ima artery. These arteries arise from the external carotid artery, the thyrocervical trunk of the subclavian artery, and the arch of the aorta, respectively. Venous drainage occurs through the superior and middle thyroid veins, which drain into the internal jugular vein, and the inferior thyroid vein, which drains into the brachiocephalic vein.

The thyroid gland receives sympathetic and parasympathetic nerve fibres, but the innervation of the gland is poor, with few fibres actually entering the substance of the thyroid, and secretion is not controlled neurologically. An important posterior relation of

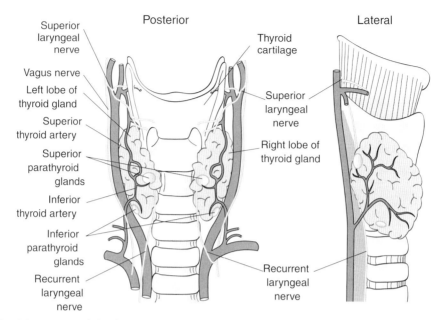

Fig. 4.1 Anatomy of the thyroid gland. Note particularly the relationship of the recurrent laryngeal nerve to the trachea and the gland.

the gland is the recurrent laryngeal nerve which lies in the groove between the trachea and the oesophagus, closely apposed to the superior thyroid artery. This nerve may be involved in thyroid malignancy and it might also be damaged during thyroid surgery, leading to various degrees of laryngeal dysfunction.

The thyroid parenchyma is largely composed of follicular cells, which surround the follicles and are responsible for formation of thyroid hormone, and parafollicular C-cells, which produce calcitonin. The follicular cells are cuboidal epithelial cells that surround the closed cavity of the follicular lumen in a single layer. The follicular cells have a basal domain that is adjacent to the extracellular matrix and is characterized by the presence of a sodium iodide transporter. The opposite end of the cell is referred to as the apical domain and faces the follicular lumen. This surface of the cell is characterized by the presence of microvilli and pseudopods that extend into the colloid. This part of the cell contains large amounts of the enzyme thyroperoxidase which is essential for the synthesis of thyroid hormone. The follicular lumen is filled with colloid. The C-cells are found as individual cells or in small groups closely associated with the follicular cells, mainly in the upper two-thirds of the lateral lobes. These cells, unlike the follicular cells, may express neuroendocrine markers, such as chromogranin, betraying their neural crest origins (Figure 4.2).

Physiology

The process of thyroid hormone synthesis commences with the uptake of iodine into the follicular cells. The sodium iodide transporter concentrates iodide from the circulation,

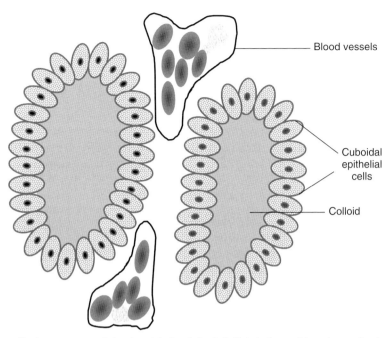

Fig. 4.2 Follicular structure of the thyroid gland. Each follicle is formed by a layer of cuboidal epithelial cells surrounding a collection of colloid.

raising the concentration within the follicular cells to approximately 30 times that of plasma. Once inside the cell, iodide diffuses to the apical membrane where it is transported into the follicular lumen. Thyroglobulin is a 660 kilodalton (kDa) protein, containing tyrosine residues, that is synthesized within the rough endoplasmic reticulum of the follicular cells. Most of the thyroglobulin is excreted into the follicular colloid by exocytosis and stored there. At the apical surface of the follicular cell, thyroperoxidase catalyses the iodination of tyrosine residues into iodothyronines on the backbone of thyroglobulin (Figure 4.3). Initial iodination of the tyrosine molecule occurs in the 3 position as the formation of mono-iodotyrosine and the addition of a second iodide in the 5 position produces 3, 5-di-iodotyrosine. Condensation of two molecules of di-iodotyrosine results in the formation of thyroxine (T_4). The coupling of one molecule each of mono-iodotyrosine and di-iodotyrosine results in the formation of T_3 (Figure 4.4). Both of these hormones remain coupled to thyroglobulin within the matrix of the colloid (Figure 4.3).

Hormone release requires the phagocytosis of iodinated thyroglobulin from the colloid into the follicular cells in the form of vesicles, which are then transported to the lysosomes. Within the lysosomes, thyroglobulin undergoes proteolytic degradation releasing T_4 and T_3, which are then transported out of the cell into the circulation (Figure 4.3). Approximately 100 nmol of T_4 and 10 nmol of T_3 are secreted by the thyroid

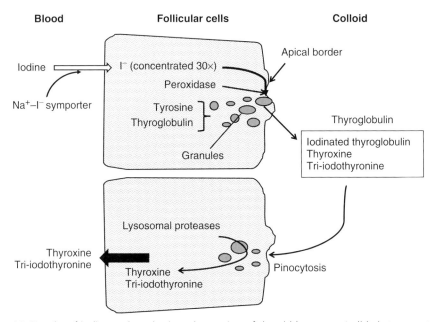

Fig. 4.3 Uptake of iodine and synthesis and excretion of thyroid hormone. Iodide is transported into the follicular cells and converted to iodine by thyroid peroxidase which also catalyses the binding of I⁻ to tyrosine residues within thyroglobulin. The thyroglobulin is stored in the colloid. Colloid is taken back into the follicular cells by pinocytosis and the thyroid hormone is cleaved from the thyroglobulin by lysosomal proteases. The thyroid hormones are then excreted into the capillaries.

gland per day and the normal total plasma T_4 is 103 nmol/L. Thyroid hormones are tightly bound to various plasma proteins and the free fraction is the important active component.

Regulation of thyroid hormone production

Thyroid-stimulating hormone (TSH) is the main regulator of thyroid function and stimulates iodine uptake, thyroglobulin production, and synthesis and release of iodothyronines. It also promotes thyroid growth by inducing hypertrophy of thyroid cells and formation of colloid. TSH is a 30 kDa glycoprotein synthesized in the anterior pituitary gland. Its production is regulated through a classic negative feedback loop and also through the action of thyrotrophin-releasing hormone (TRH) from the hypothalamus which regulates the TSH subunit gene transcription. In the feedback loop, the binding of T_3 to its receptor results in a dramatic decrease in the production of TSH and the release of TRH. Thus an increase in thyroid hormone release inhibits the release of TSH and a decrease increases TSH production.

Iodide also regulates thyroid function, inhibiting incorporation of iodide into thyroglobulin and, at high concentrations, inhibiting thyroid hormone secretion (Figure 4.5).

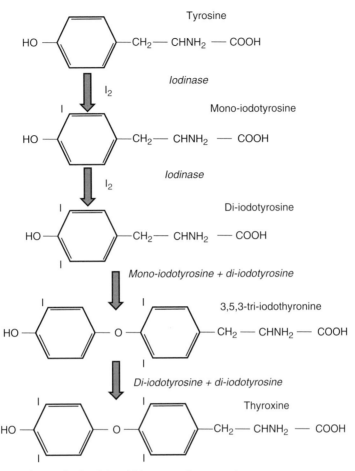

Fig. 4.4 Steps in the synthesis of thyroid hormone from tyrosine.

Actions of thyroid hormones

Thyroid hormones have a wide range of physiological functions, influencing cell differentiation and development and stimulating metabolic pathways. Failure of thyroid hormone production during fetal development and early childhood results a specific failure of brain development, leading to the syndrome of cretinism. This cannot be reversed by later hormone treatment, which indicates that there is a developmental requirement for thyroid hormone. In adults, changes in thyroid hormone production result in alterations of metabolic rate, affecting all aspects of energy production as well as the metabolism. Thus basal metabolic rate is highly responsive to the level of thyroid hormone production.

The predominant effects of thyroid hormones are exerted through modulation of gene expression, altering nuclear transcription and the synthesis of protein receptors. Thyroid

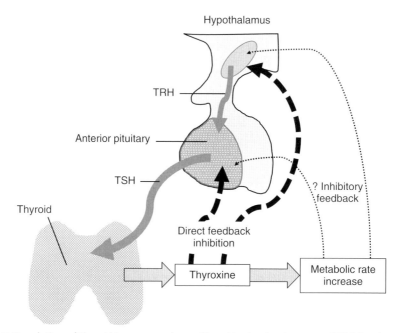

Fig. 4.5 Regulation of thyroid hormone release. Thyroid-releasing hormone (TRH) is released from the hypothalamus and conducted to the anterior pituitary gland by a network of portal capillaries. TRH then stimulates the release of thyroid-stimulating hormone (TSH) which drives the production and secretion of thyroid hormone from the thyroid gland. Thyroid hormone itself directly inhibits further production of TRH and TSH. The increase in metabolic rate caused by thyroid hormone may also exert some feedback inhibition of thyroid stimulation.

stimulation enhances the production and sensitivity of a variety of receptors, including β_1-adrenergic receptors, myosin α heavy chain and SER Ca^{2+}-ATPase (sarcoplasmic reticulum Ca^{2+} adenosine triphosphatase). This action requires the penetration of the cytosol by T_3, binding of T_3 to high-affinity nuclear receptors and the modulation of gene expression, a process that generally takes 2–6 hours before the effects are seen. Thyroid hormones cross the plasma membrane by specific processes that may be energy and/or sodium dependent. It is unlikely that significant plasma membrane transfer of hormone takes place by diffusion.[1] This process of cell penetration may be facilitated by specific thyroid hormone transporters.[2] However, thyroid hormones also exert extranuclear actions with more rapid responses, probably through the activation of G-protein-coupled receptors leading to alterations of intracellular function. Thus thyroid hormones can also exert rapid onset effects in addition to their delayed nuclear transcription activity.

Thyroid hormone increases oxygen consumption and metabolic rate, associated with an increase in heart rate and peripheral vasodilatation. It stimulates carbohydrate metabolism, increasing glucose absorption from the gut, enhancing glycolysis, and facilitating insulin secretion. It also regulates lipid metabolism, decreasing fat stores, increasing plasma free fatty acid concentrations, enhancing lipid metabolism, and reducing cholesterol.

However, it simultaneously stimulates appetite so that the consequent effects on body mass may be unpredictable. It has important effects on growth and development, stimulating growth but leading to early closure of the epiphyses. Thyroid hormones also stimulate Na^+/K^+-ATPase activity and activate mitochondrial enzymes.

The effects of thyroid hormone on the cardiovascular system are complex. Heart rate and cardiac output increase and systemic vascular resistance decreases as a consequence of the increased metabolic rate. However, thyroid hormone increases β-adrenergic activity and also has direct effects on the myocardium increasing contractility. T_3 dilates the resistance vessels in the peripheral circulation, further decreasing systemic vascular resistance. Of particular importance for the anaesthetist is the fact that thyroid hormone may modulate ion channels, leading to direct enhancement of myocardial contractility (with an increase in myocardial oxygen demand). This action is independent of adenyl cyclase and accounts for the ability of thyroxine to improve myocardial performance in the presence of β-blockade overdose. Thyroid hormone may also produce coronary artery dilatation. The vasodilatory effect activates the renin–angiotensin–aldosterone mechanism, resulting in increased sodium retention, a marked increase in blood volume and further increases in cardiac output. However, although increased T_3 concentrations can improve cardiac output and decrease systemic vascular resistance following coronary artery bypass grafting, no improvement in outcome has been demonstrated.[3]

Pathophysiology of thyroid disease

From the anaesthetic point of view, thyroid disease can be characterized into four major groups: euthyroid enlargement, thyroid malignancy, thyrotoxicosis, and hypothyroidism. Goitre is the term used to describe enlargement of the thyroid gland. Simple goitre is by far the most common condition encountered by the general anaesthetist and poses little by the way of anaesthetic problems. Thyroid malignancy may present in many different ways and, apart from the problems it may pose for airway management, may also lead to pathological fractures and frank thyrotoxicosis.

Simple thyroid goitre

The most common cause of simple goitre is iodine deficiency which leads to increased stimulation of the gland by TSH in order to maintain normal levels of hormone production. Thus simple goitre tends to occur in specific areas where there is dietary iodine deficiency. Patients with goitre generally have normal thyroid function tests, although mild, usually subclinical, hypothyroidism may occur. If left untreated, huge nodule goitres can develop (Figure 4.6), but these are generally of little functional significance unless they extend into the retrosternal area where airway compression may occur. Retrosternal goitres may produce symptoms by compression of mediastinal structures, and may lead to hoarseness of the voice, dyspnoea, dysphagia, and occasionally superior vena caval obstruction. Arterial compression or thyrocervical steal syndrome by large substernal goitres occasionally causes cerebral hypoperfusion and stroke. Nerve involvement may also occur, producing laryngeal nerve palsies, Horner's syndrome, and, very unusually,

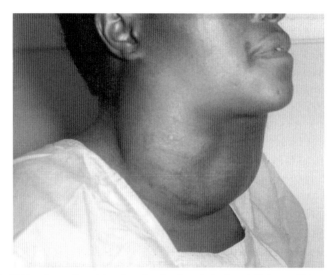

Fig. 4.6 (Plate 1) Very large thyroid goitre due to chronic iodine deficiency. This patient proved very easy to intubate.

phrenic nerve paralysis. Pleural effusions, chylothorax, and pericardial effusions may also occur.[4]

Thyroid malignancy

A full description of thyroid malignancies is beyond the scope of this chapter. The most relevant are those arising from thyroid epithelial cells: follicular tumours including papillary carcinoma (78%), follicular carcinoma which may be hormone-producing (17%), medullary carcinoma (4%), and undifferentiated (anaplastic) carcinoma (1%), which seldom produces hormone. Thyroid malignancies may impose significant airway hazard if the tumours are large or locally invasive. Medullary carcinoma arises from parafollicular calcitonin-producing C-cells and is important from an endocrine standpoint as it is a marker of the MEN 2a and 2b syndromes which may include phaeochromocytomas and parathyroid tumours. The genetic abnormality that produces medullary carcinoma has been determined.[5] If mutations of the rearranged during transfection (RET) proto-oncogene are found on the 10th chromosome then the patient has a high probability of progressing from C-cell hyperplasia to medullary carcinoma. Chromosome analysis is recommended for families of affected individuals, and this can then be used to guide the timing of thyroidectomy as determined by the type of mutation found.[6] Non-epithelial malignant disease may also occur, and various metastatic tumours from other sources (such as breast) may be found in the thyroid.

Hypothyroidism

Hypothyroidism is a graded phenomenon, ranging from very mild cases in which biochemical abnormalities are present but the individual hardly notices symptoms and signs of thyroid hormone deficiency, to very severe cases in which there is a danger of sliding down into a life-threatening myxoedema coma.[7] Worldwide, hypothyroidism is most commonly due to iodine deficiency. The minimum daily intake of iodine that is required for normal thyroid function in adults is around 150 µg, and the incidence of hypothyroidism depends largely upon the amount of iodine in the diet. However, in developed countries iodine deficiency is rare, and autoimmune thyroiditis is the most common cause followed by destructive therapy (radiation or surgery) for thyrotoxicosis or malignancy.

Hashimoto's autoimmune thyroiditis results from the production of antibodies against thyroid peroxidase and thyroglobulin, leading to inflammation and a reduction in follicular cells. Occasionally, patients may exhibit a destructive thyrotoxicosis before the advent of hypothyroidism. Goitre may occur as a result of increased TSH secretion and inflammatory swelling.

Various drugs, including lithium,[8] amiodarone, cholestyramine, and interferon, may also suppress thyroid function. Amiodarone, an iodine-rich drug, may also cause hyperthyroidism in 2–10% of patients.[9] Very rarely, hypothyroidism may have a pituitary cause with failure of TSH production. Mild subclinical hypothyroidism may occur in 7–10% of older women, as evidenced by an increased TSH. Although these patients are subclinical, treatment with thyroxine frequently results in improved cardiovascular function and feelings of wellbeing; however, an expert panel concluded that there was insufficient evidence to recommend routine thyroxine supplementation in subclinical disease.[10]

The haemodynamic changes may be subtle. The most common signs are bradycardia and mild hypertension with a narrow pulse pressure. In severe long-standing cases pericardial effusions and non-pitting oedema (myxoedema) may be seen. Cardiac output is reduced as a result of the combination of decreased ventricular filling (decreased myocardial compliance and diastolic dysfunction), bradycardia, and reduced myocardial contractility. Systemic vascular resistance may be markedly increased by as much as 50%. However, frank heart failure is uncommon. The ECG may show decreased complex size, a prolonged cardiac action potential, and a long QT interval; occasionally, this may lead to torsade de pointes. These patients may also have reduced plasma volume and impaired receptor responsiveness, making them liable to haemodynamic instability intra-operatively.

A wide range of other physiological functions may be impaired, leading to decreased ventilatory responsiveness to hypoxia and hypercapnia, impaired hepatic metabolism of various drugs, cognitive dysfunction, affective disorders, and psychosis. All these changes are reversible with adequate thyroid hormone replacement. The patients may also be anaemic. They may be very sensitive to drugs, particularly the respiratory depressant effects of opiates. The tongue may be enlarged sufficiently to make intubation difficult.

Hyperthyroidism

Thyrotoxicosis affects approximately 2% of women and 0.2% of men in the general population. The most common cause of hyperthyroidism is Graves' disease, but other causes include toxic nodular goitre, thyroiditis, follicular carcinoma, pregnancy (especially molar pregnancy), TSH-secreting pituitary adenoma, and drug-induced hyperthyroidism (e.g. during amiodarone therapy).

Hyperthyroidism produces a wide range of clinical manifestations. The metabolic consequences include weight loss, increased appetite, and diarrhoea. The often dramatic eye signs are limited to patients suffering from Graves' disease, but all patients may have hyperactivity, anxiety, nervousness, and tremor. Muscular weakness may also occur, particularly in the proximal muscle groups.

The cardiovascular consequences are probably the most important from an anaesthetic standpoint. Increased heart rate is extremely common, with sleeping heart rates greater than 90 beats/min and an exaggerated increase in heart rate with exercise. Palpitations and atrial fibrillation are also common. Cardiac output is generally elevated, but some degree of exercise impairment is frequent. There is increased flow during left ventricular ejection that may lead to an aortic flow murmur. Systolic arterial pressure may be elevated, but systemic vascular resistance is reduced, pulse pressure is wide, and diastolic pressure is often low. Although β-adrenergic blockade reduces heart rate, it does not alter the enhanced systolic and diastolic contractile function, confirming that thyroid hormone acts directly on cardiac muscle. Atrial fibrillation occurs in 5–15% of hyperthyroid patients, but may revert spontaneously to sinus rhythm when the hyperthyroid state is treated adequately. Cardiac failure may occur for a variety of reasons, including rate-related heart failure, cardiomyopathy, or ischaemic disease. Generally, the increased cardiac output is sufficient to meet the needs of the tissues, and therefore the term 'high-output cardiac failure' is not strictly accurate. Treatment with β-blockade improves the range of cardiovascular disturbances and it is not contraindicated in thyrotoxic cardiac failure.[3]

Graves' disease, or toxic diffuse goitre, is now classified as an autoimmune condition, although the ultimate cause is unknown. It is characterized by excessive thyroid hormone production, diffuse thyroid enlargement, and the characteristic ophthalmopathy, and it is five times more prevalent in women than in men. Only Graves' disease demonstrates the characteristic ophthalmic pathology, which is not a generalized feature of hyperthyroidism. The condition affects all the orbital contents, including the extra-ocular muscles, and may lead to diplopia, photophobia, and corneal abrasion. Steroids may reduce the inflammation and retrobulbar irradiation has been used to decrease intra-ocular swelling, but surgical decompression may be required if there is pressure on the optic nerve.

Diagnosis of suspected thyroid disease

Thyroid disease is suspected on clinical diagnosis, and a number of tests can be used to confirm the thyroid status.

In the case of simple goitre, subclinical hypothyroidism may be present if the patient is still receiving a potentially iodine-deficient diet. If the iodine deficiency is likely to have been corrected, no specific tests are required prior to surgery to evaluate the thyroid status.

Where hypothyroidism is suspected, a TSH estimation is usually sufficient to confirm the diagnosis unless a pituitary cause is suspected. In any patient taking thyroxine

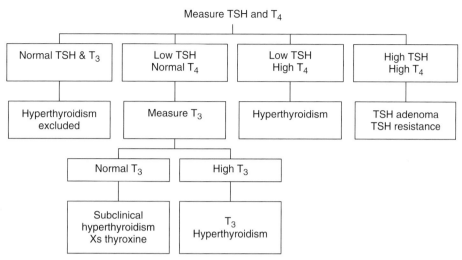

Fig. 4.7 Suggested approach to establishing the diagnosis in a patient with clinical manifestations of hyperthyroidism (modified from ref. 11).

supplements, TSH estimation should be performed as a guide to the adequacy of therapy. Overtly hypothyroid patients should be rendered euthyroid prior to surgery, but the value of thyroxine therapy in subclinical hypothyroidism remains debatable.

Hyperthyroid patients can present a significant diagnostic dilemma. A reasonable scheme for the investigation of a patient with suspected hyperthyroidism has been suggested by Weetman[11] and is illustrated in Figure 4.7. Careful clinical evaluation of the cardiovascular system of these patients is appropriate prior to surgery. As with simple goitre, hyperthyroid enlargement may indicate the need for careful pre-operative airway assessment.

Medical management

The first step in the medical management of hyperthyroidism is the use of thionamides which inhibit thyroid peroxidase and thus the synthesis of thyroid hormone. They may also diminish the autoimmune sensitivity of the gland, and may lead to long-term or even permanent remission in up to 30–40% of patients, but this may take up to 18 months to achieve. These drugs are not contraindicated in pregnancy, but the dose may need to be reduced. The most important side-effect is a reversible suppression of bone marrow function with aplastic anaemia, and regular blood counts must be performed in these patients. β-blockade may be given, particularly at the start of treatment, in order to minimize cardiovascular symptoms. Where remission is not achieved, radioactive iodine is a highly effective therapy and is no longer contraindicated in women of child-bearing age. However, it is important to ensure that the patient is not pregnant or breastfeeding and does not become pregnant during a period of treatment. In the long term, both of these therapeutic options may lead to a hypothyroid state.

Hypothyroid patients will generally require lifelong maintenance therapy with thyroxine with regular monitoring of TSH to ensure that appropriate levels of hormone are being maintained.

Pre-operative preparation

As a general principle, patients with thyroid disease should be rendered euthyroid prior to surgery. This applies equally to patients who are hypo- or hyperthyroid.

For simple goitre where hormonal dysfunction is not suspected, routine clinical evaluation together with anatomical assessment of the airway is all that is required. A chest X-ray, thoracic inlet views, or a CT scan of the neck may all be indicated in the case of a large tumour. The CT scan provides excellent views of retrosternal extension, allowing good assessment of airway distortion (Figure 4.8).

There is little evidence that pulmonary function tests are of value in predicting the risk of airway compromise. There is some controversy as to whether or not thyroid enlargement represents a predictably difficult airway (see later). Studies that have examined this issue suggest that the incidence of difficulty of intubation is no more frequent in patients with large goitres than in the general population, and that the same anatomical features that predict difficulties of laryngeal visualization can be applied. Indirect laryngoscopy and evaluation of recurrent laryngeal nerve function are advisable prior to thyroidectomy in patients with large goitres or thyroid malignancy.

Whether or not hypothyroid patients scheduled for surgery should have their operations postponed depends on a number of factors including the severity of the hypothyroidism, the presence of myocardial risk factors that might make thyroxine therapy potentially risky, and, not least, the urgency of the surgery. Mild subclinical hypothyroidism with only moderate increases in TSH levels does not present a significant

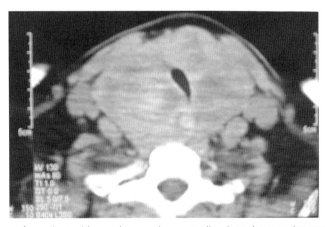

Fig. 4.8 CT scan of a patient with very large goitre extending into the superior mediastinum. Note the compression of the trachea by the mass. This patient presented a grade I view of the larynx and advancement of a 7.0 mm endotracheal tube into the trachea was straightforward.

peri-operative risk and delaying surgery to correct hypothyroidism is probably not justi-fied. However, symptomatic disease should be corrected prior to surgery wherever pos-sible. Hypothyroid patients should receive thyroxine for several days prior to surgery as the hormone has a long half-life (7 days) and its effects do not reach optimum values for some time. Tri-iodothyronine has a much shorter half-life (1.5 days), but may present a greater risk of aggravating myocardial ischaemia. In patients with adequately managed hypothyroidism, some authorities advocate omitting thyroxine on the morning of surgery, while others are happy to continue it. Either approach appears acceptable. If the patient is on T_3, the short half-life of this agent means that it is essential for the patient to take the morning dose on the day of surgery. As there is an associated risk of adrenocortical insufficiency,[12] hypothyroid patients should probably receive hydrocorti-sone cover for the peri-operative period.[13] Sedative premedication, particularly with opiates, is best avoided in this group of patients. Hypoglycaemia is a possibility during anaesthesia, and monitoring blood sugar regularly is probably a better option than blind infusion of dextrose-containing solutions. Controlled ventilation is generally preferred in these patients as they are at markedly increased risk of peri-operative hypoventilation.

Surgery is seldom, if ever, indicated nowadays as a treatment for hyperthyroidism. Once the diagnosis is established, the patient should be rendered euthyroid prior to sur-gery if it is at all possible. However, urgent surgery may be indicated in a patient who is incidentally hyperthyroid and whose medical condition requires urgent therapy. It may also be necessary to perform surgery, such as a uterine evacuation, in the presence of hyperthyroidism in a patient with a hydatidiform mole.

Hyperthyroid states should be corrected with the thionamides carbimazole (or its pre-drug methimazole) or propylthiouracil. Carbimazole has the advantage of requiring only a once daily dosage of 20–30 mg, whereas propylthiouracil requires a much larger dose of 200 mg three times daily. Propylthiouracil has the advantage of inhibiting the conversion of T_4 to T_3, but this is of little practical value in pre-operative preparation, although it may be useful in managing hyperthyroid states. In Graves' disease these drugs may also have the benefit of decreasing TSH receptor antibodies and thus encouraging remission of the disease. Both these agents take 2–4 weeks to achieve adequate control in over 90% of patients.[11] In the absence of β-blockade, clinical euthyroid states are sufficient to allow surgery to proceed; it is not necessary to establish completely normal T_4 and TSH levels prior to surgery.

Anaesthetic management

Surgical management of thyroid disease is now generally reserved for patients with malig-nancy, those in whom medical treatment has failed to produce permanent remission, or those where the size of the goitre requires surgical treatment. It may also be the preferred option in pregnancy and in patients who do not tolerate thionamides well. Occasionally, urgent surgery may be required in a patient who is incidentally hyperthyroid or whose hyperthyroid state is the result of a condition such as hydatidiform mole.

Regional anaesthesia

No specific anaesthetic technique has been demonstrated to be superior to any other for thyroid surgery. Regional anaesthesia is possible, and has been recommended for ill patients requiring thyroid surgery,[14] but the technique is not entirely satisfactory. Bilateral deep cervical plexus block carries the risk of damage to adjacent structures (including the vertebral artery and the spinal cord) and bilateral phrenic nerve paralysis. However, bilateral superficial plexus block, which does not carry these risks, has been used in situations with limited resources[15] and may be very useful for post-operative pain relief.[16] Acute airway obstruction from vocal cord dysfunction precipitated by cervical plexus block has been described.[17] The use of cervical epidural has been described,[18] but it is difficult to see how this technique can be safer than general anaesthesia.

General anaesthesia

The most popular technique for thyroidectomy is general anaesthesia with muscle relaxation and tracheal intubation. Spontaneous ventilation with a laryngeal mask airway (LMA) has been used, particularly when nerve stimulation is desired to identify the recurrent laryngeal nerve. Observation of the vocal cords through the LMA using a fibreoptic scope during nerve stimulation can assist the surgeon to identify the nerve.

Airway issues

Large thyroid goitres may distort the laryngeal inlet, produce deviation of the trachea, and erode tracheal rings. This may well lead to difficulties with airway management, particularly in the post-operative period, but the widely held perception that this will mean that there is increased potential for difficult laryngeal visualization is based more on assumption than on fact. Whilst it is well established that thyroid malignancy creates a substantial risk of difficult airway management, there are few reports of serious airway management problems at the time of intubation with benign thyroid enlargement. There have been two systematic studies looking at this particular problem. In the first of these, the incidence of increased difficulty in intubation was found to be higher amongst patients who had a goitre compared with those with no risk factors at all, but no patient presented a 'can't intubate can't ventilate' scenario. In this study of over 300 patients, there was only one failed intubation, representing a similar risk to that of the general population.[19] A second study looked at the prediction of difficult tracheal intubation in thyroid surgery in 320 consecutive patients. In this series, the authors identified the usual factors as predicting difficult and tracheal intubation, but large goitre alone was not associated with an increased incidence of difficult intubation.[20] As the thyroid gland enlarges, it usually displaces the trachea posteriorly and pushes the larynx in a cephalad direction, making the laryngeal inlet easier to view despite often significant lateral displacement (Figures 4.9, 4.10, and 4.11). These two effects have the result of presenting the larynx in a favourable position for a laryngeal visualization (Figure 4.12).

However, the lateral position of the larynx within the pharynx may be distorted, and this should be anticipated from the radiological appearances (Figure 4.9). Distortion of

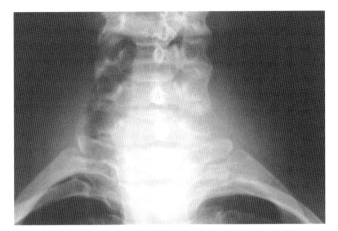

Fig. 4.9 AP X-ray of the neck in a middle-aged female with a very large goitre. Note the marked rightward displacement of the trachea, and the extension of the mass into the superior mediastinum.

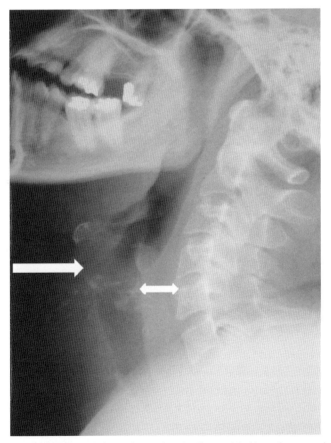

Fig. 4.10 Lateral X-ray of the neck from the patient in Figure 4.9. Note the posterior and upward displacement of the laryngeal inlet (single arrow) and the very narrow space between the larynx and the spinal column.

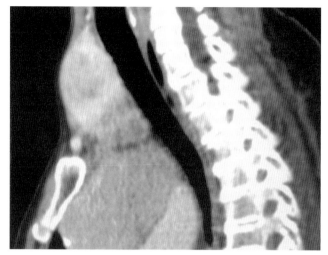

Fig. 4.11 MRI imaging of the patient in Figure 4.9, showing the large goitre anterior to the laryngeal inlet and extending into the superior mediastinum.

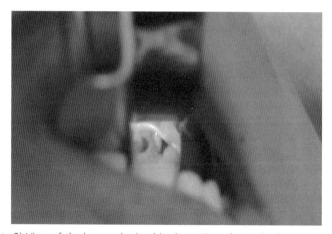

Fig. 4.12 (Plate 2) View of the larynx obtained in the patient shown in Figures 4.10 and 4.11. Note the excellent view of the laryngeal inlet, despite the lateral distortion of the larynx shown in Figure 4.10.

the trachea is frequent, and the trachea may be compressed and deviated within the thorax and thus may be at increased risk of injury from clumsy or forceful attempts at intubation. Tracheal intubation should always be performed with a flexible armoured endotracheal tube with an appropriate size selected based on the pre-operative chest X-ray views. However, it should be remembered that the gland compressing the trachea is soft and that a trachea that appears very narrow on X-ray (Figure 4.8) may be able to accommodate a fairly large endotracheal tube. Where tracheal compression is evident, particularly in the intrathoracic portion of the trachea, it is a wise precaution to have a rigid bronchoscope available in case the trachea approves impossible to intubate.

Rarely, the gland may enlarge behind the trachea, displacing the trachea anteriorly (Figure 4.13). In such circumstances, intubation may be impossible, even with fibreoptic endoscopy, since the very anterior placement of the larynx may prevent the endoscope from entering the laryngeal inlet. Under such circumstances consideration should be given to either awake thyroidectomy with regional anaesthesia or, in extreme cases, the use of an extracorporeal bypass.

Retrosternal extension of the gland frequently creates concern and raises the possibility of an anterior mediastinal compression syndrome. However, it should be remembered that the thyroid gland always enlarges into the superior mediastinum, rather than the anterior mediastinum. Thus, while thyroid enlargement may theoretically cause obstruction of venous return from the head and neck, it should not produce the problematic

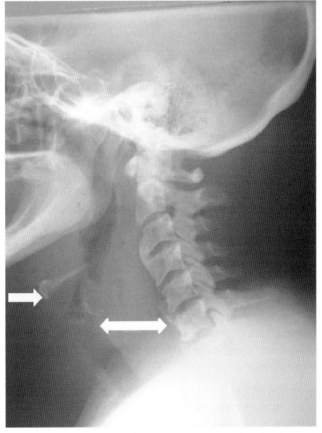

Fig. 4.13 Lateral X-ray of the neck in a patient with a posterior-placed goitre. Note the very anterior and upward position of the larynx and hyoid bone (single arrow) and the widened space between the larynx and spinal column (double arrow). This patient also had limited neck extension and laryngeal visualization was impossible.

situation of airway obstruction below the level of the carina together with the risk of right atrial inflow obstruction. Therefore these masses should not be regarded in the same light as true anterior mediastinal masses. However, retrosternal extension of a malignant thyroid tumour should always be regarded extremely seriously, and all precautions recommended for anterior mediastinal masses, including the availability of femoro-femoral bypass, should be considered based on the assessment of the pre-operative condition. The only real airway problem posed by thyroid enlargement is that the final means of establishing an emergency airway, through cryco-thyroid puncture, is not available. This means that a patient is assessed as having a difficult airway for reasons other than the enlargement of the thyroid gland (including all the usual problems of limited neck movement, limited jaw opening, short thyromental distance, and enlarged tongue or pharyngeal structures) should be taken more seriously in the presence of a large thyroid goitre than might otherwise be the case, as the option of cryco-thyroid puncture is not available. Obviously, an enlarged thyroid gland will increase the requirement for surgical manipulation, thus posing a greater risk of recurrent laryngeal nerve injury and post-operative haemorrhage, and may also present the risk of post-operative tracheomalacia with respiratory obstruction. However, whilst these airway risks must be borne in mind, they do not impose an increased risk of endotracheal tube placement.

Endotracheal intubation under direct vision is the safest and simplest approach to the placement of an endotracheal tube. Awake fibreoptic intubation is substantially less pleasant for the patient and has a higher failure rate than direct laryngeal visualization. Furthermore, fibreoptic intubation may not assist in visualizing the laryngeal inlet in cases of gross anatomical distortion. Where there is doubt, a gas induction with sevoflurane is an acceptable approach, particularly where other signs of difficulty with laryngeal visualization are present. Other alternatives to direct visualization of the larynx also have a similar lower success rate than direct laryngoscopy. Where severe difficulty is anticipated (Figure 4.13), femoro-femoral bypass may offer the only option; this is particularly true of gross anatomical distortion due to thyroid malignancy.

The introduction of sugammadex will allow rapid reversal of profound neuromuscular blockade and will considerably increase the safety margin in these patients.

Positioning

Once the airway has been secured, the patient is usually positioned with padding under the shoulders and the neck extended on a head ring. Standard sterile draping generally includes a split towel wrapped around the head, and this will require disconnection from the anaesthetic circuit and subsequently positioning of the patient. It is important to remember that this degree of patient movement may cause the endotracheal tube to be displaced, and its proper positioning must be rechecked before surgery commences. A 25° head-up tilt is frequently used to assist venous drainage and this may lead to significant hypotension; it is generally recommended that the feet should also be elevated to minimize this complication. Theoretically, this may also increase the risk of entrainment of air through an open vein in the spontaneously breathing patient, but this has never been reported. In patients who have Graves' disease, it is very important to provide full protection for the eyes.

Surgical procedure (see Chapter 11 for details)

Some surgeons choose to infiltrate the wound with adrenaline, and this is best done with the addition of bupivacaine as this will aid post-operative analgesia. Where there is retro-sternal extension of a goitre, this will generally be fairly easy to mobilize to the neck incision and sternotomy is very seldom required. Towards the end of the surgical procedure, but prior to wound closure, a Valsalva manoeuvre may help to identify sources of venous bleeding that may have been missed in the procedure. The veins of the neck are very thin-walled and collapse readily and so seldom bleed while the patient is in a head-up position. However, once the patient recovers, and particularly when they cough, quite severe bleeding can result.

Intra-operative crisis

It must be remembered that, even with good pre-operative preparation, thyroid storm may still eventuate in hyperthyroid patients. In patients at risk of thyroid storm, the crisis is likely to occur post-operatively, rather than at the time of surgery. Nevertheless, intra-operative hyperthyroid events do occur and may pose difficulties in diagnosis and management. When faced with a patient who develops signs of increasing temperature and haemodynamic stability, the anaesthetist must attempt to make a rapid diagnosis of the underlying pathology. In these circumstances, four likely conditions need to be considered, each of which requires very different and accurate management. These include malignant hyperthermia, thyrotoxic crisis, phaeochromocytoma, and sepsis. The last of these should be easy to diagnose, but the others may produce significant diagnostic dilemmas as each of them may produce an increase in body temperature, increased carbon dioxide production, and haemodynamic instability including tachycardia, arrhythmias, and hypertension. However, the pattern of the condition should assist in diagnosis as indicated in Table 4.1.

Table 4.1 Characteristics that may help to distinguish between the main differential diagnoses of an intra-operative thyroid storm

	Thyrotoxicosis	Malignant hyperthermia	Phaeochromocytoma
Rise in temperature	Early, severe	Late, severe	Early, mild to moderate
Hypertension	Moderate, wide pulse pressure	Moderate, narrow pulse pressure	Severe, mainly systolic
Tachycardia	Severe	Moderate	Severe tachycardia or bradycardia
Arrhythmia	Mainly atrial, possible atrial fibrillation	Mainly ventricular	Atrial and ventricular can occur
$Paco_2$	Moderate elevation	Severe elevation	Mild elevation
pH	Normal	Acidosis	Normal

Where there is doubt, it is important that dantrolene is administered without delay as the consequences of failing to treat malignant hyperthermia early are catastrophic. Dantrolene is very effective at reducing the increased temperature but will not ameliorate the cardiovascular disturbances. It also has significant adverse effects, including increased muscle weakness and nausea and vomiting.

Extubation

At the end of the surgical procedure, coughing at the time of extubation should be mini-mized as this may precipitate post-operative bleeding. Where the dissection has been particularly difficult, it is advisable to check vocal cord function before removing the patient from the operating room. Direct laryngoscopy at the time of extubation can be performed, but generally requires that the patient is still fairly deeply anaesthetized. A bolus dose of propofol at the time of extubation can be very useful to facilitate laryngos-copy. Alternatively, and particularly where there is serious concern, the endotracheal tube can be replaced with an LMA and vocal cord inspection conducted with a fibreoptic endo-scope through the lumen of the pharyngeal mask as the patient recovers. This provides excellent laryngeal views and allows very good assessment of recurrent nerve function.

Post-operative care

There are several post-operative problems specific to thyroidectomy. Damage to the para-thyroid glands may result in transient hypocalcaemia, although this is generally mild and of no clinical significance. Haematoma may occur and is generally benign as most bleed-ing is of venous origin. However, an arterial bleed may represent a life-threatening event that may precipitate acute airway obstruction. It is traditional to advise immediate open-ing of the wound, in the ward if necessary, in order to drain the haematoma and relieve the obstruction. However, if the haematoma has been present for any period of time, it is frequently accompanied by obstruction to the lymphatic and venous drainage of the upper airway with associated laryngeal and pharyngeal oedema. Unless tracheomalacia is present, the trachea is relatively incompressible, and if airway obstruction is present it is much more likely to be due to laryngeal and pharyngeal oedema. Consequently, simply opening the haematoma will not necessarily restore airway patency. The best strategy is to take the patient back to the operating room immediately and insert an endotracheal tube, bearing in mind that this is likely to be much more difficult than the original intubation.

Damage to the recurrent laryngeal nerve is not infrequent. Temporary unilateral vocal cord paralysis occurs in 3–4% of patients, but permanent paralysis occurs in less than 1%. Bilateral vocal cord damage is very rare, but when it occurs may lead to stridor at the time of tracheal extubation. This will require re-intubation, and tracheostomy should be considered as the problem is likely to be persistent (see Chapter 11).

Tracheomalacia is a rare complication, even in the presence of very large goitres. Long-standing pressure on the tracheal rings may lead to softening of these structures with subsequent collapse of the trachea once the supporting tumour has been removed. Flow–volume respiratory curves are of no value in predicting the risk of this complication, but surgical assessment of the trachea once the goitre has been removed may be helpful. The position of the affected tracheal rings will determine the nature of any post-operative airway obstruction. If the rings lie in the intrathoracic portion of the trachea, obstruction will occur primarily during expiration, whilst if they are in the extrathoracic portion, the obstruction will be maximum during the inspiratory phase. If it is suspected during the operation that tracheomalacia may be present, it is advisable to restore spontaneous ventilation prior to extubation of the trachea. Removal of the endotracheal tube and replacement with an LMA while the patient is still anaesthetized will allow good assessment of the risk of airway obstruction. This will also allow fibreoptic bronchoscopy to be performed so that the site of the tracheal collapse can be determined to assist the planning of further management. Where severe tracheomalacia is present, immediate tracheostomy should be performed and long-term planning for airway management should be instituted in consultation with ear, nose, and throat specialists.

Endocrine complications

These conditions are dealt with in more detail in Chapter 9, but are also mentioned here for completeness. Both carry a significant risk of morbidity and mortality and require accurate and aggressive management.

Myxoedema

Myxoedema coma is a rare life-threatening clinical condition that may occur in a fully treated or neglected hyperthyroid patient. Patients exhibit disorientation, lethargy, and psychosis which may proceed to coma. Hypothermia is common, and the precipitating event may be cold exposure. Acute stress may also precipitate this condition, and certain drugs, particularly diuretics, sedatives, and tranquillizers, also precipitate a crisis. Most cases occur in elderly females during the winter. Treatment is largely supportive, with passive rewarming, mechanical ventilation if hyperventilation is present, cautious plasma volume expansion, and correction of hypoglycaemia if it occurs. There may be an associated failure of glucocorticoid function and steroids have also been recommended. There is no consensus on the most appropriate form of thyroid hormone supplementation. Aggressive replacement with T_3 will result in abrupt increases in metabolism that may precipitate myocardial ischaemia, but too conservative an approach is also associated with poor outcome. A starting dose of thyroxine 300–500 µg followed by 50–100 µg intravenously daily until the patient can take oral medication is currently recommended. If the response is poor, 10 µg T_3 may be given intravenously every 4 hours with careful and continuous ECG monitoring until an adequate response is obtained. As adrenal cortical dysfunction may also be present, administration of hydrocortisone is recommended. The management of this condition is dealt with in more detail in Chapter 9.

Thyroid storm

Thyrotoxic crisis is now a rare complication of thyroid surgery because of the widespread use of anti-thyroid drugs. Nevertheless, it may occur following thyroid surgery and may also occur in other conditions of uncontrolled hyperthyroid states. It remains a highly dangerous condition, with mortality rates of 10–75% quoted in the literature. Severe hyperthermia, with core temperatures in the region of 40°C, can occur associated with systolic hypertension, tachycardia, and tachyarrhythmias. Mental confusion, nausea, and vomiting may complicate the condition. Treatment includes the administration of oxygen, cooling with cold intravenous fluids and body surface cooling, and appropriate supportive therapy. β-blockade is the mainstay of haemodynamic control and propranolol has the added advantage of inhibiting the conversion of T_4 to T_3, but esmolol has the advantage of being short-acting and having a more specific β_1-adrenergic blocking action. In the presence of hypertension and arrhythmias, the anti-catecholamine effect of magnesium may be of benefit. Verapamil may assist in the control of acute-onset atrial fibrillation. If sedation is necessary, chlorpromazine 5 mg is probably the drug of choice as it has central antipyretic effects as well as its excellent sedative properties. The management of this condition is dealt with in more detail in Chapter 9.

Conclusions

Most thyroid disease requiring anaesthetic management poses little by way of significant anaesthetic problems. However, disorders of thyroid hormone function require accurate and skilful management and carry a significant morbidity and mortality when the disorder is severe. Sound knowledge of the functioning of thyroid hormones and of the management options is essential.

Key clinical management points

Diagnosis

- Suspect thyrotoxicosis in younger patients with suggestive symptoms and a resting tachycardia.
- Suspect hypothyroidism in older patients, particularly those with a history of previous thyroid disease. Hypothyroidism may also occur at a subclinical level in patients with iodine-deficient goitre.

Diagnostic tests

- TSH measurement is the primary screening test for thyroid disorders and is generally all that is required for suspected hypothyroidism
- Measurement of T_4 is indicated in suspected hyperthyroidism, with T_3 estimation reserved for patients with a high index of suspicion and a normal T_4

Goitre assessment

- Careful assessment of the risks of malignancy
- Assessment of the possibility of retrosternal extension
- Airway assessment
  - Chest X-ray
  - Thoracic inlet radiological views
  - CT scans of the upper thorax and neck
  - Recurrent laryngeal nerve function
  - Standard airway assessment techniques are valid measures of risk

Pre-operative preparation

All patients should be rendered clinically euthyroid prior to surgery.

Hypothyroidism

- Correct with T_4 until TSH levels returned to normal
  - 200–500 µg daily
- Correction of subclinical hypothyroidism is controversial

Hyperthyroidism

- Carbimazole
  - 20–30 mg daily for 2–6 weeks until symptoms abate without β-blockade
- Propylthiouracil
  - 200 mg three times daily as for carbimazole

Key clinical management points (continued)

Anaesthetic management

Standard sedative premedication

Monitoring

◆ Standard anaesthetic monitoring

Anaesthetic induction

◆ Without airway problems
  • Standard intravenous induction, and neuromuscular blockade and endotracheal intubation
◆ Suspected airway difficulty
  • Awake fibreoptic intubation
  • Gas induction and attempted airway inspection
◆ Intubation with a flexible armoured tube of appropriate size

Anaesthetic maintenance

◆ Any technique is acceptable
◆ Appropriate positioning for surgery, with head and feet elevated
◆ Assess laryngeal nerve function at the end of procedure
◆ Consider superficial cervical plexus blockade for post-operative analgesia

Post-operative care

◆ Ensure adequate airway function following extubation
◆ Manage post-operative haematoma with re-intubation

References

1. Hennemann G, Everts ME, de Jong M, Lim CF, Krenning EP, Docter R (1998). The significance of plasma membrane transport in the bioavailability of thyroid hormone. *Clinical Endocrinology*, **48**, 1–8.
2. Heuer H, Visser TJ (2009). Minireview. Pathophysiological importance of thyroid hormone transporters. *Endocrinology*, **150**, 1078–83.
3. Klein I, Ojamaa K (2001). Thyroid hormone and the cardiovascular system. *New England Journal of Medicine*, **344**, 501–9.
4. Anders HJ (1998). Compression syndromes caused by substernal goitres. *Postgraduate Medical Journal*, **74**(872), 327–9
5. Marsh DJ, Mulligan LM, Eng C (1997). RET proto-oncogene mutations in multiple endocrine neoplasia type 2 and medullary thyroid carcinoma. *Hormone Research*, **47**, 168–78.

6. Frilling A, Weber F, Tecklenborg C, Broelsch CE (2003). Prophylactic thyroidectomy in multiple endocrine neoplasia: the impact of molecular mechanisms of RET proto-oncogene. *Langenbecks Archives of Surgery*, **388**, 17–26.

7. Thyroid Disease Manager. *Adult hypothyroidism*. Available at: http://www.thyroidmanager.org (accessed 14 January 2010).

8. Perrild H, Hegedus L, Baastrup PC, Kayser L, Kastberg S (1990). Thyroid function and ultrasonically determined thyroid size in patients receiving long-term lithium treatment. *American Journal of Psychiatry*, **147**, 1518–21.

9. Liang YL, Huang SM, Peng SL, *et al.* (2009). Amiodarone-induced thyrotoxicosis in a patient with autonomously functioning nodular goiter. *Annals of Pharmacotherapy*, **43**, 134–8.

10. Surks MI, Ortiz E, Daniels GH, *et al.* (2004). Subclinical thyroid disease: scientific review and guidelines for diagnosis and management. *Journal of the American Medical Association*, **291**, 228–38.

11. Weetman AP (2000). Graves' disease. *New England Journal of Medicine*, **343**, 1236–48.

12. Punj J, Arora MK (2008). Herbal intake: undiagnosed hypothyroidism leading to postoperative refractory circulatory collapse—a case report. *Middle East Journal of Anesthesiology*, **19**, 1169–77.

13. Murkin JM (1982). Anesthesia and hypothyroidism: a review of thyroxine physiology, pharmacology, and anesthetic implications. *Anesthesia and Analgesia*, **61**, 371–83.

14. Kulkarni RS, Braverman LE, Patwardhan NA (1996). Bilateral cervical plexus block for thyroidectomy and parathyroidectomy in healthy and high risk patients. *Journal of Endocrinological Investigation*, **19**, 714–18.

15. Misauno MA, Yilkudi MG, Akwaras AL, *et al.* (2008). Thyroidectomy under local anaesthesia: how safe? *Nigerian Journal of Clinical Practice*, **11**, 37–40.

16. Andrieu G, Amrouni H, Robin E, *et al.* (2007). Analgesic efficacy of bilateral superficial cervical plexus block administered before thyroid surgery under general anaesthesia. *British Journal of Anaesthesia*, **99**, 561–6.

17. Kwok AO, Silbert BS, Allen KJ, Bray PJ, Vidovich J (2006). Bilateral vocal cord palsy during carotid endarterectomy under cervical plexus block. *Anesthia and Analgesia*, **102**, 376–7.

18. Ahsan SN, Faridi S (1998). Cervical epidural anesthesia for sub-total thyroidectomy in a patient with aortic incompetence. *Journal of the Pakistan Medical Association*, **48**, 281–3.

19. Voyagis GS, Kyriakos KP (1997). The effect of goiter on endotracheal intubation. *Anesthesia and Analgesia*, **84**, 611–12.

20. Bouaggad A, Nejmi SE, Bouderka MA, Abbassi O (2004). Prediction of difficult tracheal intubation in thyroid surgery. *Anesthesia and Analgesia*, **99**, 603–6.

Chapter 5

Parathyroid disease

Philipp Riss, Eva Schaden, and Christian K Spiss

Physiology

Parathyroid gland

The parathyroid glands usually lie on the posterior surface of the thyroid gland. Most humans have four parathyroid glands, two on each side, but there is a wide variation in number (3–8 glands) and location. They can be situated intrathyroidally (intracapsularly), in the thyrothymic ligament, and intrathoracically (mediastinum, aortopulmonary window).[1] The two inferior glands originate from the third branchial pouch, whereas the superior glands descend from the fourth branchial pouch. Histologically, parathyroids consist of chief cells and oxyphil cells next to fibrovascular stroma and adipose tissue. Chief cells appear to be responsible for most of the hormone excretion. Oxyphil cells also contribute to parathyroid function, but their importance has not yet been fully examined. The number of oxyphil cells increases with increasing age.

The inferior thyroid artery provides the blood supply for the superior and inferior glands in most cases. In 15–20% of individuals the superior glands are supplied by the superior thyroid artery or by anastomoses between the superior and inferior thyroid artery. In 93% the relation of the glands to the recurrent laryngeal nerve is predictable.[2] Therefore the nerve can provide a guide to locating the parathyroid glands during surgery. Because of the variation in size, morphology, localization and number of parathyroid glands, surgery for parathyroid diseases can be challenging and requires experienced endocrine surgeons.

Parathyroid hormone

Parathyroid hormone (PTH) is a peptide hormone containing 84 amino acids, but only the first 34 seem to be essential for mineral homeostasis. Different PTH fragments are secreted in small amounts by the parathyroid glands themselves. In the Kupffer cells of the liver the whole PTH molecule undergoes rapid metabolism. The whole PTH molecule (amino acids 1–84) is split into a number of fragments.[3–6] These fragments are subsequently eliminated by the kidney. In patients with reduced renal function it is known that PTH fragments (amino acids 7–84, C-terminal fragments) accumulate.[7] C-terminal fragments may also act as antagonists to whole PTH(amino acids 1–84) regarding bone metabolism.

Mechanism of PTH excretion

Depending on the level of serum ionized calcium (iCa), the calcium-sensing receptor (CaR) is activated. This leads to mobilization of intracellular calcium stores and thus to a higher intracellular calcium level. In addition, there is a calcium influx into the parathyroid cell via transient receptor potential operated type C channels (TRPC).[8] A high intracellular calcium level inhibits PTH excretion, and vice versa. Vitamin D (1,25-dihydroxycholecalciferol, calcitriol) is also known to inhibit PTH excretion.

Effects of parathyroid hormone (Figure 5.1)

Calcium and phosphate are mobilized from the bone indirectly. PTH receptors are located on osteoblasts and stroma cells of the bone. After binding to the PTH receptor, osteoclast differentiating factor (ODF) is inserted into the plasma membrane of osteoblasts. The maturation and activation of osteclasts is induced via the receptor activator of nuclear factor κβ (RANK).

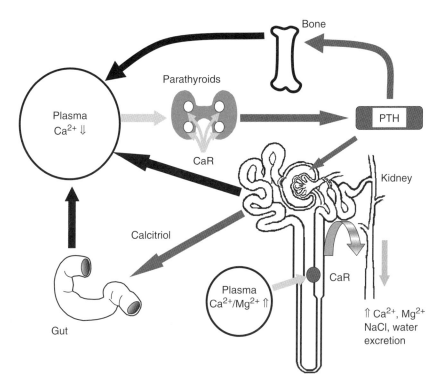

Fig. 5.1 A fall in ionized calcium activates the calcium-sensing receptor (CaR) on the parathyroid cells and initiates the release of PTH. PTH stimulates the release of Ca^{2+} from bone. At the same time PTH stimulates reabsorption of Ca^{2+} in the renal tubules and activates the conversion of vitamin D to calcitriol. Calcitriol stimulates absorption of calcium from the gut. Elevated plasma Ca^{2+} (or elevated Mg^{2+}) activates CaR on the thick ascending loop in the kidney, inhibiting Ca^{2+}, Mg^{2+}, Na^+, and water absorption, and leading to diuresis.

In the kidney, PTH blocks phosphate reabsorption in the proximal tubuli while calcium reabsorption (distal tubuli) is increased (suppression of calcium loss in urine). Furthermore, 1-α-hydoxylase is stimulated, which leads to higher levels of calcitriol.

In the small intestine, calcitriol enhances calcium absorption by synthesis of a calcium-binding protein in intestinal epithelial cells.

Calcium

Calcium is the most abundant mineral in the human body. The vast majority (99%) of the calcium is bound in the skeleton as calcium phosphate which serves as natural calcium storage. Circulating calcium is either albumin bound (50%) or ionized (iCa). Calcium homeostasis is mainly provided by parathyroid hormone (PTH) and calcitriol. Disorders in this system lead to symptomatic or asymptomatic hyper- or hypocalcaemia.

Pathology and pathophysiology

Tumour-induced hypercalcaemia

The most important differential diagnosis is paraneoplastic hypercalcaemia, which is the most common paraneoplastic metabolic syndrome and occurs in 10–20% of all patients with malignant disease.[9] It can be caused by tumour-induced osteolysis (bone metastasis) or PTH-related protein (PTHrP), which is directly secreted from the tumour cells.[10] Important parts of PTHrP are similar to PTH and make binding to the PTH receptor possible. Paraneoplastic hypercalcaemia is diagnosed by elevated serum calcium levels and suppressed PTH levels (negative feedback to parathyroid glands). PTHrP is elevated or bone metastasis can be diagnosed by whole-body scintigraphy. In patients with parathyroid carcinoma, PTH and calcium are elevated (equal to those seen in primary hyperparathyroidism (PHPT)).

Primary hyperparathyroidism

PHPT is a very common endocrine disorder. It affects more women than men, with a peak incidence in the fifth and sixth decades.[11] It is characterized biochemically by elevated total calcium and PTH. Patients are classified as asymptomatic, minimally symptomatic (osteopenia, high blood pressure, hypercalcaemic syndrome), or symptomatic (renal manifestation, osteoporosis, hypercalcaemic crisis). Surgery with complete excision of hyperfunctioning tissue is the only curative treatment. In up to 20%, more than one parathyroid gland is affected and has to be removed (double adenoma, 5%; four gland hyperplasia, 15%). Intra-operative PTH monitoring and post-operative calcium measurements confirm cure.[12] Because of the autonomous PTH secretion there is always a negative calcium balance in bone in patients with PHPT.[13] PHPT is diagnosed biochemically (elevated serum calcium *and* PTH on three different days). [^{99m}Tc]Sestamibi scanning (single-photon emission computed tomography (SPECT)) or high-resolution ultrasound are only performed as pre-operative localization studies.

Hereditary conditions are rare causes of PHPT. In multiple endocrine neoplasia 1 (MEN 1) all patients develop PHPT until the age of 25 years. PHPT occurs in 20–30% of patients with MEN 2a. There are also non-MEN-associated forms of PHPT.

Renal hyperparathyroidism (RHPT)

External stimulation of the parathyroids with hyperfunction of the gland is referred to as 'secondary hyperparathyroidism' and is usually caused by chronic renal failure. A low serum calcium level combined with low calcitriol levels (decreased 1-α-hydroxylase activity) acts as a permanent stimulus to the parathyroid cells. The low serum calcium levels are due to a failure of calcitriol production in the failing kidney which leads to a failure of intestinal absorption of calcium, while poor renal tubular function results in inadequate reabsorption of calcium from the urine. Secondary hyperparathyroidism may require parathyroidectomy to protect the bone against demineralization. In tertiary hyperparathyroidism, PTH excretion becomes autonomous as a result of hyperplasia of all parathyroid glands because of this chronic stimulation. This condition frequently arises after successful renal transplantation and re-establishment of calcium homeostasis. This results in hypercalcaemia, putting the transplanted kidney at risk of nephrocalcinosis. Parathyroidectomy is frequently required for tertiary hyperparathyroidism to protect the kidney.

In recent years, medical therapy with cinacalcet, a 'calcimimetic' drug, has been developed. Cinacalcet binds directly at the CaR and increases the sensitivity of the receptor for extracellular calcium which leads to decreased PTH excretion. However, adverse reactions (nausea, vomiting, dizziness, paraesthesia, myalgia, and diarrhoea) occur in some patients, while others do not show the desired effect. Therefore increasing numbers of patients with PHPT are submitted to surgery. Its effective use with acceptable levels of side-effects has been described in patients with intractable PHPT.[14]

Reactive HPT

Patients with increased bone turnover (osteoporosis, osteopenia), low vitamin D levels, or decreased calcium intake may show a normocalcaemic hyperparathyroidism which is a physiological reaction and therefore is not an indication for surgery.

Parathyroid carcinoma

Carcinoma of the parathyroid glands is responsible for 0.5–2% of PHPT. Biochemical and clinical presentation in the early stage is similar to that of PHPT. However, PTH values can be much higher than in patients with benign PHPT. A radical surgical procedure, including functional cervical lymph node dissection, is required. Patients with recurrent or metastatic disease may profit from a calcimimetic therapy with cinacalcet.

Critically ill patients

Critically ill patients have to be considered separately.[15] A number of hormonal changes, including PTH changes, are relatively common in these patients (see Chapter 1).[16] Up to

88% develop hypocalcaemia at some stage, and 15–32% develop hypercalcaemia during their stay in the intensive care unit (ICU).[17–19] Calcium status should be evaluated by iCa levels in this patient population.[20,21]

Hypocalcaemia in ICU patients

Hypocalcaemia correlates with the severity of disease, and not with disease *per se* (i.e. sepsis etc.)[19] and is a common state in critically ill patients. The aetiology of this phenomenon is not totally clear but some (possible) mechanisms have been found. In septic and shocked patients the inflammatory response (elevated interleukin 6 and tumour necrosis factor α) leads to increased PTH-resistance in bone and kidney.[22] Furthermore, because of altered calcium sensing, PTH secretion in the parathyroid glands is suppressed.[23]

In patients with acute pancreatitis, as outlined in the mechanism described above, endotoxinaemia *per se* leads to hypocalcaemia.[24] Elevated calcitonin in these patients (or elevated pro-calcitonin as a sign for systemic inflammatory disease) seems not to influence the calcium levels but contributes to the derangement of gut barrier functions.[25] Hypocalcaemia is an early predictive marker for multi-organ failure in patients with acute necrotizing pancreatitis.[26]

Overall, low iCa together with elevated PTH is an early predictor of mortality in critically ill surgical patients.[27–29] Calcium is significantly decreased in non-survivors.[30] There is an inverse correlation between iCa and the APACHE II score.[19,27] There also seems to be a higher mortality in patients with elevated PTH but normal iCa.[31]

Hypercalcaemia in ICU patients

Hypercalcaemia occurs in at least 15–32% of ICU patients.[17,18] The most important reason is parathyroid overactivity (stimulated after prolonged hypocalcaemia). It has been postulated as 'new kind of hyperparathyroidism'.[18] Severity of illness is the best predictor for later hypercalcaemia.[17] In about 18% of these patients parenteral nutrition contributes to hypercalcaemia (connected with hypophosphataemia).[32] An important cause of hypercalcaemia is immobilization (together with low PTH and calcitriol).[33,34] It has been described in patients with acute renal failure,[17] in burn ICUs,[33,35] and in patients without a critical disease but with prolonged immobilization.[34]

Hypercalcaemic crisis

Hypercalcaemic crisis is an uncommon but severe symptom of (primary) hyperparathyroidism and a medical emergency. Currently, intravenous application of bisphosphonates combined with aggressive fluid replacement (NaCl) is the standard therapy for hypercalcaemic crisis.[35–37] The use of loop diuretics should be restricted to those patients who are in danger of fluid overload. Loop diuretics are not effective in promoting significant renal calcium excretion, and may provoke volume depletion when used in patients whose volume deficit has not been reversed and who are not fully rehydrated.[36,38] In severe cases, especially in patients with acute renal failure, haemodialysis may also be helpful. There is no indication for emergency parathyroidectomy, as rehydration, calciuresis, and bisphosphonate therapy provide an effective bridge to parathyroidectomy[39] (see also Chapter 9).

Evaluation and pre-operative preparation

Patients with PHPT may have a higher cardiovascular risk depending on the progress of the disease. In particular, high blood pressure is common and myocardial dysfunction must be evaluated by pre-operative chest X-ray, a 12-lead ECG and optionally by echocardiography. Hypercalcaemic crisis may need urgent surgical treatment in an emergency setting.

In patients with renal failure (secondary or tertiary hyperparathyroidism) a careful evaluation and preparation of the patient is necessary. As these patients are often under surveillance of nephrologists, peri-operative treatment with dialysis can be sometimes necessary.

Surgery

Primary hyperparathyroidism

Surgery with complete removal of hyperfunctioning tissue is the only curative treatment of PHPT. In patients with localized single-gland disease minimally invasive surgery (open or video-assisted) with removal of the hyperfunctioning gland is performed ('targeted exploration'). Intra-operatively, blood is drawn at defined time-points and PTH is analysed using a quick PTH assay (analysis time 15 minutes). Different criteria are used to interpret the intra-operative PTH curve. Frequently used criteria are the Miami and the Vienna criteria.[12] If no gland can be localized pre-operatively or if localization studies or intra-operative PTH monitoring indicate multiple-gland disease a bilateral neck exploration is performed with visualization of all parathyroid glands and removal of those that are macroscopically enlarged. This procedure is also necessary when bilateral or contralateral thyroid surgery is performed simultaneously.

Renal hyperparathyroidism

As all parathyroid glands are affected in RHPT, one of two different surgical techniques are performed in the majority of patients: total parathyroidectomy with immediate autotransplantation of parathyroid tissue (with or without transcervical thymectomy and central neck dissection) or subtotal parathyroidectomy (removal of 3½ parathyroid glands). Explanted parathyroid tissue is cryopreserved for delayed autotransplantation. This is necessary in non-functioning grafts to prevent permanent hypoparathyroidism.

Anaesthetic management

Surgery is performed under either general anaesthesia or a superficial cervical plexus block,[40,41] depending on the relative experience of the anaesthetist and surgeon as well as patient preference.

The determination of the calcium homeostasis is of particular interest in the peri-operative period. Hypercalcaemia associated with severe primary hyperparathyroidism can lead to potentially life-threatening disturbances of cardiac rhythm which increase the anaesthetic risk.[41,42] Invasive arterial blood pressure monitoring via a peripheral artery catheter is mandatory and offers the possibility of repeated electrolyte measurements during surgery. In addition, there is increasing evidence that hypercalcaemia may antagonize the effect of non-depolarizing muscle relaxants.[43] Therefore continuous monitoring of neuromuscular blockade is recommended. In an emergency setting (hypercalcaemic crisis), high-capacity intravenous access should be obtained. If a central venous line is necessary, the subclavian vein is preferred to the internal jugular vein to ensure that surgical access to the neck is unimpeded (see Chapter 9).

At the end of the surgical procedure, in agreement with the surgeon, positive end-expiratory pressure (PEEP) may be increased stepwise up to a level of 30 mmHg. This provides maximum filling of the cervical veins (venous congestion) and leads to augmentation of occult bleeding.

During extubation, especially in patients after bilateral neck exploration or re-operation in the neck, special attention should be paid to a possible injury of the recurrent laryngeal nerve (vocal cord palsy). If there is bilateral damage of the laryngeal nerve immediate re-intubation is required (see also Chapter 4).

Excessive coughing after extubation leads to cervical venous congestion and may be the reason for early secondary haemorrhage. If there is tracheal obstruction due to a haematoma, revision surgery and evacuation of the haematoma may become necessary to facilitate re-intubation. Atropine is the emergency medication for antagonizing bradycardia and even asystole because of the extensive vagal stimulation occurring in this situation.

Post-operative care

In low-risk patients, only routine monitoring in the recovery room is required. Cooling the operating wound to reduce post-operative swelling may help to maintain airway patency.

However, admittance to a high care facility should be considered for patients with cardiovascular risk, elderly patients, or patients with pre-operative hypercalcaemic crisis.

Day case procedure

In the case of minimally invasive surgery (with or without local anaesthesia) a day case procedure can be planned, and discharge after a short recovery period is possible. Discharge criteria include vital signs, orientation, surgical concerns, and other necessary prerequisites, and are defined in current guidelines.[44] Scoring systems such as the Post-Anaesthesia Recovery Score modified for day surgery[45] are widely used for this purpose.

Hypocalcaemia

Normally functioning parathyroid glands can be suppressed by a high functioning adenoma. After removal of the adenoma, recovery of parathyroid hormone excretion by the remaining normal glands may be delayed and this may lead to transient hypoparathyroidism.

In regions where goitre is endemic[46] surgery for thyroid and parathyroid disease is often performed simultaneously. A common cause of hypocalcaemia is iatrogenic removal or devascularization of the (normal) parathyroid glands during thyroid surgery[47] or extensive bilateral neck exploration. It may be transient or may require life-long medical treatment. Thus, measurement of serum calcium and PTH on the first post-operative day is mandatory. Neuromuscular effects, such as paraesthesia of the distal extremities (always bilateral) and peri-oral area, are the predominant symptoms. Chvostek and Trousseau signs, muscle cramps, laryngospasm, tetany, and seizures may also occur.[48] Acute symptomatic hypocalcaemia is treated with an immediate intravenous infusion of calcium. Calcium gluconate is available in 10% ampoules (940 mg per unit) and should be preferred to calcium chloride for peripheral injection as it is less likely to cause tissue necrosis if extravasation occurs. If calcium chloride (which contains three times the amount of elemental calcium as the gluconate) is used, it should always be given through a central vein. One or two ampoules in 100 ml sodium chloride should be given over 4–20 minutes, depending on the severity of the symptoms. Attention should be paid to hypomagnesaemia which should be treated simultaneously.

Follow-up

In the hands of experienced endocrine surgeons over 98% of patients with primary hyperparathyroidism can be cured by the initial operation.[46] However, total cure from symptoms can be achieved in only 80% of symptomatic patients.[49]

The rate of persistent or recurrent disease is higher after surgery for renal hyperparathyroidism. Nevertheless, re-operation based on meticulous localization studies gives good results.[49,50] After autotransplantation of parathyroid tissue into the brachioradial muscle, a simple test helps to diagnose the site of recurrence (temporary implantectomy; Casanova's test).[51] Overall, most patients with renal hyperparathyroidism benefit from improvement of symptoms and signs (skin itch, bone pain, weakness, hypercalcaemia).

In all patients, follow-up examination (PTH, electrolytes, kidney function, symptoms, clinical presentation) should be performed at 6 weeks, 6 months, 12 months, and then annually to exclude persistent or recurrent disease.

Key clinical management points

Diagnosis

- PHPT: elevated serum calcium (ionized calcium) and PTH in three tests
- RHPT and tertiary HPT: patients with chronic renal failure not responding to medical treatment—elevated PTH with normal total and ionized calcium

Key clinical management points (continued)

Pre-operative preparation

◆ No special preparation necessary in most patients

◆ Hypercalcaemic crisis: saline infusion and (rarely) intravenous bisphosphonates, electrolyte replacement

◆ Assessment of fitness for anaesthesia

  • Cardiovascular risk factors

  • Volume status in patients with disequilibrium

  • Longer history of disease → more symptomatic, higher risk

  • Haemodialysis in patients with RHPT (in consultation with nephrologist)

Post-operative problems

◆ May develop acute hypocalcaemia, hypokalaemia, hypophosphataemia, and hypomagnesaemia (hungry bone syndrome)

◆ Requires ICU admission and aggressive electrolyte replacement

References

1. Clark OH, Duh QY, Kebebew E (2005). *Textbook of Endocrine Surgery*, 2nd edn. WB Saunders, Maryland Heights, MO.

2. Pyrtek L, Painter RL (1964). An anatomic study of the relationship of the parathyroid glands to the recurrent laryngeal nerve. *Surgery, Gynecology and Obstetrics*, **119**, 509–12.

3. Pillai S, Zull JE (1986). Production of biologically active fragments of parathyroid hormone by isolated Kupffer cells. *Journal of Biological Chemistry*, **261**, 14919–23.

4. Bringhurst FR, Segre GV, Lampman GW, Potts JT (2002). Metabolism of parathyroid hormone by Kupffer cells: analysis by reverse-phase high-performance liquid chromatography. *Biochemistry*, **21**, 4252–8.

5. Habener JF, Rosenblatt M, Potts JT, Jr. (1984). Parathyroid hormone: biochemical aspects of biosynthesis, secretion, action, and metabolism. *Physiological Reviews*, **64**, 985–1053.

6. Potts JT, Jr., Kronenberg HM, Rosenblatt M (1982). Parathyroid hormone: chemistry, biosynthesis, and mode of action. *Advances in Protein Chemistry*, **35**, 323–96.

7. Kaczirek K, Riss P, Wunderer G, *et al.* (2005). Quick PTH assay cannot predict incomplete parathyroidectomy in patients with renal hyperparathyroidism. *Surgery*, **137**, 431–5.

8. Braänström R, Lu M, Berglund E, Forsberg L, Farnebo L-O (2009). Evaluation of the endogenous expression of TRCP channels in human parathyroid. *Langenbeck's Archives of Surgery*, **394**, 411.

9. Mundy GR, Martin TJ (1982). The hypercalcemia of malignancy: pathogenesis and management. *Metabolism*, **31**, 1247–77.

10. Burtis WJ (1992). Parathyroid hormone-related protein: structure, function, and measurement. *Clinical Chemistry*, **38**, 2171–83.

11. Niederle B, Stamm L, Langle F, Schubert E, Woloszczuk W, Prager R (1992). Primary hyperparathyroidism in Austria: results of an 8-year prospective study. *World Journal of Surgery*, **16**, 777–82.

12. Riss P, Kaczirek K, Heinz G, Bieglmayer C, Niederle B (2007). A 'defined baseline' in PTH monitoring increases surgical success in patients with multiple gland disease. *Surgery*, **142**, 398–404.

13. Ambrogini E, Cetani F, Cianferotti L, *et al.* (2007). Surgery or surveillance for mild asymptomatic primary hyperparathyroidism: a prospective, randomized clinical trial. *Journal of Clinical Endocrinology and Metabolism*, **92**, 3114–21.

14. Marcocci C, Chanson P, Shoback D, *et al.* (2009). Cinacalcet reduces serum calcium concentrations in patients with intractable primary hyperparathyroidism. *Journal of Clinical Endocrinology and Metabolism*, **94**, 2766–72.

15. Baker SB, Worthley LI (2002). The essentials of calcium, magnesium and phosphate metabolism. Part I: Physiology. *Critical Care and Resuscitation*, **4**, 301–6.

16. Wuster C (1997). Parathyroid hormone—a new prognostic marker of mortality? *European Journal of Clinical Investigation*, **27**, 982–3.

17. Lind L, Ljunghall S (1992). Critical care hypercalcemia—a hyperparathyroid state. *Experimental and Clinical Endocrinology*, **100**, 148–51.

18. Forster J, Querusio L, Burchard KW, Gann DS (1985). Hypercalcemia in critically ill surgical patients. *Annals of Surgery*, **202**, 512–18.

19. Zivin JR, Gooley T, Zager RA, Ryan MJ (2001). Hypocalcemia: a pervasive metabolic abnormality in the critically ill. *American Journal of Kidney Disease*, **37**, 689–98.

20. Dickerson RN, Alexander KH, Minard G, Croce MA, Brown RO (2004). Accuracy of methods to estimate ionized and 'corrected' serum calcium concentrations in critically ill multiple trauma patients receiving specialized nutrition support. *Journnal of Parenteral and Enteral Nutrition*, **28**, 133–41.

21. Byrnes MC, Huynh K, Helmer SD, Stevens C, Dort JM, Smith RS (2005). A comparison of corrected serum calcium levels to ionized calcium levels among critically ill surgical patients. *American Journal of Surgery*, **189**, 310–14.

22. Lind L, Carlstedt F, Rastad J, *et al.* (2000). Hypocalcemia and parathyroid hormone secretion in critically ill patients. *Critical Care Medicine*, **28**, 93–9.

23. Carlstedt E, Ridefelt P, Lind L, Rastad J (1999). Interleukin-6 induced suppression of bovine parathyroid hormone secretion. *Bioscience Reports*, **19**, 35–42.

24. Ammori BJ, Barclay GR, Larvin M, McMahon MJ (2003). Hypocalcemia in patients with acute pancreatitis: a putative role for systemic endotoxin exposure. *Pancreas*, **26**, 213–17.

25. Ammori BJ, Becker KL, Kite P, *et al.* (2003). Calcitonin precursors: early markers of gut barrier dysfunction in patients with acute pancreatitis. *Pancreas*, **27**, 239–43.

26. Kawa S, Mukawa K, Kiyosawa K (2000). Hypocalcemia <7.5 mg/dl: early predictive marker for multisystem organ failure in severe acute necrotizing pancreatitis, proposed by the study analyzing post-ERCP pancreatitis. *American Journal of Gastroenterology*, **95**, 1096–7.

27. Carlstedt F, Lind L, Rastad J, Stjernstrom H, Wide L, Ljunghall S (1998). Parathyroid hormone and ionized calcium levels are related to the severity of illness and survival in critically ill patients. *European Journal of Clinical Investigation*, **28**, 898–903.

28. Burchard KW, Gann DS, Colliton J, Forster J (1990). Ionized calcium, parathormone, and mortality in critically ill surgical patients. *Annals of Surgery*, **212**, 543–9.

29. Cherry RA, Bradburn E, Carney DE, Shaffer ML, Gabbay RA, Cooney RN (2006). Do early ionized calcium levels really matter in trauma patients? *Journal of Trauma*, **61**, 774–9.

30. Ward RT, Colton DM, Meade PC, *et al.* (2004). Serum levels of calcium and albumin in survivors versus nonsurvivors after critical injury. *Journal of Critical Care*, **19**, 54–64.

31. Carlstedt F, Lind L, Wide L, *et al.* (1997). Serum levels of parathyroid hormone are related to the mortality and severity of illness in patients in the emergency department. *European Journal of Clinical Investigation*, **27**, 977–81.

32. Martinez MJ, Martinez MA, Montero M, Campelo E, Castro I, Inaraja MT (2006). Hypophosphatemia in postoperative patients with total parenteral nutrition: influence of nutritional support teams. *Nutrición Hospitalaria*, **21**, 657–60.

33. Peralta MC, Gordon DL (2002). Immobilization-related hypercalcemia after renal failure in burn injury. *Endocrine Practice*, **8**, 213–16.

34. Cheng CJ, Chou CH, Lin SH (2006). An unrecognized cause of recurrent hypercalcemia: immobilization. *Southern Medical Journal*, **99**, 371–4.

35. Sam R, Vaseemuddin M, Siddique A, *et al.* (2007). Hypercalcemia in patients in the burn intensive care unit. *Journal of Burn Care Research*, **28**, 742–6.

36. LeGrand SB, Leskuski D, Zama I (2008). Narrative review: furosemide for hypercalcemia: an unproven yet common practice. *Annals of Internal Medicine*, **149**, 259–63.

37. Mundy GR, Guise TA (1997). Hypercalcemia of malignancy. *American Journal of Medicine*, **103**, 134–45.

38. Pecherstorfer M, Brenner K, Zojer N (2003). Current management strategies for hypercalcemia. *Treatments in Endocrinology*, **2**, 273–92.

39. Phitayakorn R, McHenry CR (2008). Hyperparathyroid crisis: use of bisphosphonates as a bridge to parathyroidectomy. *Journal of the American College of Surgery*, **206**, 1106–15.

40. Pintaric TS, Hocevar M, Jereb S, Casati A, Jankovic VN (2007). A prospective, randomized comparison between combined (deep and superficial) and superficial cervical plexus block with levobupivacaine for minimally invasive parathyroidectomy. *Anesthesia and Analgesia*, **105**, 1160–3.

41. Miccoli P, Barellini L, Monchik JM, Rago R, Berti PF (2005). Randomized clinical trial comparing regional and general anaesthesia in minimally invasive video-assisted parathyroidectomy. *British Journal of Surgery*, **92**, 814–18.

42. Papadima A, Lagoudianakis EE, Markogiannakis H, Pappas A, Georgiou L, Manouras A (2008). Anaesthetic considerations in parathyrotoxic crisis. *European Journal of Anaesthesiology*, **25**, 772–4.

43. Al Mohaya S, Naguib M, Abdelatif M, Farag H (1986). Abnormal responses to muscle relaxants in a patient with primary hyperparathyroidism. *Anesthesiology*, **65**, 554–6.

44. British Association of Day Surgery. *Guidelines about the Discharge Process and the Assessment of Fitness for Discharge*. Available online at: http://www.daysurgeryuk.org/bads/joomla/index.php/bads-handbooks (accessed 14 January 2010).

45. Aldrete JA (1995). The post-anesthesia recovery score revisited. *Journal of Clinical Anesthesiology*, **7**, 89–91.

46. Prager G, Czerny C, Kurtaran A, *et al.* (2001). Minimally invasive open parathyroidectomy in an endemic goiter area: a prospective study. *Archives of Surgery*, **136**, 810–16.

47. Wilson RB, Erskine C, Crowe PJ (2000). Hypomagnesemia and hypocalcemia after thyroidectomy: prospective study. *World Journal of Surgery*, **24**, 722–6.

48. Bushinsky DA, Monk RD (1998). Electrolyte quintet: calcium. *Lancet*, **352**, 306–11.

49. Niederle B, Roka R, Woloszczuk W, Klaushofer K, Kovarik J, Schernthaner G (1987). Successful parathyroidectomy in primary hyperparathyroidism: a clinical follow-up study of 212 consecutive patients. *Surgery*, **102**, 903–9.

50. Chou FF, Lee CH, Chen HY, Chen JB, Hsu KT, Sheen-Chen SM (2002). Persistent and recurrent hyperparathyroidism after total parathyroidectomy with autotransplantation. *Annals of Surgery*, **235**, 99–104.

51. Casanova D, Sarfati E, De FA, Amado JA, Arias M, Dubost C (1991). Secondary hyperparathyroidism: diagnosis of site of recurrence. *World Journal of Surgery*, **15**, 546–9.

Chapter 6

Anaesthetic management of patients with carcinoid tumours

Anis S Baraka

Over 100 years ago, Lubarsh[1] described multiple tumours found in the distal ileum of two patients on autopsy as carcinoid tumours.[1] Oberndorfer,[2] in 1907, was the first to use the term *Karzinoid* to denote the less-aggressive behaviour of carcinoid-like tumours.

Carcinoid tumours are derived from neurochromaffin cells and can be found in any tissue derived from endoderm, although the gastrointestinal tract is the most common site. Carcinoid tumours are neuroendocrine tumours, and therefore are part of the APUD (amine precursor uptake and decarboxylation) system.[3]

Incidence

Carcinoid tumours are relatively rare, with a reported prevalence of 1.0–2.5 per 100 000 population. However, autopsy studies indicate that the incidental finding of carcinoid tumours can be as high as 8%. Geographical variation was seen in the incidence of carcinoid tumours, being 1–2 cases per 100 000 in the USA compared with 8.4 cases per 100 000 in Sweden.[4]

Classification

Carcinoid tumours have been traditionally classified according to the embryonic site of origin as foregut, midgut, and hindgut.[5,6] The foregut is represented by the thymus, lung, stomach, pancreas, and proximal duodenum, the midgut is represented by the distal duodenum, jejunum, appendix, and proximal colon, and the hindgut is represented by the distal colon and rectum (Table 6.1).

A more recent classification limits the term carcinoid tumour to midgut carcinoids, and other carcinoids are named neuroendocrine tumours of the anatomical location (e.g. neuroendocrine tumour of the bronchus, ovary, etc).[7] Some foregut carcinoids lack the aromatic amino acid decarboxylase, and these tumours produce 5-hydroxytryptophane (and histamine) instead of serotonin. Hindgut carcinoids cannot convert tryptophan into serotonin and its subsequent metabolites, and they are not associated with the carcinoid syndrome even when they metastasize to the liver.

Over 75% of carcinoid tumours originate in the gastrointestinal tract, principally in the appendix, ileum, and rectum. The lung is the most common non-gut site (more than 22% of cases) for carcinoid tumours. Although usually found in adults of middle to old

Table 6.1 Carcinoid tumour classification

Foregut	Lung, thymus, stomach, pancreas, proximal duodenum
Midgut	Distal duodenum to proximal colon
Hindgut	Distal colon including rectum

Table 6.2 Products of carcinoid tumours

Amines
Serotonin
5-Hydroxy tryptophan
Histamine
Polypetides
Kallikrein
Pancreatic polypeptides
Bradykinin
Prostaglandins E and F

age, carcinoid tumours have been described in children, where they are most common in the appendix.

Carcinoid mediators[8–12]

Carcinoid tumours release a variety of amines and peptides from either the primary tumour or the liver metastases. As many as 40 secretory products have been identified (Table 6.2).

Serotonin is the most common secretory product. It is produced from tryptophan by hydroxylation and decarboxylation. In normal subjects, only 1% of dietary tryptophan is converted to serotonin; however, in the carcinoid patient this value may increase up to 70% or more. Adrenergic stimulation causes the release of serotonin into the circulation where it is broken down to 5-hydroxy-indole acetic acid (5-HIAA). Urinary and plasma 5-HIAA is used for diagnosis and to monitor disease progress (Figure 6.1).

Carcinoid syndrome[8–12]

Carcinoid syndrome is a variable collection of signs and symptoms associated with the release of a variety of vasoactive amines and neuropeptides into the systemic circulation by the primary carcinoid tumour or the liver metastasis. The development of the carcinoid syndrome generally indicates the presence of hepatic or pulmonary metastasis, as the liver normally metabolizes these mediators before they reach the systemic circulation. However, in some rare cases carcinoid mediators may gain access to the systemic circulation without hepatic metastasis.

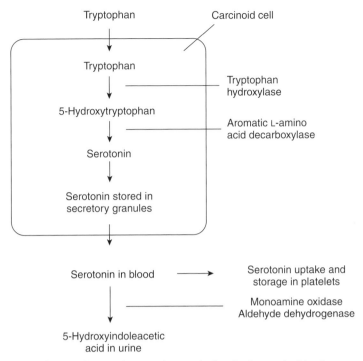

Fig. 6.1 Pathway of tryptophan and serotonin metabolism in the carcinoid cell.

About 15–18% of patients with carcinoid tumours develop carcinoid syndrome. At the time of diagnosis, only 20–30% of patients have disseminated disease and present with carcinoid syndrome because the liver and lungs inactivate the bioactive products of the tumour. Hence patients with carcinoid disease may not develop the syndrome.

Manifestations of carcinoid syndrome[8–12]

Manifestations of the carcinoid syndrome include the 'classic' triad of cutaneous flushing, diarrhoea, and heart disease, and less commonly telangiectasis, wheezing, and paroxysmal hypotension. While flushing is the most common sign (84%), diarrhoea is the most commonly occurring symptom (70%), varying from slight alterations in bowel habit to torrential diarrhoea unresponsive to fasting and associated with dehydration, hyponatraemia, hypokalaemia, and hypochloraemia.

Manifestations of the carcinoid syndrome occur when the output of the vasoactive mediators overwhelms the ability of liver and lungs to inactivate them. Serotonin can cause vasoconstriction or vasodilatation, so that both hypertension and hypotension are seen. Serotonin also increases gut motility and the accumulation of water, sodium, chloride, and potassium by the small intestine. Vomiting, bronchospasm, and hyperglycaemia may also occur. Prolonged drowsiness following anaesthesia in carcinoid sufferers has been attributed to elevated levels of serotonin. Histamine release is predominantly seen in patients with gastric carcinoid tumour. This amino acid is thought to be responsible for flushing and bronchospasm. Kallikreins are protease enzymes that generate kinins from kininogens. Bradykinin and its associated family produce profound vasomotor relaxation, causing severe hypotension and flushing, probably via nitric oxide synthesis. Bradykinin also causes bronchospasm, particularly in asthmatic subjects and in the presence of cardiac disease. Lysosomal kallikrein release is triggered by sympathetic stimulation. Tachykinins (e.g. neuropeptide K, neurokinin A, vasoactive intestinal polypeptide, and substance P) may be involved with flushing and are the possible cause of fibrotic processes in the heart.

Cutaneous flushing

Cutaneous flushing is the most common symptom, occurring in 84% of patients, and is considered the hallmark of the syndrome. Flushing begins suddenly and lasts from 30 seconds to 30 minutes, involving the face, neck, and upper chest. The colour of the flushing changes from an initial red to purple, and is associated with a mild burning sensation. Severe flushes are accompanied with a fall in blood pressure and rise in pulse rate. As the disease progresses, the episodes may last longer and the flushing may be more diffuse and cyanotic. Serotonin does not cause the flushing, which may be mediated by bradykinin (which is a potent vasodilator) and/or histamine.

Venous telangiectasia

Venous telangiectases are purplish vascular lesions, appearing late in the course of carcinoid syndrome. They are due to prolonged vasodilatation, and occur mostly on the nose, upper lip, and malar areas.

Diarrhoea

Diarrhoea occurs in 80% of the cases, and is usually unrelated to the flushing episodes. It is caused by water secretion and is watery and non-bloody; it is the most debilitating symptom of the disease since up to 30 episodes occur per day. The diarrhoea may result in severe dehydration and electrolyte abnormalities. Serotonin is the most likely cause of the diarrhoea since it stimulates intestinal secretion and motility and inhibits intestinal absorption.

Bronchospasm

Bronchospasm occurs in 20% of patients. It manifests as wheezing and dyspnoea, often associated with the flushing episode. Carcinoid bronchospasm must be differentiated from traditional bronchial asthma because treatment with β-adrenergic agonists can worsen, rather than relieve, the bronchospasm.

Tryptophan deficiency

In normal subjects only 1% of dietary tryptophan is converted to serotonin, but in carcinoid patients up to 70% is converted into serotonin, resulting in tryptophan deficiency which is manifested by pellagra, dermatitis, diarrhoea, and dementia. Muscle wasting may also occur as a result of poor protein synthesis.

Regional carcinoid diseases

Carcinoid tumours of the small intestine

Small bowel carcinoid tumours make up approximately one-third of small bowel tumours. They are often located in the distal ileum and are usually multicentric. Patients with small bowel carcinoids generally present in the sixth or seventh decade of life, most commonly with abdominal pain or small bowel alteration. Because standard imaging techniques, such as computed tomography (CT) and barium studies, rarely identify the primary tumour, the pre-operative diagnosis of small bowel carcinoid is difficult, and patients frequently have vague abdominal pain for several years before diagnosis.

The majority of patients present with metastasis to the lymph nodes or the liver; only 5–7% present with the carcinoid syndrome. Tumour size is an unreliable predictor of metastasis. Long-term survival correlates closely with the stage of the disease. The 5 year survival rate is 65% among patients with localized or regional disease, but is only 36% among those with distant metastasis.

Patients in whom metastatic disease is suspected should be evaluated with abdominal CT to rule out liver metastasis. Liver function tests are an unreliable indicator of metastatic involvement of the liver. Carcinoid liver metastases are often hypervascular and may appear isodense relative to the liver after the administration of intravenous contrast material (Figure 6.2). The liver is a fertile site for metastases, and hepatic spread results in the release of excessive amounts of mediators into the systemic circulation, resulting in the development of carcinoid syndrome as well as carcinoid heart disease.

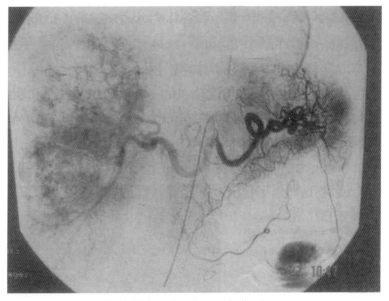

Fig. 6.2 Angiogram for selective right hepatic artery embolization.

Carcinoid heart disease[13–17]

Once the carcinoid syndrome has developed, approximately 50% of patients manifest carcinoid heart disease. Clinically, the period between onset of symptoms and diagnosis of carcinoid heart disease is generally around 1–2 years and may be as long as 5 years. However, carcinoid heart disease may be the first sign of a carcinoid tumour. The cardiac manifestations of carcinoid syndrome are caused by the paraneoplastic effects of vasoactive substances such as serotonin or other tumour by-products released from hepatic metastases rather than direct carcinoid or metastatic involvement of the heart. While the vasoactive tumour products are usually inactivated by the liver and lungs, the presence of hepatic metastases may allow large quantities of the mediators to reach the right side of the heart.

The preferential right heart involvement is most likely related to inactivation of the vasoactive substances by the lung before they reach the left atrium. However, in 5–10% of cases the left side of heart is involved, and where this occurs one should suspect extensive liver metastases, or bronchial carcinoid whose mediators bypass the pulmonary circulation, or a right-to-left shunt such as a patent foramen ovale.

The structural carcinoid heart lesions are characterized by plaque-like fibrous endocardial thickening which classically involves the tricuspid valve, the pulmonary valve, and the endocardium. The development of these lesions appears to be mediated by serotonin receptors subtype 1b. The endocardial lesions result from myofibril proliferation, which causes tricuspid valve regurgitation and less frequently valvular stenosis (Figure 6.3).

The pulmonary valve is also commonly affected, resulting in a combination of stenosis and regurgitation. However, haemodynamically relevant pulmonary stenosis occurs more frequently than tricuspid stenosis because the orifice of the pulmonary valve is much smaller.

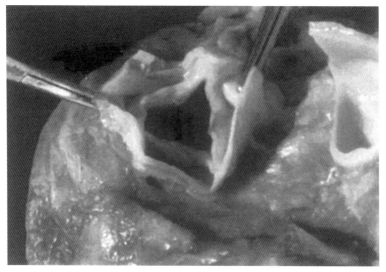

Fig. 6.3 (Plate 3) Endocardial carcinoid lesions on the tricuspid valve.

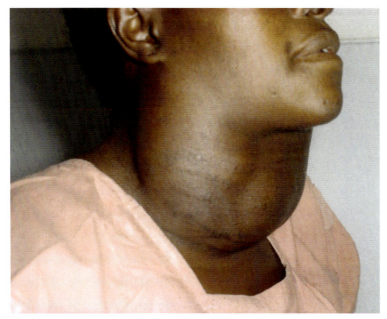

Plate 1 Very large thyroid goitre due to chronic iodine deficiency. This patient proved very easy to intubate. (See Chapter 4, p. 82.)

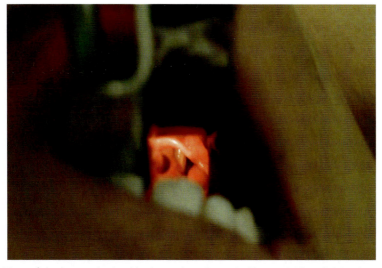

Plate 2 View of the larynx obtained in the patient shown in Figures 4.10 and 4.11. Note the excellent view of the laryngeal inlet, despite the lateral distortion of the larynx shown in Figure 4.10. (See Chapter 4, p. 90.)

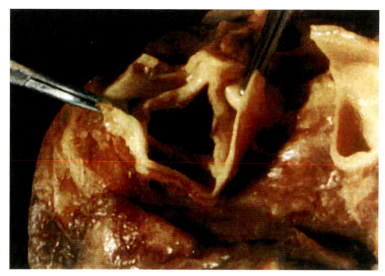

Plate 3 Endocardial carcinoid lesions on the tricuspid valve. (See Chapter 6, p. 116.)

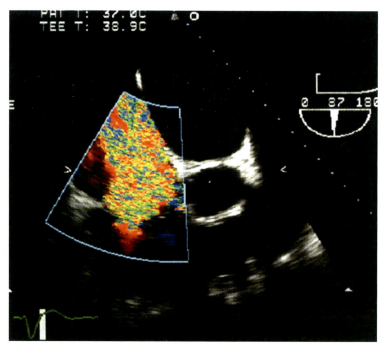

Plate 4 Colour flow Doppler assessment of the hepatic veins showing systemic flow reversal, consistent with severe tricuspid regurgitation secondary to carcinoid heart disease. (See Chapter 6, p. 117.)

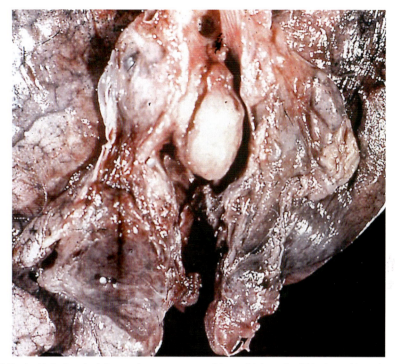

Plate 5 Typical lobulated pink-purple appearance of bronchial carcinoid lesions. (See Chapter 6, p. 120.)

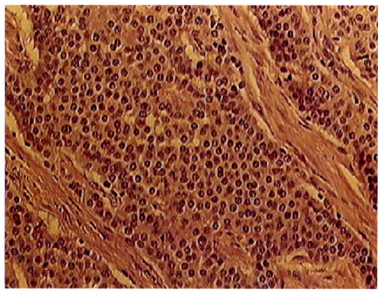

Plate 6 Histological appearance of ileal carcinoid. (See Chapter 6, p. 122.)

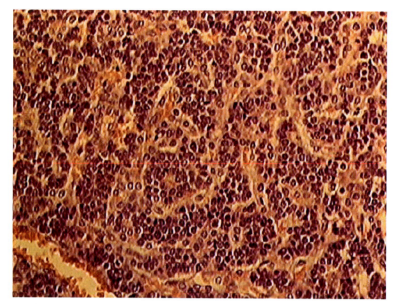

Plate 7 Histological appearance of hepatic carcinoid metastasis. (See Chapter 6, p. 123.)

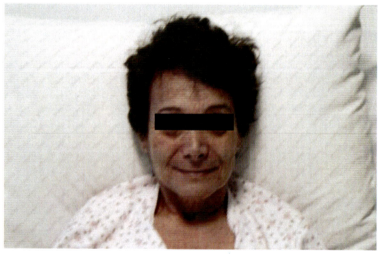

Plate 8 Typical flushed appearance of a patient experiencing carcinoid symptoms. The thin lined appearance is indicative of weight loss. (See Chapter 6, p. 130.)

The diagnosis of carcinoid heart disease may be delayed by the fact that cardiac symptoms and signs are often absent or subtle early in the course of cardiac involvement. Right-sided valvular heart disease first presents with easy fatiguability and exertional dyspnoea.

On physical examination, a palpable right heart ventricular impulse may indicate cardiac involvement. Cardiac murmurs are audible in more than 90% of cases at the time of diagnosis of carcinoid heart disease. Tricuspid regurgitation can produce a systolic murmur along the left sternal edge, and murmurs of pulmonary valve disease can be heard over the left second and third interspaces.

Distension of the jugular veins associated with an early large V wave may be the first finding suggestive of significant tricuspid regurgitation; the liver may also be enlarged and pulsatile. With progressive right-sided heart failure, the patient develops worsening dyspnoea, peripheral oedema, and ascites. ECG or chest X-ray is of limited value in the diagnosis of carcinoid heart disease. Echocardiography is the key element in the diagnostic evaluation and in the assessment of the disease severity of carcinoid heart disease. On two-dimensional echocardiography, the tricuspid leaflets are typically thickened and shortened. With progression of the disease, the leaflets become increasingly retracted with reduced motility. Colour flow Doppler assessment of the hepatic veins may show systemic flow reversal consistent with severe tricuspid regurgitation (Figure 6.4).

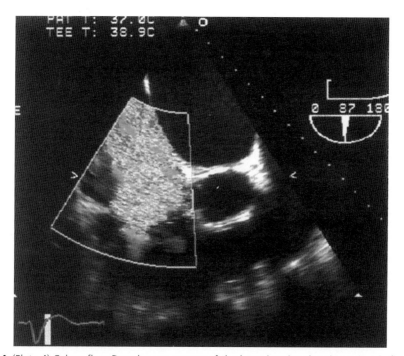

Fig. 6.4 (Plate 4) Colour flow Doppler assessment of the hepatic veins showing systemic flow reversal, consistent with severe tricuspid regurgitation secondary to carcinoid heart disease.

Medical treatment of heart failure, such as salt and water restriction and the use of diuretics, may improve the symptoms of oedema. However, with advanced right ventricular failure and reduction of cardiac output, depletion of intravascular volume by these therapeutic measures may further aggravate the hemodynamic situation, leading to increased fatigue and dyspnoea. Cardiac surgery is the only therapeutic option which avoids this vicious circle in advanced stages of carcinoid heart disease.

The timing of cardiac surgery has to be individualized. The indications for cardiac valve replacement surgery in patients with carcinoid heart disease are symptoms of right ventricular failure with progressive fatigue, significantly impaired exercise capacity, progressive right ventricular enlargement, or decrease in right ventricular systolic function.

Tricuspid valve replacement is the operation of choice to treat the dysfunctional tricuspid valve. Valve repair is not an option because of the severe retraction and fixation of the leaflets. For pulmonary valve stenosis, a mean transpulmonary gradient of more than 10 mmHg is considered an indication for valve surgery. The choice of valve prosthesis should be individualized in patients with carcinoid heart disease. The use of mechanical prosthesis versus bioprosthesis is controversial. The bioprosthesis may be less durability and have a less favourable haemodynamic profile than a mechanical prosthesis because of premature bioprosthesis degeneration attributed to the deposition of carcinoid plaques. However, the potential degeneration of the bioprosthesis may be prevented by systemic and regional therapy against the carcinoid disease. In contrast with the bioprosthesis, the mechanical prosthesis has a long life, but unfortunately it requires continuous anticoagulation therapy which represents a considerable bleeding risk in patients with malignant carcinoid tumours because of the potential development of hepatic dysfunction due to advanced liver metastasis. The advantages and disadvantages of each form of valve prosthesis should be discussed with the patient.

Bronchial carcinoids[18–20]

Pulmonary carcinoids make up approximately 2% of primary lung tumours. Bronchial carcinoids are considered as a distinct and well-defined group in the neuroendocrine scale. In this scale, typical carcinoids represent the best-differentiated form, while small cell carcinoma is the most undifferentiated form. There is no apparent correlation between the formation of bronchial carcinoid and family history, age, tobacco use, and environmental exposure.

Symptoms of bronchial carcinoid are related to bronchial irritation and obstruction which depend on the central or peripheral location of the tumour. The most frequent symptoms are persistent irritative or productive cough, haemoptysis, and recurrent pulmonary infections, as well as asthma-like symptoms.

PA chest X-rays and CT screening are the most useful techniques for diagnosis. A CT scan is necessary for evaluating the lesion, especially for its extension of the lesion and for the prediction of lymph node metastasis (Figure 6.5).

Patients with typical pulmonary carcinoid (i.e. well-differentiated pulmonary neuroendocrine tumours) usually present in the fifth decade of life. These tumours may have a

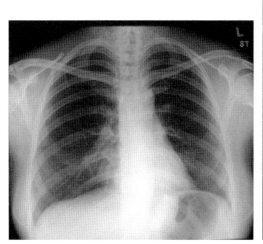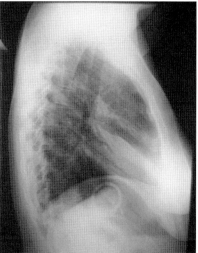

Fig. 6.5 Chest X-ray showing right pulmonary infiltration secondary to bronchial carcinoid.

variety of neuroendocrine manifestations. Ectopic secretion of corticotrophin accounts for 1% of all cases of Cushing's syndrome. Acromegaly due to ectopic secretion of growth hormone-releasing hormone has also been reported. Approximately one-third of pulmonary carcinoids have atypical histological features. Atypical carcinoids have an aggressive clinical course, metastasizing to mediastinal lymph nodes in 30–50% of cases.

Rigid or flexible bronchoscopy is a major diagnostic tool. Distinguishing a benign tumour from a malignant tumour can be achieved by bronchoscopic biopsy. A lobulated pink-purple appearance is typical (Figure 6.6). They are also highly vascularized, so that taking a biopsy may cause major bleeding.

Conservative surgery is the treatment of choice of bronchial carcinoids which are histologically typical and anatomically endobronchial. Bronchotomy with simple excision or sleeve resection is effective, especially for polypoid type carcinoids and selected sessile types. Sleeve resections with or without lobectomy rather than pneumonectomy have been considered as the operation of choice for central carcinoids. However, the adequacy of conservative resection in patients with atypical carcinoid has been questioned.

Gastric carcinoid tumours[8]

Gastric carcinoid tumours make up less than 1% of gastric neoplasms. They can be classified into three distinct groups on the basis of clinical and histological characteristics. Those associated with chronic atrophic gastritis type A may be accompanied by pernicious anaemia, while those associated with Zollinger–Ellison syndrome occur almost exclusively in patients with multiple endocrine neoplasm type 1 as well as sporadic gastric carcinoid tumours.

Sporadic carcinoid gastric tumours have been associated with an atypical carcinoid syndrome that is manifested primarily by flushing and is thought to be mediated by

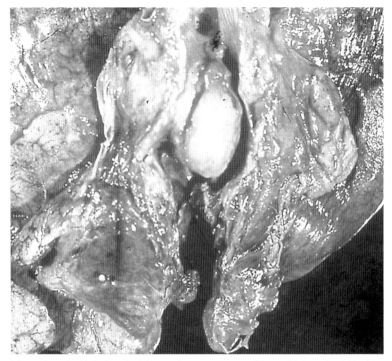

Fig. 6.6 (Plate 5) Typical lobulated pink-purple appearance of bronchial carcinoid lesions.

histamine.[19] In patients with the gastric syndrome variant, the flushes are patchy, sharply demarcated, serpigious, and cherry red; they are also intensely pruritic. Diarrhoea or cardiac lesions are unusual. The secreted histamine may account for the characteristic flush as well as the increased prevalence of peptic ulcer.

Appendiceal carcinoid tumours[8,21]

Carcinoid tumours are the most common tumours of the appendix. Thus greater frequency in women has been attributed to an increased incidental appendectomy in women undergoing cholecystectomy or operations such as hysterectomy, oophorectomy, and Caesarean section. Recently, however, incidental appendectomy has become less common, and most appendiceal carcinoids are found during surgery for acute appendicitis, which is similar among men and women.

Less than 10% of appendiceal carcinoids cause symptoms, because approximately 75% are located in the distal third of the appendix where they are unlikely to cause obstruction. Most of the remainder are located in the middle third and less than 10% at the base. The size of the tumour is the best predictor of prognosis in patients with appendiceal carcinoid tumours. Over 95% of the tumours are less than 2 cm in diameter. Although metastases from tumours of this size have been reported, they are rare and are usually diagnosed at the time of surgery.

Diagnosis of carcinoid disease

Most carcinoid tumours are discovered incidentally during endoscopic or radiographic procedures planned for other purposes, especially if they are non-functional. They can be an incidental intra-operative or post-operative finding during abdominal surgery for other lesions.

When symptoms occur, they are caused by:

◆ local tumour effects

◆ action of the secreted bioactive products on different organs, resulting in the carcinoid syndrome which includes the carcinoid heart disease

◆ tryptophan deficiency syndrome.

The local symptoms of carcinoid tumours are non-specific and include abdominal pain, diarrhoea, intermittent intestinal obstruction, and gastrointestinal bleeding. These are often vague and generalized signs and symptoms, and hence there is a delay in diagnosis in many patients. Although symptoms may be caused by the mechanical effects of the tumour, most of the symptoms of carcinoid tumours are caused by the effects of the mediators secreted by the tumour and released into the systemic circulation, resulting in the carcinoid syndrome as discussed above. The presence of these symptoms and signs should lead to consideration of carcinoid disease in the differential diagnosis, and usually leads to biochemical screening by measuring the 24-hour urinary excretion of 5-HIAA. Urinary 5-HIAA determination is the most useful and readily available initial diagnostic test.

Biochemical testing

Carcinoid tumour cells take up the amino acid tryptophan and convert it into the biologically active metabolic derivative serotonin. Serotonin is secreted into the circulation, and is then metabolized mainly in the liver and lung by monoamine oxidase (MAO) and aldehyde dehydrogenase into 5-HIAA.

Measurement of 24-hour urinary 5-HIAA excretion (normally 2–8 mg/day) has a sensitivity of 75% and a specificity up to 100% for the diagnosis of carcinoid disease. Urinary 5-HIAA is a reliable marker not only for the presence but also for the activity of the carcinoid tumour. However, certain drugs and serotonin-containing foods can interfere with the determination of urinary 5-HIAA, causing false-positive results (Table 6.3).

Table 6.3 Foods and drugs that affect serotonin concentration

Foods with a high serotonin content
Spinach, cheese, wine, caffeine, tomatoes, kiwi fruit, bananas, pineapples, avocados, walnuts
Drugs that increase plasma serotonin
Isoniazid, phenothiazines, phenacetin, monoamine oxidase inhibitors, acetaminophen (paracetamol), fluorouracil, iodine solutions

If measurement of urinary 5-HIAA is inconclusive, determination of blood serotonin concentration, as measurements of alternative biochemical markers such as plasma chromogranin A, can be helpful and is also an important prognostic indicator, with high levels indicating numerous metastatic tumours and a worse prognosis.

Localization

Once the biochemical diagnosis of the carcinoid syndrome is confirmed, the tumour must be localized by CT and octreotide scans.

- Abdominal CT scan with intravenous and oral administration of radiographic contrast agents has a sensitivity of 87%.
- Octreotide imaging (indium-111): 80% of carcinoid tumours have type 2 somatostatin receptors and can be localized by scintigraphy with radioactive-labelled octreotide.

Pathology

Carcinoids arise from enterochromaffin cells and stain with potassium dichromate, a feature of cells that contain serotonin. On gross appearance, carcinoid tumours are well circumscribed round submucosal lesions, and the cut surface appears yellow because of their high lipid contents.

Carcinoid tumours have been classified based upon their histological characteristics as 'typical' or 'atypical'. Five distinct histological patterns have been recognized: insular, trabecular, glandular, undifferentiated, and mixed (Figures 6.7 and 6.8).

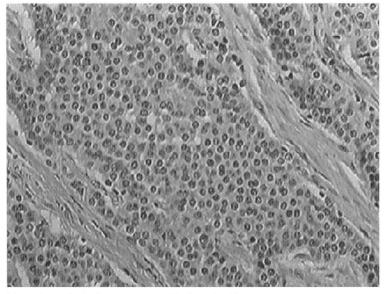

Fig. 6.7 (Plate 6) Histological appearance of ileal carcinoid.

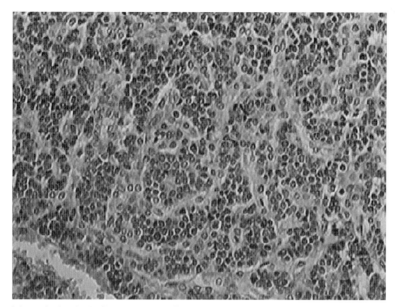

Fig. 6.8 (Plate 7) Histological appearance of hepatic carcinoid metastasis.

Compared with typical tumours, atypical carcinoids have increased nuclear atypia and greater mitotic activity, and contain areas of necrosis. Despite these histological distinctions, the biological behaviour of carcinoid tumours does not always correspond to their histological characteristics. The distinction between benign and malignant carcinoid is based upon the presence or absence of metastasis rather than histology alone. The metastatic potential of carcinoids correlates with the size and site of the primary tumour.

Medical treatment

The aim of medical treatment of patients with carcinoid disease is to control symptoms and avoid precipitating factors. It consists of symptomatic (palliative) treatment, carcinoid mediator antagonists, chemotherapy, and somatostatin analogue biotherapy.

Symptomatic (palliative) treatment

- Avoid conditions that causes anxiety
- Dietary supplementation with nicotinamide
- Treat heart failure with diuretics
- Treat wheezing by non-catecholamine bronchodilators
- Control diarrhoea

Carcinoid mediator antagonists

- 5-Hydroxytryptamine (5-HT) antagonists
  - 5-HT$_1$ and 5-HT$_2$ receptor antagonists (methysergide, cyproheptodine, ketanserin) have all been used to control diarrhoea, but usually do not decrease flushing
  - 5-HT$_3$ receptor antagonists, such as ondansetron, can control nausea and diarrhoea, and occasionally ameliorate the flushing
- A combination of histamine H$_1$ and H$_2$ receptor antagonists (diphenylhydramine, cimetidine, or ranitidine) may control flushing
- Aprotonin, a bradykinin inhibitor, can be used for flushing and intra-operative hypotension
- Codeine can be used for diarrhoea

Chemotherapy

Several systemic chemotherapeutic protocols have been evaluated. Only a third of patients with metastatic diseases had an objective response, and the effect on survival was minimal. Leucocyte interferon decreased tumour size in approximately 20% and decreased 5-HIAA excretion in about 50%.

Somatostatin analogues[9,22–27]

Somatostatin analogues have become the cornerstone of the treatment of carcinoid syndrome. They inhibit the synthesis and release of the bioactive mediators, and may block the action of the vasoactive mediators on their target organs.

Although initially described as a hypothalamic substance that inhibits growth hormone release, it is now clear that somatostatin is also present in other tissues such as the gastrointestinal tract and the pancreas, where it inhibits the release of certain gastrointestinal and pancreatic hormones. Five types of somatostatin receptor have been identified.

Carcinoid tumours are particularly rich in type 2 receptors. Somatostatin is a naturally occurring inhibitory peptide found in two forms: somatostatin-14 and somatostatin-28. It has diverse effects, including regulation of growth hormone and thyrotrophin secretion and a regulatory function in the gastrointestinal tract and pancreas. The half-life of somatostatin is 3 minutes and therefore it is not well suited for effective treatment of carcinoid episodes. Also, rebound hypersecretion of growth hormone insulin and glucagon occur after discontinuation of somatostatin infusion. The synthetic somatostatin analogues, octreotide and lanreotide, have a longer half-life (100–120 minutes), and do not exhibit rebound hypersecretion after discontinuation of therapy (Table 6.4).

Somatostatin analogues bind to somatostatin receptors on the surface of carcinoid tumour cells and inhibit the release of vasoactive substances that provoke the carcinoid syndrome. These drugs have been shown to relieve symptoms in a high proportion of patients who have carcinoid syndrome and they also frequently reduce 5-HIAA levels.

Two different versions of somatostatin analogues are currently used. Subcutaneous octreotide acetate is a short-acting formulation that is usually administered three

Table 6.4 Properties of somatostatin and octreotide

Somatostatin	Octreotide
14 amino acid peptide	8 amino acid peptide
Inhibits adenylcyclase and voltage-dependent Ca^{2+} channels	Somatostatin analogue
Short half-life (2 minutes)	Long half-life (90 minutes)
Lacks inhibitory selectivity	Selectivity enhanced
Rebound hypersecretion when discontinued	No rebound hypersecretion

times daily. In 1994, octreotide acetate long-acting release (LAR), a microencapsulated formulation, became available. The LAR form, injected once a month as an intramuscular depot, has been shown to control symptoms of carcinoid syndrome as effectively as the short-acting octreotide.

The predominant effect of somatostatin analogues is symptomatic relief. Octreotide controls symptoms, including diarrhoea and flushing, in over 50% of patients and produces a decrease of more than 50% in urinary 5-HIAA in 70% of patients. However, stabilization of tumour growth is achieved only in about 50% of the patients, with a duration ranging between 8 and 16 months, and tumour regression is rarely obtained.

Pre-operative and intra-operative somatostatin analogues are valuable for the prevention and management of carcinoid crisis during surgery, anaesthesia, chemotherapy, or stress. If indicated, catecholamines may also be administered under the umbrella of somatostatin analogues. Patients with mild to moderate symptoms should initially be treated with octreotide 100 µg subcutaneously every 8 hours. However, individual variations occur and doses as high as 3000 µg/day have been given.

Anaesthesiologists must be aware that octreotide inhibits the secretion of many hormones, including insulin and glucagon. Thus it is essential to monitor blood glucose levels intra-operatively and during the early post-operative period in order to maintain normoglycaemia.

Surgical treatment

The treatment of carcinoid syndrome is largely palliative, while the treatment of carcinoid tumour is surgical. Resection of the primary carcinoid tumour is the rule. In the presence of liver metastasis, liver resection is indicated as a curative or as a palliative treatment which improves the symptoms of the carcinoid syndrome. Liver transplant may even be indicated in some patients.[28] Surgery is also indicated for the palliative treatment of intestinal obstruction secondary to the carcinoid tumour, and for correction of valvular heart lesions in patients with severe right ventricular failure.

Resection with a curative intent is done when complete tumour clearance is possible. Where this can be achieved by complete resection of the primary tumour and hepatic metastasis, 5 year survival is around 40%. Resection of the primary should be done if the tumour is discovered incidentally during laparotomy to avoid future symptoms such as intestinal obstruction.

Palliative cyto-reduction resection is justified if medical treatment fails to control symptoms or improve the quality of life. Reduction of the tumour load by more than 90% is usually considered to be an effective modality of treatment and offers good quality of life.

Hepatic artery embolization and chemotherapy have been used to reduce tumour tissue and alleviate symptoms. Arterial occlusion by gelfoam embolization provides transient relief of symptoms in approximately 90% of patients. Its success depends on the fact that the hepatic artery supplies nearly all the blood to the tumour and less than half to the normal hepatic tissues.[29,30]

Carcinoid crisis (see also Chapter 9)

Carcinoid crisis is the result of a massive release of serotonin and other mediators, such as histamine and kallikreins. Patients at risk are those with pre-existing carcinoid syndrome and those with liver metastasis, as well as patients with carcinoid tumour whose venous blood drains directly the systemic circulation. As well as mechanical stimulation of the tumour, a carcinoid crisis can be triggered during surgery and anaesthesia by stress, tracheal intubation, inadequate analogues, hypercapnia, hypothermia, hypertension, and in general all situations associated with catecholamine release. An acute intra-operative carcinoid crisis characteristically presents with hypotension, tachycardia, flushing, diarrhoea, bronchoconstriction, acidosis, and even cardiac arrest.

Anaesthetic management[4,12,17,31–40]

Introduction

The anaesthesiologist should be aware of the features of carcinoid syndrome as the presence of an occult carcinoid tumour may become biochemically evident during non-carcinoid surgery. In this situation, a patient who has not received any pre-operative preparation may develop a catastrophic carcinoid crisis which can result in a high mortality rate similar to that observed in a non-prepared phaeochromocytoma patient.

In patients undergoing carcinoid surgery, anaesthesia and surgery can be a trigger for development of carcinoid crisis. This life-threatening complication may result in profound hypotension, paroxysmal hypertension, severe flushing, bronchoconstriction, and arrhythmia. The crisis can be triggered by stress related to pre-operative anxiety, intra-operative light anaesthesia, or post-operative pain. It can also be triggered by sympathomimetic agents or histamine-releasing drugs, since adrenergic stimulation and histamine can activate the synthesis of serotonin and enhance its release into the circulation. In addition to adrenergic and histaminergic stimuli, manipulations of the carcinoid tumour either directly or by chemotherapy and/or hepatic artery embolization can result in a serious carcinoid crisis.

Special considerations in the anaesthetic management of patients with carcinoid disease include pre-operative optimization of carcinoid syndrome control, intensified pre-operative and intra-operative blockade of serotonin release by somatostatin analogues,

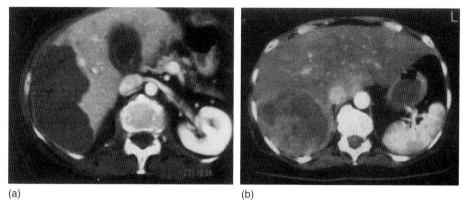

(a)   (b)

Fig. 6.9 CT scans of metastatic liver: (a) before hepatic artery embolization; (b) after embolization showing marked decrease of vascularity.

and avoidance of drugs that can stimulate the release of vasoactive substances from tumour cells.

In carcinoid patients undergoing liver resection for hepatic metastases, the patient can be prepared for surgery by gelfoam embolization of the hepatic artery in order to decrease the hepatic hypervascular lesions (Figure 6.9). The combination of pre-operative gelfoam embolization and octreotide therapy can decrease carcinoid symptoms such as flushing, diarrhoea, and bronchospasm pre-operatively. In addition, it will decrease the incidence of peri-operative carcinoid crisis, and decrease bleeding during hepatic secretion.

Catecholamines are not recommended for the treatment of hypotension and bronchospasm triggered by the carcinoid crisis, as they may paradoxically increase the hypotension. Administration of catecholamines may lead to release of kallikrein, which activates bradykinins and may aggravate the hypotension. However, octreotide administration can decrease the release of mediators by catecholamines. Thus catecholamines may be cautiously administered whenever indicated under the umbrella of octreotide. There have been no reports of carcinoid crisis triggered by catecholamines in patients who have received a somatostatin analogue.

Patients with carcinoid heart disease may be more vulnerable to the symptoms of carcinoid crisis, since the combination of severe tricuspid regurgitation, pulmonary stenosis, and right ventricular failure can limit the compensatory mechanisms, resulting in a vicious circle which further exacerbates the tricuspid regurgitation and worsens the ventricular failure. There are currently no risk factors that indicate which patients will develop intra-operative carcinoid crisis. The 5-HIAA levels and the severity of pre-operative symptoms and do not predict the development of peri-operative complications.

Somatostatin analogues are becoming the mainstay of carcinoid disease treatment. Octreotide has been successfully used for both prevention and acute management of carcinoid crisis by inhibiting release of vasoactive substances from the carcinoid tumour. In a retrospective review of pre-anaesthetic risks and outcomes of abdominal surgery for metastatic tumours, Kinney *et al.*[40] suggested that no operative complications occurred in patients who received octreotide intra-operatively.

Pre-operative preparation

Pre-operative preparation of patients with carcinoid disease is aimed at optimization of the patient for surgery by relief of carcinoid symptoms and correction of fluid and electrolyte abnormalities secondary to diarrhoea. In patients with carcinoid heart disease who have symptoms of right ventricular failure, general measures such as salt and water restriction and the use of diuretics may improve symptoms.

Combination therapy with histamine H_1 and H_2 receptor antagonists, such as diphenylhydramine and ranitidine, can inhibit flushing and other histamine-induced symptoms. Histamine release is more likely to occur with gastric carcinoids, and anti-histamines may not be needed for carcinoid tumours originating in other areas. Other drugs used for the peri-operative management of patients with carcinoid syndrome include steroids, ketanserin, and the serotonin receptor antagonists cyproheptadine and methysergide. However, the introduction of the somatostatin analogue octreotide has rendered the administration of antihistaminics and antiserotonin drugs superfluous.

Octreotide should be given 100 µg subcutaneously three times daily for 2 weeks prior to surgery, followed by 100 µg intravenously at induction of anaesthesia to reduce mediator release. Octreotide is even beneficial if administered within 24 hours prior to surgery. All usual pre-operative medications should be continued until the time of surgery. Intravenous octreotide may be slowly infused during surgery at a rate of 50–100µg/hour in order to prevent or ameliorate intra-operative carcinoid crisis. If more octreotide is required, intravenous bolus doses (25–100 µg) can be administered until the desired effect is achieved.

Pre-operative stress and anxiety can cause catecholamine release, which is a potent trigger to carcinoid mediator release. Another pre-operative consideration is the patient's need for emotional support, especially for those with gastrointestinal diseases who have had to endure the psychosocial trauma of having to face such a prospect. An anxiolytic premedication such as a benzodiazepine should be prescribed.

Anaesthetic considerations

In addition to the routine monitoring (ECG, pulse oximetry, and temperature monitoring), carcinoid patients must be monitored by invasive continuous intra-arterial blood pressure and central venous pressure monitoring to provide rapid continuous and accurate assessment of haemodynamics. Pulmonary artery catheterization and oesophageal echocardiography may also be indicated in the carcinoid cardiac patient, although the advisability of passing a pulmonary artery catheter in a patient with valvular lesions can be debated.

The anaesthesiologist should avoid anxiety, light anaesthesia, hypercapnia, hypothermia, and hypotension, all of which may release catecholamines and trigger release of carcinoid mediators. Drugs that might stimulate release of vasoactive substances from tumour cells also have to be avoided. For instance, mediator release has been reported to be triggered by administration of histamine-releasing neuromuscular relaxants (atracurium, mivacurium, D-tubocurarine), and opioids (morphine, meperidine).

Induction of anaesthesia should be smooth to avoid catecholamine release. Propofol may be suitable for induction of anaesthesia in patients with carcinoid disease, since it obtunds the pressor response to tracheal intubation and causes negligible histamine release compared with thiopental and etomidate. However, hypotension may follow propofol administration. Suxamethonium is preferably avoided for neuromuscular blockade as it may provoke histamine release and peptide release from the liver. Although pancuronium has been used safely, caution should be exercised with respect to the elevation of blood pressure secondary to its sympathomimetic effects. Rocuronium, vecuronium, and cisatracurium are better alternatives. Morphine can induce serotonin and histamine release; hence fentanyl and its analogues are the most commonly used opioid drugs. Patients with high serum serotonin concentrations are prone to delayed recovery following general anaesthesia; therefore short-acting drugs such as remifentanil, propofol, and the rapidly eliminated volatile anaesthetics such as sevoflurane are preferred.

Vigorous surgical preparation of the abdomen or manipulation of the tumour by the surgeon may exert mechanical pressure on the tumour and trigger release of vasoactive substances with resultant hypotension. The administration of octreotide prior to such manoeuvres may prevent or attenuate untoward haemodynamic responses.

The use of regional anaesthesia is controversial, as the sympathetic blockade produced by spinal or epidural anaesthesia may increase the severity of hypotension, although the enhanced post-operative pain relief may be advantageous. Close monitoring of cardiovascular parameters and the level of regional blockade are necessary.

Post-operative management

Patients with carcinoid tumours require close haemodynamic monitoring in the post-operative period as secretion of vasoactive substances from the residual tumour or metastasis can occur. Thus, all pre-operative drug therapy including octreotide should be continued into the post-operative period, and the patient should be weaned slowly over the first post-operative week. Effective post-operative analgesia with non-histamine-releasing opioids is vital to ameliorate emotional and physical stress that may trigger substance release from the carcinoid tumour. Post-operative regional analgesia with opioids may be used. Ondansetron, a serotonin antagonist, is be the first choice as an anti-emetic agent.

Typical case presentation[12]

The following case report reviews the anaesthesia management of a patient with a carcinoid tumour of the ileum associated with metastases to the liver. The patient was a 50-year-old married female, known to be hypothyroid and on Eltroxin therapy, who was

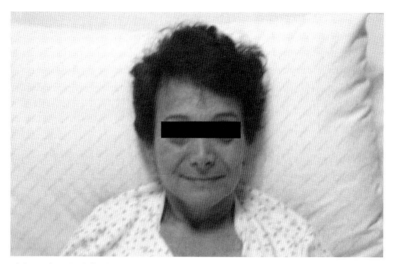

Fig. 6.10 (Plate 8) Typical flushed appearance of a patient experiencing carcinoid symptoms. The thin lined appearance is indicative of weight loss.

having cardiac arrhythmias as diagnosed by Holter monitoring. Two years previously, the patient had started to suffer from hot flushes and facial telangiectasis (Figure 6.10), which were attributed to the menopause and treated by hormone replacement therapy, but to no avail. Ten months prior to admission to the American University of Beirut Medical Centre (AUBMC), the patient started to have severe voluminous diarrhoea (six to seven times daily), that was watery, non-bloody, non-mucoid, and occasionally associated with nausea, vomiting, and intermittent right upper quadrant pain. The patient's body weight decreased by 10 kg in 1 year, despite there being no history of diet or exercise changes.

Physical examination, chest X-ray, ECG, laboratory tests, stool study, colonoscopy, and gastrin levels were all normal. However, 24-hour urine analysis showed a significant elevation of 5-HIAA (56.1 mg, normal range 2–8 mg). The symptomatology, facial telangiectasis, voluminous diarrhoea, and the increase in 5-HIAA in the urine suggested the diagnosis of carcinoid syndrome. A CT scan of the abdomen showed multiple heterogeneous hypervascular lesions in the liver, the largest of which was 8 × 7 cm, and 1 × 1 cm lesion in the pancreas.

The patient was admitted to AUBMC, and was scheduled for partial hepatectomy and pancreatic exploration. Pre-operatively, she was prepared for surgery by gelfoam embolization of the hypervascular hepatic lesion in segment 5 of the liver. A repeat CT scan 1 month later showed a marked decrease in the vascularity of the previous liver lesions except for that seen in segment 2, and one mass showed central necrosis with linear areas of free air. The patient was discharged home on octreotide (50 µg three times daily). Following gelfoam embolization and octreotide therapy, flushing decreased, the diarrhoea stopped, and electrolytes, blood pressure (130/80 mmHg), and heart rate

(78 beats/min) were normal. The patient was admitted one month later for open abdominal exploration, right hepatectomy, and left partial hepatectomy.

Anaesthesia management

The patient was premedicated 1 hour before surgery with 10 mg of diazepam orally. Standard intra-operative monitoring techniques (ECG, non-invasive blood pressure, and pulse oximetry) were applied pre-operatively. Two intravenous large-bore cannulas (18 gauge and 16 gauge), an arterial line, and a central venous line were inserted via the internal jugular approach. After 3 minutes of pre-oxygenation with 100% oxygen, anaesthesia was induced with midazolam 2 mg, propofol 120 mg, fentanyl 150 µg, lidocaine 100 mg, and cisatracurium 10 mg. Endotracheal intubation did not provoke any bronchospasm or haemodynamic changes. Anaesthesia was maintained with isoflurane in oxygen–air mixture, cisatracurium 6 mg/hour, and fentanyl 50 µg/ hour. After anaesthetic induction, a Foley catheter was inserted. Temperature and end-tidal capnography ($ETco_2$) monitoring were added.

Throughout surgery, which lasted for 7 hours, oxygen saturation (Spo_2) was maintained at 99%, and $ETco_2$ was maintained at 29–30 mmHg (4 kPa). Central venous pressure (CVP) was maintained at 5–6 cm H_2O to reduce blood loss. During liver resection, systolic blood pressure was maintained between 100 and 120 mmHg and heart rate at 70–80 beats/minute. Total blood loss was around two units and the patient received two units of packed red blood cells, 4 L of lactated Ringer's solution, 1 L of Haemaccel®, and two units of fresh frozen plasma. Hourly urine output was maintained between 100 and 300 mL/hour.

Surgical management

The patient had a large hepatic tumour with a neighbouring smaller one involving segments 5, 6, 7, and 8, in addition to two other nodules involving segments 2 and 3 as shown by the triphasic CT scan. Intra-operative ultrasound confirmed the tumours described above with no additions. A bilateral subcostal incision was used, and unexpectedly the primary tumour was found in the terminal ileum and was resected with small bowel end-to-end anastomosis; a right hepatectomy was performed following inflow control to segments 5, 6, 7, and 8 by extra-hepatic dissection. Outflow control was achieved by securing proximal control around the right hepatic vein. The liver parenchyma was mobilized from the retro-hepatic inferior vena cava. The liver tissue was divided using a cavitron ultrasonic surgical aspirator (CUSA) and an argon beam coagulator. The two lesions in segments 2 and 3 were excised. Post-operative pathology confirmed the diagnosis of primary carcinoid tumour in the ileum with liver metastasis.

At the end of the operation, the patient's temperature was 35.4°C, and she was transferred intubated to the recovery room. Post-operatively, she developed a few episodes of hypoglycaemia and transient mental confusion. Three months later, the patient presented to follow-up, symptom free.

Key clinical management points

Diagnosis

◆ Suspect the diagnosis of carcinoid syndrome by the classic triad of episodic facial flushing, diarrhoea, and cardiac arrhythmia

Diagnostic tests

◆ Urinary 5-hydroxy-indole acetic acid

◆ Octreotide scan

Pre-operative preparation

◆ Somatostatin analogues are becoming the main drug for pre-operative preparation

◆ Octreotide should be given 100 µg subcutaneously three times daily for 2 weeks prior to surgery, followed by 100 µg intravenously at induction of anaesthesia

◆ Others

• Histamine H_1 and H_2 receptor antagonists

• Serotonin receptor antagonists

• Hepatic artery gelfoam embolization to decrease the excessive hepatic secretions

Anaesthetic management

◆ Adequate sedation

◆ Monitoring

• Standard anaesthetic monitoring

• Direct arterial pressure monitoring

• Central venous pressure

• Cardiac carcinoid

▪ Pulmonary artery catheterization

▪ Transoesophageal echocardiography

Anaesthetic technique

◆ Propofol for induction of anaesthesia

◆ Vecuronium, rocuronium, or cisatracurium for muscle relaxation

◆ Fentanyl or remifentanil for analgesia

◆ Volatiles: isoflurane or sevoflurane

Key clinical management points (continued)

Carcinoid crisis (flushing, severe hypotension, and arrhythmia)

- ◆ Can be triggered by:
  - Tumour manipulations, organic surgical preparation of the abdomen
  - Sympathomimetic drugs or stimuli
  - Histamine-releasing drugs
  - Stress, pre-operative anxiety
  - Intra-operative light anaesthesia
- ◆ Management of carcinoid crisis
  - Avoid carcinoid triggering factors or drugs
  - Intravenous octreotide
    - Bolus100 µg
    - Intravenous infusion 50–100 µg/hour, supplemented by intravenous bolus doses (25–100 µg) until control of the crisis is achieved

Post-operative care

- ◆ High-care unit admission
- ◆ Close haemodynamic monitoring
- ◆ Maintain octreotide infusion
- ◆ Provide adequate post-operative analgesia

Follow-up

The possibility of residual primary tumour or liver metastasis dictates follow-up by looking for carcinoid syndrome and monitoring urinary 5-HIAA volumes.

References

1. Lubarsch O (1888). Über den primaren Krebs des ileum, nebst Bemerkungen über das gleichzeitige Vorkommen von Krebs und Tuberkolose. *Virchows Archiv für pathologische Anatomie und Physiologie und für klinische Medizin*, **111**, 280–317.

2. Oberndorfer S (1907). Karzinoide: tumoren des dünndarms. *Frankfurter Zeitschrift für Pathologie*, 1, 425–9.

3. Shebani KO, Souba WW, Finkelstein DM, *et al.* (1999). Prognosis and survival in patients with gastrointestinal tract carcinoid tumors. *Annals of Surgery*, 229, 815–21.

4. Dierdorf SF (2003). Carcinoid tumor and carcinoid syndrome. *Current Opinion in Anaesthesiology*, 16, 343–7.

5. Williams ED, Sandler M (1963). The classification of carcinoid tumours. *Lancet*, i, 238–9.

6. de Vries H, Verschueren RC, Willemse PH, Kema IP, de Vries EG (2002). Diagnostic, surgical and medical aspect of the midgut carcinoids. *Cancer Treatment Reviews*, 28, 11–25.

7. Oberg K (2002). Carcinoid tumors: molecular genetics, tumor biology, and update of diagnosis and treatment. *Current Opinion in Oncology*, 14, 38–45.

8. Pernow B, Waldenstrom J (1954). Paroxysmal flushing and other symptoms caused by 5-hydroxytryptamine and histamine in patients with malignant tumours. *Lancet*, 267, 951.

9. Vinik AI, Thompson N, Eckhauser F, Moattari AR (1989). Clinical features of carcinoid syndrome and the use of somatostatin analogue in its management. *Acta Oncologica*, 28, 389–402.

10. Modlin IM, Sandor A (1997). An analysis of 8305 cases of carcinoid tumors. *Cancer*, 79, 813–29.

11. Kulke MH, Mayer RJ (1999). Carcinoid tumors. *New England Journal of Medicine*, **340**, .858–68

12. Jabbour-Khoury S, Dabbous A, al Jazzar M, *et al.* (2003). Anesthetic management of a patient having a carcinoid syndrome. *Middle East Journal of Anesthesiology*, **17**, 435–47.

13. Bernheim AM, Connolly HM, Hobday TJ, Abel MD, Pellikka PA (2005). Carcinoid heart disease. *Progress in Cardiovascular Diseases*, **49**, 439–51.

14. Botero M, Fuchs R, Paulus DA, Lind DS (2002). Carcinoid heart disease: a case report and literature review. *Journal of Clinical Anesthesiology*, **14**, 57–63.

15. Connolly HM, Pellikka PA (2006). Carcinoid heart disease. *Current Cardiology Reports*, **8**, 96–101.

16. Fox DJ, Khattar RS (2004). Carcinoid heart disease: presentation, diagnosis, and management. *Heart*, **90**, 1224–8.

17. Weingarten TN, Abel MD, Connolly HM, Schroeder DR, Schaff HV (2007). Intraoperative management of patients with carcinoid heart disease having valvular surgery: a review of one hundred consecutive cases. *Anasthesia and Analgesia*, **105**, 1192–9.

18. Chughtai TS, Morin JE, Sheiner NM, Wilson JA, Mulder DS (1997). Bronchial carcinoid: twenty years' experience defines a selective surgical approach. *Surgery*, **122**, 801–8.

19. Fischer S, Kruger M, McRae K, Merchant N, Tsao MS, Keshavjee S (2001). Giant-bronchial carcinoid tumors: a multidisciplinary approach. *Annals of Thoracic Surgery*, **71**, 386–93.

20. Filosso PL, Rena O, Donati G, *et al.* (2002). Bronchial carcinoid tumors: surgical management and long-term outcome. *Journal of Thoracic and Cardiovascular Surgery*, **123**, 303–9.

21. Roggo A, Wood WC, Ottinger LW (1993). Carcinoid tumors of the appendix. *Annals of Surgery*, **217**, 385–90.

22. Roy RC, Carter RF, Wright PD (1987). Somatostatin, anaesthesia, and the carcinoid syndrome. Peri-operative administration of a somatostatin analogue to suppress carcinoid tumour activity. *Anaesthesia*, **42**, 627–32.

23. Parris WC, Oates JA, Kambam J, Shmerling R, Sawyers JF (1988). Pre-treatment with somatostatin in the anaesthetic management of a patient with carcinoid syndrome. *Canadian Journal of Anaesthesia*, **35**, 413–16.

24. Kvols LK (1994). Metastatic carcinoid tumors and the malignant carcinoid syndrome. *Annals of the New York Academy of Science*, **733**, 464–70.

25. Lamberts SW, van der Lely AJ, de Herder WW, Hofland LJ (1996). Octreotide. *New England Journal of Medicine*, **334**, 246–54.

26. Arnold R, Simon B, Wied M (2000). Treatment of neuroendocrine GEP tumours with somatostatin analogues: a review. *Digestion*, **62** (Suppl), 184–91.

27. de Herder WW, Lamberts SW (2002). Somatostatin and somatostatin analogues: diagnostic and therapeutic uses. *Current Opinion in Oncology*, **14**, 53–7.

28. Claure RE, Drover DD, Haddow GR, Esquivel CO, Angst MS (2000). Orthotopic liver transplantation for carcinoid tumour metastatic to the liver: anesthetic management. *Canadian Journal of Anaesthesia*, **47**, 334–7.

29. Ruszniewski P, Rougier P, Roche A, *et al.* (1993). Hepatic arterial chemoembolization in patients with liver metastases of endocrine tumors: a prospective phase II study in 24 patients. *Cancer*, **71**, 2624–30.

30. Eriksson BK, Larsson EG, Skogseid BM, Lofberg AM, Lorelius LE, Oberg KE (1998). Liver embolizations of patients with malignant neuroendocrine gastrointestinal tumors. *Cancer*, **83**, 2293–301.

31. Banzali FM, Jr., Tiwari AK, Frantz R, D'Attellis N (2007). Valvular heart disease caused by carcinoid syndrome: emphasis on the use of intraoperative transesophageal echocardiography. *Journal of Cardiothoracic and Vascular Anesthesia*, **21**, 855–7.

32. Balestrero LM, Beaver CR, Rigas JR (2000). Hypertensive crisis following meperidine administration and chemoembolization of a carcinoid tumor. *Archives of Internal Medicine*, **160**, 2394–5.

33. Farling PA, Durairaju AK (2004). Remifentanil and anaesthesia for carcinoid syndrome. British Journal of Anaesthesia, **92**, 893–5.

34. Mason RA, Steane PA (1976). Carcinoid syndrome: its relevance to the anaesthetist. *Anaesthesia*, **31**, 228–42.

35. Vaughan DJ, Brunner MD (1997). Anesthesia for patients with carcinoid syndrome. *International Anesthesiology Clinics*, **35**, 129–42.

36. Propst JW, Siegel LC, Stover EP (1994). Anesthetic considerations for valve replacement surgery in a patient with carcinoid syndrome. *Journal of Cardiothoracic and Vascular Anesthesia*, **8**, 209–12.

37. Marsh HM, Martin JK, Jr., Kvols LK, *et al.* (1987). Carcinoid crisis during anesthesia: successful treatment with a somatostatin analogue. *Anesthesiology*, **66**, 89–91.

38. Neustein SM, Cohen E (1995). Anesthesia for aortic and mitral valve replacement in a patient with carcinoid heart disease. *Anesthesiology*, **82**, 1067–70.

39. Quinlivan JK, Roberts WA (1994). Intraoperative octreotide for refractory carcinoid-induced bronchospasm. *Anasthesia and Analgesia*, **78**, 400–2.

40. Kinney MA, Warner ME, Nagorney DM, *et al.* (2001). Perianaesthetic risks and outcomes of abdominal surgery for metastatic carcinoid tumours. *British Journal of Anaesthesia*, **87**, 447–52.

Chapter 7

Adrenal cortex

WJ Russell and MFM James

A normal person has two adrenal glands with a total weight of about 10–20 g sited immediately superior to each kidney. Corticosteroid production occurs in the more superficial two-thirds of these glands. The outer 10–15%, the zona glomerulosa, produces aldosterone, and deep to this the zona fasciculata manufactures cortisol[1] while the deepest layer of the cortex, the zona reticularis, produces the androgens (Figure 7.1). The adrenal medulla manufactures, stores, and releases catecholamines (see Chapter 8). The main source of production of the steroid hormones is cholesterol, which is obtained mainly from the diet; the remainder is synthesized from acetate. About 80% of the cholesterol required for steroid synthesis is captured from the blood by low-density lipoprotein receptors and the remaining 20% is synthesized from acetate within the adrenal cells. The core of cholesterol and all steroid hormones is the cyclopentanoperhydrophenanthrine nucleus (Figure 7.2) which is modified through the cytochrome P450 enzymes to make progesterone and finally corticosterone, which is hydroxylated to either aldosterone or cortisol (Figure 7.3).

The steroid hormones have wide-ranging physiological effects. The androgens exert masculinizing effects. Testosterone is the most active form of androgen, but only 20% of total androgen activity depends on the adrenal-derived hormones. Abnormalities of these hormones may produce a number of clinical syndromes, including pseudohermaphroditism, but these are generally of little importance in anaesthetic practice and will not be considered further.

Aldosterone is the principal hormone regulating sodium and potassium balance. It binds to the type I mineralocorticoid receptor located in the distal cortical collecting principal cells of the renal tubule to increase the number of 'open' sodium channels, resulting in increased reabsorption of sodium. The resultant reabsorption of sodium produces a negative electrical gradient in the tubular lumen, resulting in potassium and hydrogen ion secretion to maintain electrical neutrality. Unlike the other adrenal hormones, aldosterone is only minimally regulated by pituitary function, although adrenocorticotrophic hormone (ACTH) exerts a small effect on aldosterone release. Regulation of aldosterone release occurs primarily through the renin–angiotensin mechanism. Renin is released from the juxtaglomerular apparatus of the renal tubule in response to a variety of stimuli, including a drop in plasma sodium concentration, an increase in plasma potassium concentration, a drop in arterial pressure, hypovolaemia, constriction of the renal arteries, and the level of sympathetic activity. The sensory mechanism is probably

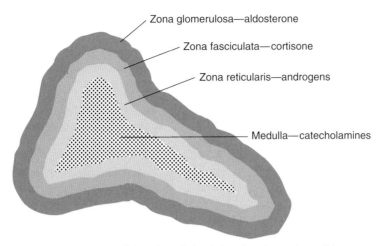

Fig. 7.1 Diagrammatic structure of the adrenal gland showing the regions of hormone formation.

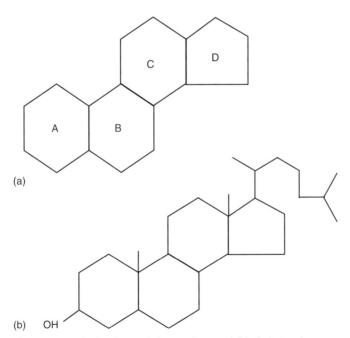

Fig. 7.2 (a) Cyclopentanoperhydrophenanthrine nucleus and (b) cholesterol.

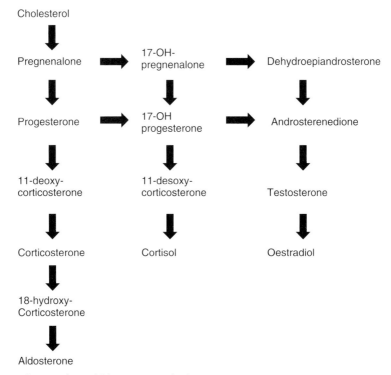

Cholesterol

Pregnenalone → 17-OH-pregnenalone → Dehydroepiandrosterone

Progesterone → 17-OH progesterone → Androsterenedione

11-deoxy-corticosterone   11-desoxy-corticosterone   Testosterone

Corticosterone   Cortisol   Oestradiol

18-hydroxy-Corticosterone

Aldosterone

Fig. 7.3 Pathways of steroid hormone synthesis.

driven by the rate of transport of chloride ions, or possibly sodium ions, across the portion of the distal tubule related to the macula densa. Renin cleaves the decapeptide angiotensin I from a much larger glycoprotein known as angiotensinogen. Angiotensin-converting enzyme, largely in the lung but also found elsewhere in the body, converts angiotensin I to the octapeptide angiotensin II. Angiotensin II is one of the most potent vasoconstrictors known, but has a half life of only 1–2 minutes; it acts directly on the adrenal cortex to increase the release of aldosterone (Figure 7.4). A rise in plasma potassium concentration also directly stimulates the release of aldosterone from the adrenal cortex.

The glucocorticoids exert wide-ranging physiological effects and are critical to the hormonal response to stress (see Chapter 1). In anabolic phases, glucocorticoids increase amino acid absorption, stimulate protein synthesis, and have a moderate stimulant effect on fat synthesis. In catabolic conditions, the glucocorticoids drive gluconeogenesis through proteolysis and the release, deamination, and conversion of amino acids to new sugars. They also inhibit glucose uptake, stimulate lactate release in metabolism, and increase lipolysis. They are critical in the regulation of the stress response (see Chapter 1), limiting the actions of cytokines and other inflammatory mediators, moderating the inflammatory process. The interaction of glucocorticoids and catecholamines is also

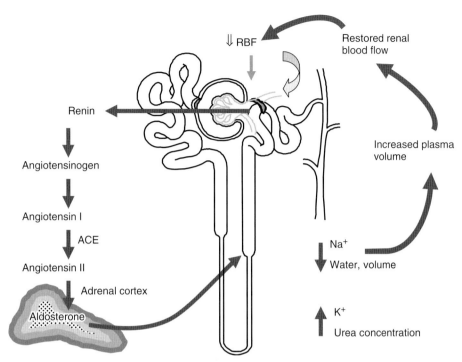

Fig. 7.4 Regulation of aldosterone release through the renin–angiotensin mechanism. A fall in renal perfusion pressure (and other related stimuli) activates the release of renin, which in turn releases angiotensin I. Angiotensin-converting enzyme converts angiotensin I to angiotensin II and stimulates the release of aldosterone from the adrenal cortex. Restoration of renal blood flow consequent on reabsorption of sodium and water completes a feedback inhibitory loop. RBF, renal blood flow, ACE, angiotensin converting enzyme.

important as glucocorticoids are required for the synthesis of adrenaline (see Chapter 8) and provide important permissive actions that are necessary for the effectiveness of catecholamines in inotropic, vasopressor, and bronchodilatory roles.

Cortisol levels are controlled through corticotrophin-releasing hormone (CRH) from the hypothalamus and this in turn regulates the output of ACTH from the anterior pituitary gland. Ultimately, control of normal corticosterone production depends on negative feedback through the hypothalamic–pituitary–adrenal (HPA) axis (Figure 7.5). Cortisol has a negative feedback effect on CRH from the hypothalamus and ACTH from the pituitary.[2] The amount of feedback control through the CRH from the hypothalamus may be less than that produced by the ACTH from the anterior pituitary.

The main negative feedback is from cortisol itself. This control of cortisol is influenced by many factors. In the normal person there is a diurnal fluctuation with the predominant release of pulses of ACTH occurring in the early morning before awakening. However, under stress of severe illness such as septicaemia, burns, trauma, or surgery, the diurnal fluctuation is lost and cortisol production may increase as much as sixfold.[3] In addition, the levels of free cortisol may rise, as normally about 80% is reversibly bound

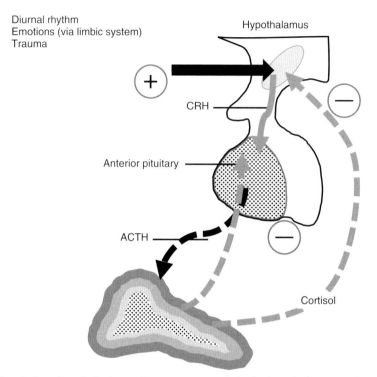

Diurnal rhythm
Emotions (via limbic system)
Trauma

Hypothalamus

CRH

Anterior pituitary

ACTH

Cortisol

Fig. 7.5 Regulation of cortisol release. Neurosecretory cells in the hypothalamus produce corticotrophin-releasing hormone (CRH) in response to a variety of stimuli. CRH is carried to the anterior pituitary gland through a portal capillary system. This stimulates the release of adrenocorticotrophic hormone (ACTH) which stimulates the release of cortisol from the adrenal gland. Cortisol exerts a negative feedback on both the hypothalamus and the anterior pituitary, regulating further hormone release.

to the globulin transcortin and a small amount (about 10%) is bound to albumin. However, the transcortin levels do not rise with stress, and may even fall, so that the free cortisol rises markedly.[4]

Diseases of the adrenal cortex and implications for anaesthesia

Given the central role of adrenal cortical hormones in physiology, and particularly in the stress response, it is not surprising that the implications of adrenal cortical disease for anaesthetic practice are considerable.

Underproduction

Failure of the adrenal glands to produce appropriate levels of hormones may be due to a failure of pituitary drive, suppression of the HPA axis, or damage to the adrenal gland itself.

Addison's disease

Thomas Addison lived from 1793 to 1860. He graduated as a Doctor of Medicine at Edinburgh University in 1812 and then moved to London. In 1817 he began his association with Guy's Hospital which lasted until his retirement in 1860. He died a few months later from a fall, probably suicide. Addison recognized a debilitating disease associated with the supra-renal capsules which had a fatal outcome. He identified the disease with anaemia, languor, debility, and a peculiar change of skin colour. He described 11 cases in his publication *On the constitutional and local effects of disease of the supra-renal capsules*. In 10 of these cases, the adrenal damage was confirmed at post mortem.[5]

Cortisol deficiency

In addition to adrenal gland failure, cortisol deficiency can also occur as a failure of stimulation by the hypothalamus or the pituitary. Hypothalamic damage is uncommon, but tumours can occur in this area. Direct trauma is unlikely because the hypothalamus is a deeply placed structure, but any damage may impede release of corticotrophic hormone.

Pituitary tumours are also uncommon but will disrupt the production of ACTH. This can also occur if there is damage to the pituitary, for example by development of cysts,[6] and will also occur with necrosis or bleeding in the pituitary such as occurs in postpartum Sheehan's syndrome and may occur with meningococcal infections, creating the Waterhouse–Friderichsen syndrome.[7]

Patients who are on long-term glucocorticoids may have a suppressed ACTH feedback. Under stress, their increased requirement may not be met and a relative deficiency may arise.[8] The likelihood of HPA axis suppression depends on the dose and duration of steroid therapy. Patients receiving standard physiological levels of steroid supplementation of less than 5 mg prednisone or the equivalent are very unlikely to have any significant risk of HPA suppression. Approximate physiological equivalents of various steroids are given in Table 7.1. Doses between this level and 20 mg prednisone daily may be associated with HPA suppression if treatment is continued daily for more than 4 weeks. Alternate-day regimens are much less likely to cause HPA suppression and are now widely used

Table 7.1 Approximate equivalence between different steroid preparations, together with their relative glucocorticoid and mineralocorticoid actions

Steroid	Glucocorticoid effect	Mineralocorticoid effect	Half-life (hours)	Routes
Hydrocortisone	1	1	6–8	PO, IV, IM
Prednisone	4	0.1–0.2	18–36	PO
Methylprednisolone	5	0.1–0.2	18–36	IV
Dexamethasone	30	< 0.1	36–54	PO, IV
Fludrocortisone	0	20	18–36	PO

PO, oral; IV, intravenous; IM, intramuscular.

where long-term steroid therapy is envisaged, particularly in children. There is a definite risk of HPA suppression if steroid therapy of >20 mg prednisone or equivalent is continued daily for longer than 5 days.[9] If therapy at these levels is continued for 1 month, HPA suppression is likely to last for 6–12 months after cessation of therapy.[10] Recovery from HPA suppression is slow, but pituitary function normalizes first with the secretion of ACTH returning to normal within a few weeks. However, adrenocortical function recovers much more slowly and is responsible for the majority of their delayed recovery.

Patients who are on substantial doses (e.g. 400 mg or more of hydrocortisone or equivalent daily) are well covered and stress is not likely to cause a relative deficiency.

Direct damage to the adrenal glands may result in primary adrenal insufficiency and cause cortisol deficiency. However, this requires damage to both adrenals as the hypothalamic feedback of CRH and the anterior pituitary feedback of ACTH will normally adjust to the loss of a single adrenal gland. Such loss of function may arise because of damage to the adrenals from, for example, infection, classically tuberculosis, amyloid disease, secondary carcinoma, or infarction. HIV infection is emerging as an important cause of primary adrenal insufficiency, and up to 30% of patients with advanced HIV will exhibit some degree of adrenal cortical failure.[11] Surgical bilateral adrenalectomy will also lead to adrenocortical failure and will require life-long supplementation of both glucocorticoids and mineralocorticoid. Patients with primary adrenal insufficiency may have aldosterone deficiency, complicating the failure of cortisol production.

Management during anaesthesia

Clinical suspicion of adrenal suppression may be raised by either a history of high-dose steroid intake in the previous 6–12 months or the presentation of findings consistent with adrenal insufficiency, such as hyponatraemia, hyperkalaemia, hypotension, and eosinophilia. Patients who are suspected of having a deficient response can be tested with intravenous cosyntropin, a synthetic form of ACTH (also known as short ACTH). In this test, exogenous glucocorticoids are withheld for 24 hours. Baseline sampling of plasma cortisol is followed by intravenous or intramuscular administration of 250 µg cosyntropin. A normal response is a cortisol rise of 18–35µg/L within 60 minutes, although there is some debate on this.[3,9] Since the hypothalamic and pituitary components of the HPA pathway recover early, an adequate response to cosyntropin indicates that the response to surgical stress is likely to be normal. An extensive review of the need for peri-operative steroid supplementation and methods of assessing the patient's stress response was reported in 1998.[12]

The expectation is that there will be a rise in cortisol and aldosterone levels during anaesthesia and surgery. Clinically, the absence of a steroid response may be experienced as hypotension, a diminished response to vasopressors, and a low cardiac output. This may be exacerbated by hyperkalaemia. A guideline to suitable replacement for adults during the post-operative phase, if a diminished or absent adrenocortical response is found, is given in Table 7.2.

Table 7.2 Guidelines for peri-operative supplementation in patients currently taking glucocorticoids or at risk of HPA suppression

Degree of surgical stress	Type of surgery	Glucocorticoid dose
Minor	Procedure under local anaesthesia and procedures lasting <1 hour	Hydrocortisone 25 mg or equivalent
Moderate	Peripheral vascular surgery, joint replacement, cholecystectomy	Hydrocortisone 50–75 mg or equivalent *or* Continue usual steroid dose if equivalent supplemented by 50 mg hydrocortisone on induction
Major	Cardiopulmonary bypass, abdominal aortic aneurysm repair, thoracic surgery etc.	Hydrocortisone 50 mg 8 hourly from induction for 48–72 hours Ensure that at least the usual steroid dose is administered

Doses should be tapered rapidly but never to below the baseline steroid requirement in patients on current therapy. If steroid provision is longer than 48 hours, consider switching to a steroid with a lower mineralocorticoid activity such as methylprednisolone.[9]

Patients who are Addisonian or have suppression because of regular steroid medication may be at risk if they develop an acute illness or severe trauma which would normally induce an increased level of cortisol. Failure to respond with a sufficient rise can be lethal, and it is essential to identify the suppression and provide the increased cortisol support.[13] The management of an Addisonian crisis is discussed in detail in Chapter 9.

Pharmaceutical adrenal suppression

In 1984, Watt and Ledingham[14] reported a retrospective review of 428 patients in intensive care. The mortality fluctuated between 19% and 29% in the 12 years from 1969 to 1980, but rose to 47% in the following 2 years without a change in the average injury severity score. They identified that over the 4 years from 1979 to 1982, there were 50 patients who were given morphine with or without benzodiazepine as analgesia/sedation and had a mortality of 28%, whereas the 27 patients given morphine and etomidate sedation had a mortality of 77%, with similar injury severity scores in both groups. They hypothesized that this was caused by the inhibition of mitochondrial hydroxylation caused by etomidate. This is now an accepted fact, and indeed etimodate has been used as the primary suppression drug in the acute phase of Cushing's disease.[15] Despite the attractiveness of the cardiostability offered by etomidate, this agent should be avoided in the population of patients who have any degree of HPA suppression or adrenal dysfunction.[10] The recent development of methoxycarbonyl-etomidate, an esther-containing form of the drug which is rapidly metabolized and does not produce prolonged adrenocortical suppression after bolus administration, may resolve this issue, but this agent is still at an early stage of development. Animal studies so far are promising.[16]

Overproduction

Over production of corticosteroids can be caused by a tumour in the adrenal cortex or from uncontrolled stimulation by corticotrophin. However, probably the most common cause of 'overproduction' is when a patient is given high-dose steroids for other diseases such as rheumatoid arthritis. The high level of corticosteroid is very likely to create a diabetic tendency, as well as muscle weakness and susceptibility to infection. The change in appearance to a 'moon face' is well recognized, but has not usually been associated with problems in ventilation or intubation. However, increased neck size secondary to the facial changes may increase the risk of difficulty in intubation.[17]

Cushing's disease/syndrome

The overproduction of corticosteroid is the characteristic of Cushing's disease which occurs with basophilic adenoma of the pituitary. It is ironic that Cushing, who was a neurosurgeon, never operated on a patient with this problem. In the 1930s these patients were treated by radiotherapy, not open surgery. Cushing saw his first tumour when one of his patients died in 1935, and at his request the family allowed an autopsy which found a well-circumscribed basophilic adenoma.[18]

The term Cushing's syndrome should be restricted to those patients in whom there is overproduction of corticosteroid from adrenal tumours or aberrant neoplasms, or where the syndrome has been created by continued administration of a high quantity of corticosteroid.

A hyperglycaemic and hypertensive patient is no novelty for the anaesthetist. These two aspects of excess corticosteroid tend to dominate, but electrolyte abnormalities, acid–base disturbances, and fluid excess may also be present and require pre-operative treatment with the aldosterone antagonist spironolactone.

In addition to the biochemical abnormalities, these patients may also display thin fragile skin, osteoporosis (which may render them liable to pathological fractures), and immunocompromise. Part of the peri-operative care of these patients must include careful attention to positioning to avoid the risk of fracture, great care in the placement of adhesive dressings to avoid skin damage, and scrupulous attention to aseptic techniques, particularly if neuraxial blockade or central venous cannulation is contemplated. If adrenalectomy is to be performed laparoscopically, the anaesthetist must be aware of the risk of diaphragmatic injury and the possibility of tension pneumothorax. Careful haemodynamic monitoring is appropriate, and consideration should be given to the use of dynamic measures of plasma volume expansion, such as stroke volume variation or corrected flow time, to allow careful and accurate maintenance of circulating volumes, and this should be continued into the early post-operative period. After tumour removal, steroid replacement should initially be given at a dose of about 300 mg daily for a 70 kg adult, in three or four divided doses, and reduced to 100 mg over the following 2 days. The exact initial dose and decrement are widely debated and there are few data to support any specific recommendation. Where bilateral adrenal removal is performed, patients will need life-long cortisol support and will also need mineralocorticoid supplementation, usually administered as oral fludrocortisone in a dosage range of 0.05–0.1 mg/day (range, 0.1 mg three times weekly to 0.2 mg/day).

Conn's syndrome

This was first described by Professor J.W. Conn of Michigan in his Presidential Address to the Central Society for Clinical Research in 1954 and subsequently published in 1955.[19] The excessive production of aldosterone causes hypertension, with hypokalaemia. In some of these patients there is a genetic tendency to develop hyperaldosteronism.[20] Conn's syndrome is usually the result of a single adrenal adenoma, and adrenalectomy is a highly effective treatment.

These patients often suffer from muscular weakness and may have cardiac dysfunction secondary to the hypertension. The chronic sodium retention usually results in hypervolaemia. Consideration may be given to the use of spironolactone in a daily dosage of 100–400 mg to antagonize the excessive aldosterone, but this is seldom sufficient on its own to control the hypertension associated with this condition and additional antihypertensive agents are frequently required. Pre-operative replacement of potassium and magnesium is usually indicated. Apart from the risk of excessive bleeding and pleural tearing with an adrenalectomy, the anaesthetic management of these cases is unremarkable.[21] Hyperventilation should be avoided, as respiratory alkalosis may worsen the hypokalaemia. Direct arterial pressure monitoring and volume monitoring appear to be indicated, as for adrenalectomy for Cushing's syndrome.

Summary

Deficiencies of corticosteroids are not generally an anaesthetic problem provided that the condition is recognized and appropriately treated before surgery. Tumours stimulating the release of corticosteroids or secreting cortisol or aldosterone are not associated with unstable anaesthesia.

Key clinical management points

Adrenal cortical insufficiency (Addison's disease, pituitary ACTH failure, iatrogenic HPA suppression)

Diagnosis

- Clinical suspicion.
  - The presence of unexplained nausea, vomiting, hypotension, orthostasis, change in mental status, hyponatraemia, or hyperkalaemia warrant investigation
  - History of steroid therapy
    - Less than 5 mg prednisone or equivalent—HPA suppression unlikely
    - 5–20 mg prednisone or equivalent—HPA suppression possible if daily dose for more than 4 weeks; less likely with alternate daily dosing
    - More than 20 mg prednisone or equivalent for more than 5 days—HPA suppression likely
      - Recovery within 3 months if therapy is less than 1 month
      - Recovery 6–12 months if therapy is more than 1 month

Diagnostic tests: (where required)

- Random plasma cortisol
- Short ACTH (cosyntropin) test

Pre-operative preparation

- Ensure adequate steroid cover (with fludrocortisone if necessary for adrenal failure)
- Continue standard steroid cover if currently receiving treatment

Anaesthetic management

Sustain normal steroid cover

- Minor surgery
  - If not currently receiving steroids, 25 mg hydrocortisone or equivalent on induction
- Moderate surgery
  - Hydrocortisone 50–75 mg on induction of anaesthesia
- Major surgery:
  - Hydrocortisone 50 mg 8 hourly from induction for 48–72 hours
  - Taper back to previous dosage rapidly
  - If high dose is required for more than 48 hours, consider steroid with low mineralocorticoid activity (e.g. methylprednisolone) in equivalent doses

Key clinical management points (continued)

Post-operative care

◆ Ensure re-establishment of pre-operative level of steroid therapy following surgery

Steroid hormone excess

Diagnosis

◆ Clinical suspicion
  • Plasma cortisol, ACTH, or aldosterone as appropriate
◆ Biochemical profile
  • Glycaemic control, sodium and potassium concentrations

Pre-operative preparation

◆ Correct biochemical profile
◆ Antihypertensive medication
◆ Spironolactone for Conn's syndrome

Anaesthetic management

◆ Cushing's syndrome/disease
  • Care to avoid physical injury and infection
  • Control blood sugar appropriately
  • Avoid hyperventilation
  • Careful fluid balance and volume monitoring
  • Be aware of pneumothorax risk
  • For bilateral adrenalectomy:
    ▪ Hydrocortisone 50 mg 8 hourly from gland removal for 48–72 hours
    ▪ Fludrocortisone (may be started later)
◆ Conn's syndrome
  • Control hypertension appropriately
  • Avoid hyperventilation

Post-operative care

◆ Steroid replacement should initially be given in a dose of about 300 mg daily for a 70 kg adult in three or four divided doses and reduced to 100 mg over the following 2 days
◆ Careful fluid balance monitoring for 24 hours
◆ Blood sugar control

References

1. Pocock G, Richards CD (2006). *Human Physiology: The Basis of Medicine*, 3rd edn. Oxford Medical Publications.
2. Bouillon R (2006). Acute adrenal insufficiency. *Endocrinology and Metabolism Clinics of North America*, **35**, 767–75.
3. Cooper MS, Stewart PM (2003). Corticosteroid insufficiency in acutely ill patients. *New England Journal of Medicine*, **348**, 727–34.
4. Langouche L, Van den BG (2006). The dynamic neuroendocrine response to critical illness. *Endocrinology and Metabolism Clinics of North America*, **35**, 777–91.
5. Wehner C (2009). Addison,T. On the constitutional and local effects of disease of the supra-renal capsules. Available online at: http://wehner.org/addison/cv/index.htm (accessed 17 January 2010).
6. White SM, Campbell DJ (2009). Primary hypopituitarism and peri-operative steroid supplementation. *Anaesthesia*, **64**, 336–7.
7. Cotran RS, Kumar V, Robbins SL (1989). *Robbins Pathologic Basis of Disease*, 4th edn. WBSaunders, Philadelphia, PA.
8. James ML (1970). Endocrine disease and anaesthesia. A review of anaesthetic management in pituitary, adrenal and thyroid diseases. *Anaesthesia*, **25**, 232–52.
9. Axelrod L (2003). Perioperative management of patients treated with glucocorticoids. *Endocrinology and Metabolism Clinics of North America*, **32**, 367–83.
10. Kohl BA, Schwartz S (2009). Surgery in the patient with endocrine dysfunction. *Medical Clinics of North America*, **93**, 1031–47.
11. Connery LE, Coursin DB (2004). Assessment and therapy of selected endocrine disorders. *Anesthesiology Clinics of North America*, **22**, 93–123.
12. Nicholson G, Burrin JM, Hall GM (1998). Peri-operative steroid supplementation. *Anaesthesia*, **53**, 1091–1104.
13. Smith MG, Byrne AJ (1981). An Addisonian crisis complicating anaesthesia. *Anaesthesia*, **36**, 681–4.
14. Watt I, Ledingham IM (1984). Mortality amongst multiple trauma patients admitted to an intensive therapy unit. *Anaesthesia*, **39**, 973–81.
15. Dabbagh A, Sa'adat N, Heidari Z (2009). Etomidate infusion in the critical care setting for suppressing the acute phase of Cushing's syndrome. *Anesthesia and Analgesia*, **108**, 238–9.
16. Cotten JF, Husain SS, Forman SA, *et al.* (2009). Methoxycarbonyl-etomidate: a novel rapidly metabolized and ultra-short-acting etomidate analogue that does not produce prolonged adrenocortical suppression. *Anesthesiology*, **111**, 240–9.
17. Brodsky JB, Lemmens HJ, Brock-Utne JG, Vierra M, Saidman LJ (2002). Morbid obesity and tracheal intubation. *Anesthesia and Analgesia*, **94**, 732–6
18. Fulton J (1946). *Harvey Cushing: A Biography*, Charles C Thomas, Springfield, IL.
19. Conn JW (1955). Primary aldosteronism. *Journal of Laboratory and Clinical Medicine*, **45**, 661–4.
20. Gordon RD, Klemm SA, Tunny TJ, Stowasser M (1992). Primary aldosteronism: hypertension with a genetic basis. *Lancet*, **340**, 159–61.
21. Finch JS (1969). Primary aldosteronism. Review of the anaesthetic experience in sixty patients. *British Journal of Anaesthesia*, **41**, 880–3.

Chapter 8

Adrenal medulla

The anaesthetic management of phaeochromocytoma

MFM James

Physiology

The adrenal medulla is a modified sympathetic ganglion comprising approximately 28% of the total mass of the adrenal gland. It contains two types of secretory cells, 90% of which produce adrenaline and the remainder noradrenaline. A third catecholamine, dopamine, is also produced in the adrenal medulla. The catecholamines are synthesized from phenylalanine in the process illustrated in Figure 8.1. All sympathetic nerve terminals are capable of the synthetic process up to the point of the formation of noradrenaline. However, the enzyme phenylethanolamine-N-methyl transferase (PNMT) is almost exclusively found in the adrenal medulla and requires high levels of glucocorticoids to be effective. These high concentrations of glucocorticoids are provided by a portal system delivering glucocorticoids directly from the adrenal cortex to the adrenal medulla. For this reason, the adrenal gland is virtually the only source of adrenaline, whereas the other catecholamines can be produced by all the other parts of the sympathetic nervous system.

Under normal circumstances, the plasma concentrations of noradrenaline are in the region of 200–400 pg/mL, and this concentration represents spillover from resting sympathetic discharge. At these concentrations, noradrenaline has no hormonal activity as the concentrations required for hormonal activity of noradrenaline are in excess of 2000 pg/mL. Dopamine and adrenaline are found in concentrations that reflect hormonal activity, both in the range of 40–80 pg/mL. However, these levels can fluctuate widely depending on the state of sympathetic activity. Increasing sympathetic activity not only releases noradrenaline from peripheral sympathetic nerve terminals, but also increases the release of adrenaline from the adrenal medulla.

Catecholamines are metabolized mainly intraneurally and within the adrenal medulla through the enzymes catechol-O-methyl transferase (COMT) and monoamine oxidase (MAO). Metabolites are also produced within catecholamine-secreting tumours. Sympathetic nerves contain MAO, but not COMT. Thus intraneuronal metabolism of noradrenaline leads to production of the deaminated metabolite dihydroxyphenylglycol (DHPG), but not of the O-methylated metabolite normetadrenaline (normetanephrine).

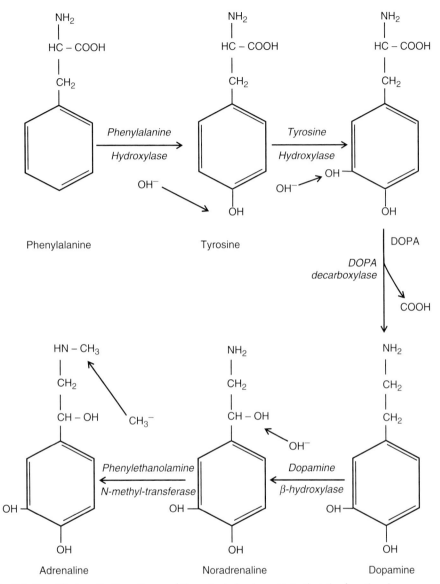

Fig. 8.1 Simplified synthetic pathway of the catecholamines. Note that the functional catecholamines commence with the decarboxylation of DOPA, producing an amine from the preceding amino acid.

Consequently, almost all the DHPG in plasma has a neuronal source, whereas normetadrenaline and metadrenaline are derived exclusively from non-neuronal sources (Figure 8.2).[1] These non-neuronal sources include chromaffin cells in the adrenal medulla. This means that metadrenalines are extraneuronal O-methylated metabolites of noradrenaline and adrenaline; thus measurements of their plasma concentrations enable

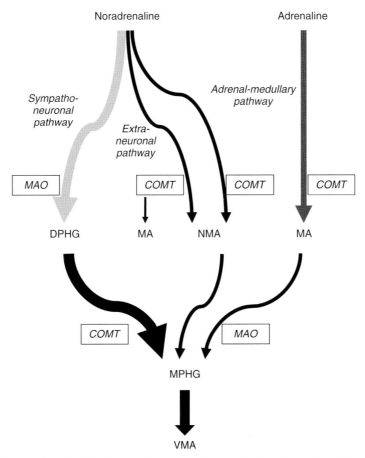

Fig. 8.2 Diagram showing the three main pathways for metabolism of noradrenaline and adrenaline derived from sympathoneuronal or adrenal medullary sources. The sympathoneuronal pathway (light grey) is the major pathway of catecholamine metabolism and involves intraneuronal deamination of noradrenaline leaking from storage granules or of noradrenaline recaptured after release by sympathetic nerves. The extraneuronal pathway (black) is a relatively minor pathway of metabolism of catecholamines released from sympathetic nerves or the adrenal medulla, but is important for further processing of metabolites produced by neuronal and adrenal medullary pathways. The adrenal medullary pathway (dark grey) involves O-methylation of catecholamines leaking from storage granules into the cytoplasm of adrenal medullary cells. Metabolism by sulphate conjugation which operates as part of the extraneuronal pathway is not shown. MA, metadrenalines; NMA, normetadrenaline.[1] Redrawn from Eisenhofer G, Kopin IJ, Goldstein DS (2004). Catecholamine metabolism: a contemporary view with implications for physiology and medicine. *Pharmacol Rev*, **56**(3), 331–49, with permission.

examination of the extraneuronal uptake and metabolism of catecholamines. These are particularly useful in the diagnosis of phaeochromocytoma, as they are consistently produced within the tumour and are less dependent on periodic release than other measures such as plasma catecholamines and vanillyl mandillic acid (VMA).

Pathophysiology

Phaeochromocytomas are uncommon catecholamine-secreting tumours derived from neural crest tissues and may arise from either the adrenal medulla or other neural crest derivatives, mainly the sympathetic chain. True phaeochromocytomas are those arising from the adrenal medulla, whereas those arising from the sympathetic chain are generally referred to as paraganglionomas or extra-adrenal phaeochromocytomas. This latter group can arise from many locations, from the base of the skull to the urinary bladder, with the most common extra-adrenal site being the organ of Zuckerkandl in the para-aortic area. Catecholamine-producing tissues contain chromaffin cells, so named because of the characteristic staining pattern seen when they are exposed to potassium dichromate. The cells are rich in chromogranin A, a polypeptide chain that appears to be crucial for the formation of secretory granules and sequestration of hormones in neuroendocrine cells. However, chromogranin A estimations in phaeochromocytoma patients do not appear to have the same diagnostic and prognostic relevance that they have in carcinoid disease.[2] Less commonly, catecholamine-secreting tumours may arise from other tissues, including ganglioneuroblastoma, ganglioneuroma, and neuroblastoma. Phaeochromocytoma has been referred to as the '10% tumour' because, for example, 10% are extra-adrenal and of those, 10% are extra-abdominal, 10% are malignant, 10% are found in patients who do not have hypertension, and finally 10% are hereditary. However, this simple view is misleading, since over 80% of phaeochromocytomas are isolated single adrenal tumours. The extra-adrenal tumours are more likely to be multiple and malignant, while the familial forms more frequently present without hypertensive episodes. Familial phaeochromocytoma is inherited as an autosomal dominant trait alone or as a component of the multiple endocrine neoplasia type 2 syndromes (MEN 2a and MEN 2b), von Hippel–Lindau disease, or, in rare cases, neurofibromatosis type 1.[3,4] The remaining 90% of phaeochromocytomas are classified as sporadic or non-syndromic. However, recent evidence has suggested that there may be a genetic or familial basis for the development of phaeochromocytoma in up to 25% of affected individuals.[5] Germ-line mutations in the RET proto-oncogene have been associated with MEN 2, but more recently the gene encoding succinate dehydrogenase subunit D (SDHD) and SDHB have been associated with autosomal dominant familial paraganglionomas and glomus tumours.[6] In a recent study, a large cohort of patients with non-syndromic phaeochromocytoma from registries in Germany and Poland were screened for the germ-line mutations together with the tumour-suppressor gene VHL associated with the von Hippel–Lindau syndrome.[5] This study suggests that a significant proportion of previously classified non-syndromic phaeochromocytoma probably has a genetic basis.[7]

Phaeochromocytomas are associated with numerous other conditions including MEN 2a (medullary thyroid carcinoma, phaeochromocytoma, and parathyroid hyperplasia) and MEN 2b (MEN 2a together with marfanoid habitus and vascular neuromas, particularly of the face). In von Hippel–Lindau disease there is an incidence of approximately 20% of phaeochromocytoma. There is a weak association with von Recklinghausen's neurofibromatosis; about 1% of these patients have phaeochromocytoma. Malignant tumours are more likely to occur in association with the genetically determined forms of phaeochromocytoma, and are also more common in association with extra-adrenal phaeochromocytoma.

Malignancy is difficult to diagnose histologically, as the tumours are well differentiated and there are no specific histological appearances that define malignancy. The diagnosis depends on the behaviour of the tumour, particularly on the development of metastatic disease, and tumour occurrence in sites not associated with neuroendocrine crest tissue. Metastatic lesions have a predilection for bone, particularly the vertebral bodies. Pathological fractures commonly occur with secondary lesions, but these are usually seen late in the course of the illness and are seldom the presenting event.

Although catecholamine excess is the hallmark of phaeochromocytoma, an array of other neuropeptides may be found in association with these tumours, including parathyroid hormone, adrenocorticotrophic hormone (ACTH), tachykinins, and neuropeptide Y. The last of these may contribute to hypertension, particularly during a crisis, and may contribute to hypertension that is partially resistant to α-adrenergic blockade.

Diagnosis

The clinical features of phaeochromocytoma are frequently diagnostic, but these tumours may also present with a bewildering variety of symptoms (Table 8.1).[8] At least one of a triad of excessive sweating, headaches, and palpitations occurs in over 90% of patients on careful inquiry, but may not be the presenting symptom. Personal experience suggests

Table 8.1 Signs and symptoms of phaeochromocytoma (in order of frequency).

Symptoms	Signs
Headaches	Hypertension
Palpitations	Sustained
Sweating	Episodic
Anxiousness	Postural hypotension
Tremor	Hyperglycaemia
Abdominal pain	Arrhythmias
Weakness and fatigue	Weight loss
Nausea and vomiting	

Adapted from Eisenhofer G, Goldstein DS, Walther MM *et al.* (2003). Biochemical diagnosis of pheochromocytoma: how to distinguish true- from false-positive test results. *Journal of Clinical Endocrinology and Metabolism*, **88**, 2656–66.

that all three symptoms occur together in less than 50% of patients. Patients may present with anxiety, tremor, nausea and vomiting, weight loss, chest and abdominal pain, peripheral vascular disease, cardiac failure, and cerebral vascular accident. Hypertension is classically episodic, but may be sustained in up to 50% of patients. Heart rate may be normal, rapid, or slow, and arrhythmias may or may not be present. Abdominal pain, presumably due to bowel ischaemia, together with chronic constipation and pseudo-obstruction may lead to an erroneous diagnosis of an acute abdomen. Phaeochromocytoma crisis may present with severe pounding headache, sweating, pallor, palpitations, and a feeling of impending doom. The onset may be sudden, but the duration is generally short. However, only a minority of patients with phaeochromocytoma will have experienced such a crisis. Metabolic problems, including weight loss and frank diabetes mellitus, may be presenting signs, and occasionally patients may present in diabetic ketoacidotic coma.[9] Surprisingly, hypoglycaemia with severe hypertension has also been reported as a presenting event.[10]

Traditionally, diagnosis of phaeochromocytoma relied on the measurement of catecholamine metabolites VMA and metadrenaline in a 24-hour urine sample. However, VMA measurements have a sensitivity of only 60%, and should never be relied upon as a screening test. At the very least, they should be combined with metadrenaline estimations on three separate occasions before the diagnosis is excluded in a patient with suggestive symptomatology. This combination should give a sensitivity and specificity of above 90%. The development of reliable high-pressure liquid chromatography (HPLC) with electrochemical detection techniques allows the estimation of plasma and urine catecholamines, providing greater specificity (95%) but without improvement in sensitivity, as sampling during periods of tumour quiescence may miss the diagnosis. Plasma adrenaline concentrations >400 pg/ml and plasma noradrenaline concentrations >2000 pg/ml are generally diagnostic. However, there may be overlap, particularly at these marginal values, between patients with high-catecholamine hypertension and patients with phaeochromocytoma. In these cases, the clonidine suppression test, in which plasma catecholamines are estimated before and after an oral dose of 0.3 mg clonidine, may be a useful differentiating test.[11] A fall in plasma noradrenaline of 30% or to <500 pg/ml implies that the elevated catecholamines are unlikely to be derived from a phaeochromocytoma.[12] An improvement in sensitivity has been offered by the development of HPLC measurement of free metadrenalines within the plasma. These metabolites are produced continuously from the tumour cells, regardless of the level of catecholamine secretion, and are thus less likely to produce false negatives. In a large prospective study, measurement of plasma free metadrenaline produced a 99% sensitivity, although the specificity was only 89%.[13] This implies that a negative result on this estimation virtually excludes the diagnosis of phaeochromocytoma. Plasma or urine fractionated metadrenalines should now be considered as the principal screening test for phaeochromocytoma.[14,15] The ratio of 24-hour urinary metadrenaline production to creatinine secretion may improve the sensitivity of this estimation.

Tumour imaging is another important component of the diagnosis. Once the diagnosis is suspected, CT scanning of both adrenals should be performed.[16] MRI does not appear to offer better tumour visualization. It should be remembered that ionized contrast media can precipitate a phaeochromocytoma crisis, and intravenous contrast should only be used if the patient has received appropriate adrenergic blockade. If CT scanning of the adrenals fails to demonstrate a lesion, or if malignancy or multiple tumours are suspected, radionuclide scanning with meta-iodo-benzylguanethidine (MIBG) should be performed, preferably using the [^{123}I]MIBG isotope, as it has a shorter half-life than the older [^{131}I]MIBG and can be given in larger doses. The tricyclic antidepressants guanethidine and labetalol may interfere with the test, but propranolol, α-blocking drugs, and calcium antagonists do not. Occasionally, octreotide scintigraphy has revealed small tumours not detected with MIBG.[17] In cases where biochemistry suggests the presence of a phaeochromocytoma, but other imaging tests have failed, positron emission tomographic scanning using the imaging agent 6-[^{18}F]fluorodopamine as a substrate for the noradrenaline transporter offers a highly effective method of tumour localization.[18,19]

Evaluation

Patient evaluation should include a detailed cardiovascular assessment, looking particularly for evidence of catecholamine-induced cardiomyopathy. A chest X-ray and 12-lead ECG should be performed and evidence of myocardial dysfunction evaluated. Personal experience suggests that left atrial enlargement secondary to catecholamine-induced left ventricular diastolic dysfunction (Figure 8.3) is quite common (around 20%), but seldom poses a management problem unless accompanied by left ventricular systolic dysfunction.

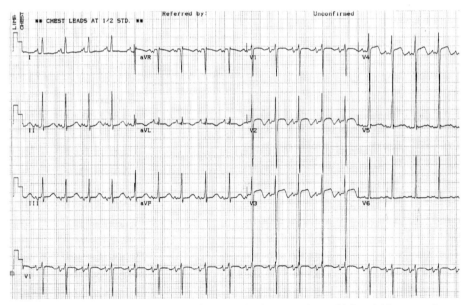

Fig. 8.3 ECG of a patient with marked left ventricular hypertrophy and left atrial hypertrophy. Note the typical 'P-mitrale' pattern in leads II and V$_1$. Echocardiography showed this patient to have a normal mitral valve.

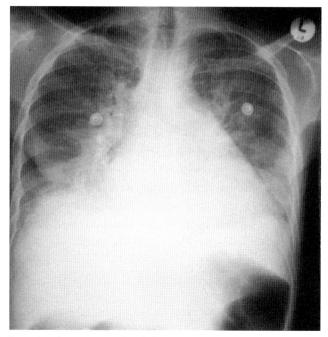

Fig. 8.4 Chest X-ray showing gross cardiac failure with pulmonary oedema in a patient with catecholamine-induced cardiomyopathy. This patient had an ejection fraction of 24%.

Left ventricular hypertrophy is frequently seen, as are ST and T-wave abnormalities, but there appears to be little advantage in attempting to correct these by medical management prior to tumour excision. These changes generally regress once the excess catecholamines source is removed. Left ventricular failure and pulmonary oedema may be present, particularly if the patient has developed signs of a catecholamine-induced cardiomyopathy (Figure 8.4). An array of vascular pathology may be seen, as discussed above.

Pre-operative preparation

As most phaeochromocytomas are benign, treatment is almost invariably surgical. Medical management, prior to surgery, predominantly with α-adrenergic blockade is generally regarded as desirable,[20] but is by no means universally accepted as essential. The rarity of these tumours means that large randomized prospective controlled trials on pre-operative preparation are unlikely to be performed. Two small trials have been conducted. In the first, six patients received phenoxybenzamine, 28 patients received prazosin, and the remaining 29 patients received no pre-operative α blockade; there were no discernible differences between the groups in terms of outcome.[21] In the other study, phenoxybenzamine appeared to provide better haemodynamic stability during the peri-operative period than either prazosin or labetalol, but only 14 patients were studied in total.[22] Phenoxybenzamine is a non-competitive non-selective α-adrenergic blocking agent that has the advantage of forming an irreversible covalent bond with the α-adrenergic receptor, and thus the blockade cannot be overcome during a surge of catecholamine release. For this reason, it is generally the favoured agent for pre-operative haemodynamic control.[23] However, it produces significant postural hypotension, lethargy, and nasal congestion that patients find unpleasant, and in high doses can result in post-operative hypotension. Alternative approaches have been suggested, including the use of selective α_1-blocking drugs such as prazosin and, more recently, the longer-acting agent doxazosin. Good results have been reported with doxazosin.[24] The supposed advantage of α_1-selective agents—that they allow inhibition of further catecholamine release through the unblocked α_2-receptors—is unfounded as these receptors are ineffective in phaeochromocytomas (see the clonidine suppression test, discussed above). The place of β-adrenergic blockade is even more controversial, and it is the author's personal practice to avoid using these drugs if at all possible. It seems sensible to avoid β-adrenergic blockade at the time of tumour removal, and therefore long-acting β-blockers should be withdrawn at least three half-lives prior to surgery. Where necessary, intra-operative β-blockade can be provided with the short-acting agent esmolol, although this is very infrequently required. Extra-adrenal tumours are very unlikely to produce adrenaline, and there is little place for β-blockade in the pre-operative preparation of patients with these tumours. Calcium-channel blockers have a theoretical appeal in that they not only produce peripheral arteriolar vasodilatation, but may also inhibit calcium-mediated release of catecholamines and other neurotransmitter substances. They have been beneficial in the control of blood pressure in patients with moderate hypertension[25] and have been used intra-operatively with some success. However, failure of haemodynamic control with these drugs has also been reported, and as the experience with them is less extensive than that with the α-adrenergic blocking agents, they cannot be regarded as first-line therapy for pre-operative preparation at the present time.

Fitness for surgery

There are no absolute guidelines as to the adequacy of preparation of a patient prior to surgery. Suggested guidelines have included the following:[26]

- supine arterial pressure not greater than 160/90 mmHg
- orthostatic hypotension, with the arterial pressure not falling below 85/45 mmHg
- ECG free of ST segment and T-wave changes for at least 2 weeks
- no more than one premature ventricular contraction every 5 minutes.

None of these criteria has been adequately validated, although they are largely sensible. Paradoxically, failure to achieve adequate control by medical means, particularly in patients with large tumours, may be an indication for relatively urgent surgery as the only mechanism for controlling the excessive catecholamine production. There is little evidence to support the recommendation on reversal of ECG changes, as these seldom resolve within the relatively short time frame that is now thought appropriate for pre-operative preparation, and may take months to return to baseline. It is probably more appropriate to proceed with anaesthesia and surgery unless the patient clearly has myocardial ischaemia.

Satisfactory expansion of blood volume is difficult to estimate. There is little evidence that patients with relatively stable disease have significantly diminished blood volume, but patients who have recently suffered a hypertensive crisis may well have markedly diminished blood volume. In these circumstances, regular monitoring of haematocrit may be helpful. There is no accepted rule regarding the duration of adequate pre-operative preparation, with most centres opting for 7–14 days of pre-operative preparation;[23] however, the study by Russell *et al.*[22] suggested that 5–7 days should generally be sufficient. The author's practice is to increase α-blockade on a daily basis until adequate haemodynamic control is achieved and then to proceed to surgery, rather than use any predetermined time period. Where phenoxybenzamine is not available, doxazocin is an acceptable alternative and provides reasonable control, although current evidence suggests that phenoxybenzamine will result in fewer intra-operative haemodynamic fluctuations. Either agent is given in increasing doses to a target value, as indicated in the section on key clinical management points, depending on the quality of blood pressure control.

Anaesthetic management

Various approaches to the management of anaesthesia have been recommended. Most anaesthetic agents have been used with relative safety, although it is generally recommended that agents releasing histamine should be avoided, as should agents that might induce tachycardia such as atropinics (Table 8.2). Droperidol inhibits the re-uptake of catecholamines, and is probably best avoided.[27] Oral premedication with a benzodiazepine is generally all that is required. Where phenoxybenzamine has been used, it should be omitted on the morning of surgery as it has a very long half-life. β-blockade,

Table 8.2 Drugs to consider avoiding in a patient with a phaeochromocytoma

Anticholinergics (drugs with anticholinergic effects)
Atropine
Pancuronium
Histamine-releasing agents
Suxamethonium
Atracurium
Morphine
Mivacurium, atracurium, cisatracurium
Droperidol
Catecholamine-sensitizing anaesthetic agents
? Halothane
? Desflurane

where utilized, should also be withdrawn in good time, so that the patient is not under β-blockade at the time of tumour excision. Morphine may release histamine and should probably be avoided. Fentanyl and sufentanil have been widely used with good results, but remifentanil is a potent venodilator and may be associated with greater haemodynamic instability than the other opiates.[28] Whether or not epidural anaesthesia is performed as part of the anaesthetic technique is largely a matter of choice, although the presence of additional sympathetic blockade will not enhance haemodynamic control because of catecholamine release and may make management of hypotension after tumour extirpation more difficult. Theoretically, desflurane, which may stimulate sympathetic discharge, and halothane, which may predispose to ventricular arrhythmia, should be avoided, but there is no scientific evidence to support either of these suggestions.

Prior to induction of anaesthesia, good high-capacity intravenous access should be obtained and direct arterial pressure monitoring established. Once the patient is stabilized, central venous access should be established for both monitoring and drug administration purposes. There is little evidence to support the use of pulmonary artery catheters in these patients, even where cardiomyopathy has been shown to be present pre-operatively. However, transoesophageal echocardiography can be extremely valuable, particularly in terms of assessing adequate ventricular filling and myocardial performance.[29,30] Assessment of volume status can be very difficult, and static pressure measurements of central venous pressure or pulmonary capillary wedge pressure are of little value. Dynamic techniques, such as stroke volume variation, pulse pressure variation, or recruitable stroke volume, are all appealing but none have been studied in this setting. Personal experience suggests that systolic pressure variation is a useful guide, and a difference in systolic pressure between peak inspiration and expiration of more than 10 mmHg strongly suggests inadequate volume status regardless of the actual value of the arterial pressure. Blood loss is frequently significant, particularly with open procedures, as these are very vascular tumours. Properly prepared patients with good α-adrenergic blockade tolerate volume loss poorly and it must be recognized that the viscosity provided by red cells is an important component of peripheral vascular resistance in a vasodilated patient. Blood transfusion should probably be used earlier in these patients than would normally be the case in order to maintain peripheral resistance, particularly following tumour excision.

No one anaesthetic technique has been shown to be superior to any other, and a variety of induction agents and muscle relaxants have been used. Both anaesthetic induction and tracheal intubation may be accompanied by a surge in blood pressure, but a substantial fall in blood pressure may also occur during surgical preparation after induction. A range of pharmacological agents to handle either of these eventualities should be immediately to hand. However, it is unwise to administer indirect-acting vasopressor agents (such as ephedrine) at this time. If vasopressor support is required prior to the start of surgery, phenylephrine is probably the agent of choice as it is direct acting and of short duration.

Intra-operative haemodynamic control has been performed with a variety of α-adrenergic blocking agents, β-adrenergic blocking agents, and direct-acting vasodilators.

Sodium nitroprusside has been the most widely used vasodilator, although it may be difficult to titrate the infusion with sufficient accuracy to control the very rapid changes in blood pressure that frequently occur during tumour handling. Theoretically, agents that cause venodilation may increase reflex hypertensive responses and worsen haemodynamic instability; thus both sodium nitroprusside and glyceryl trinatrate may be less useful than pure arteriolar-dilating agents. Phentolamine has been used, but has also proved difficult to control adequately. On the basis that calcium antagonism will oppose both the release of catecholamines and their peripheral effects, calcium-channel blockers have recently been used for intra-operative control with considerable success, particularly nicardipine[31,32] at a rate of 2–6 µg/kg/min, often with accompanying β-adrenergic blockade. Calcium-channel blockers produce mainly arteriolar vasodilation with minimal venodilation, and this may make them theoretically preferable to general vasodilators.

A similar rationale applies to the use of magnesium sulphate, given as an initial bolus of 2–4 g with an infusion of 2 g/hour and intermittent 2 g boluses to a maximum of 30 g. Good results have been achieved with this technique, often as a sole vasodilator agent and in emergency situations where other agents such as sodium nitroprusside have failed.[20,25,26,33–41] Magnesium has the additional advantage that an immediate antagonist is available in the form of calcium chloride.

Venous drainage of the tumours can be very extensive, and unexpected recurrence of hypertension may occur despite apparent ligation of the main venous drainage of the tumour. The only reliable sign that no further catecholamine release will occur is complete detachment of the tumour from the surrounding tissues. Until that time, the anaesthetist must remain vigilant and be prepared to manage further hypertensive episodes. Once the tumour is removed, vasodilator therapy should be withdrawn and aggressive volume expansion undertaken with a combination of colloids and red blood cells as indicated. Brief periods of adrenergic support, particularly with phenylephrine, may be necessary immediately after tumour excision, but it should be possible to withdraw adrenergic support by the end of the procedure. Persistent requirements for haemodynamic support should alert the attending clinicians to the possibility of occult haemorrhage. Blood sugar monitoring should be performed at hourly intervals throughout the procedure and for the first 24 hours post-operatively as the withdrawal of catecholamines may result in increased sensitivity to insulin.

A range of surgical approaches are available, and the surgical technique should be determined by the size and location of the tumour, the possibility of multiple tumour sites, and the skill and experience of the operator and the anaesthetist. Laparoscopic removal of small tumours has received considerable recent support,[31,42–50] but in at least one report the creation of a capnoperitoneum has been associated with increased haemodynamic instability[31,44] leading to the abandonment of the procedure.[51] Nevertheless, laparoscopic resection has now become the technique of choice for single moderately sized adrenal tumours (up to 7–10 cm in diameter) in view of the better post-operative recovery afforded with similar peri-operative haemodynamic problems.[52] Intra-abdominal pressure should be maintained at the lowest level possible for good surgical access, and most authorities recommend that the capnoperitoneum is limited to a pressure of 10 mmHg.[53] There is no doubt that a laparoscopic technique is more demanding of both anaesthetist and surgeon,[54] but current literature suggests that the morbidity is extremely low and that the increased operative demands are worth while in terms of earlier hospital discharge of the patient and lower morbidity (see Chapter 11).

Post-operative care

Post-operatively, patients should be admitted to a high-care facility for continuing monitoring. Ventilatory support should not be necessary, unless dictated by the nature of surgery and the site and size of the tumour. Provided that adequate haemodynamic control was established intra-operatively, post-operative haemodynamic instability should not occur, and if hypotension is problematic, the possibility of bleeding should be considered. Elevated blood pressures, together with persistently elevated plasma catecholamines, may be seen for several days following surgery, presumably because of uptake and storage of catecholamines in sympathetic nerve terminals with subsequent release, and does not necessarily imply incomplete tumour excision. Withdrawal of catecholamines may produce marked alterations in insulin sensitivity, and blood sugar monitoring should be performed on an hourly basis for 24 hours as dangerous hypoglycaemia may occur in the post-operative period.[55,56] Post-operative analgesia can be provided using any technique with which the practitioners are familiar.

Follow-up

The long-term prognosis is generally good, with 75% of patients returning to normal haemodynamic states. Catecholamine-induced cardiomyopathy has a surprisingly good prognosis, and normal myocardial performance architecture can be re-established following complete tumour removal (Figure 8.5). Unfortunately, some patients in whom the diagnosis of phaeochromocytoma has been missed have undergone heart transplantation for catecholamine-induced cardiomyopathy. Some patients will remain persistently hypertensive, but the hypertension is not paroxysmal and can be regarded as 'essential' hypertension. Patients with paraganglionomas, multiple tumours, or multiple endocrine neoplasias have an increased risk of tumour recurrence and should be monitored on an annual basis for at least 5 years following tumour excision. However, recurrence of tumours as late as 15 years after original excision has been reported.

Malignant disease

The diagnosis of malignant disease depends largely on tumour behaviour and location as the histology of these tumours is usually well differentiated and malignancy cannot be diagnosed with confidence on histological examination alone. Multiple lesions do not necessarily imply malignancy as paraganglionomas can occur in any location within the sympathetic chain or extensions of the neural crest. Local invasion of the tumour across tissue planes, or occurrence of the tumour in abnormal sites, strongly suggests malignancy. Phaeochromocytomas typically metastasize to bone, with the vertebral bodies being a particularly common site. Long-bone metastases also occur and may lead to pathological

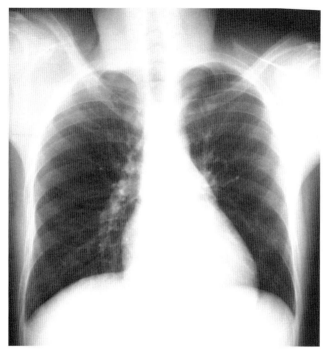

Fig. 8.5 Chest X-ray of the patient in Figure 8.4, 6 months after tumour excision. This patient had completely recovered from the cardiomyopathy and had an ejection fraction of 75% at this time.

fractures requiring orthopaedic fixation. Secondaries can also occur in the lung. Secondary tumours produce mainly noradrenaline and can result in persistent hypertension that is difficult to control. However, they are generally devoid of neuronal connections and therefore do not produce severe responses to surgical stress. Unless the nature of the tumour requires direct tumour manipulation, surgery poses much less of an anaesthetic problem than it does in cases where neuronal connections exist or where direct tumour handling is required. Considerable experience of the management of bony metastases, in which the involved bone can be exercised without handling the tumour, suggests that routine anaesthetic care as for any hypertensive patient is acceptable for most of these patients, although the anaesthetist should be fully prepared to manage a crisis should it occur.

The tumours are generally highly differentiated and very slow growing, and are consequently resistant to radiation therapy and chemotherapy. Treatment with $[^{131}I]$MIBG can produce some improvement and delay tumour expansion. However, a hypertensive crisis may occur, particularly at the first time of exposure to this agent, and the patient should be carefully monitored during treatment. Clinical management involves appropriate antihypertensive treatment and may require not only high doses of α-adrenergic blockade, but other hypotensive medication in addition. A prognosis of 10 years or more is not unusual in patients even with widely disseminated malignant phaeochromocytoma.

Key clinical management points

Diagnosis

◆ Suspect the diagnosis in young patients with atypical hypertension

◆ The classical triad of sweating, headaches, and palpitations only occur together in 15% of patients, but one of these is often present (>70%).

Diagnostic tests

◆ Plasma or urinary metadrenalines; ratio of urine metadrenalines to creatinine is often helpful

◆ CT adrenals

◆ An isolated adrenal mass together with a suggestive clinical picture and positive metadrenalines is diagnostic

◆ Further tests are only necessary where multiple tumours are suspected

  • Children (50% bilateral)

  • MEN syndromes

  • Paraganglionomas

Pre-operative preparation

α-adrenergic blockade is recommended until the patient is haemodynamically stable (normally after 5–10 days).

◆ Phenoxybenzamine

  • Generally preferred

  • Non-competitive blockade; hence provides stability during catecholamine surges

  • Dosage

    ▪ Start at 25 mg daily, increasing daily until adequate blockade is established

    ▪ Dosage limit 250 mg/day

  • Side-effects:

    ▪ Postural hypertension (desirable endpoint)

    ▪ Nasal stuffiness (indicator of adequate blockade)

    ▪ Impotence

    ▪ Drowsiness

Key clinical management points (continued)

- Doxazocin
  - Competitive α-adrenergic antagonist
  - May allow 'breakthrough' hypertensive episodes
  - Dosage
    - Start at 2mg daily increasing daily to maximum of 8mg bd
  - Side-effects similar to, but less severe than, phenoxybenzamine
- Others
  - Calcium-channel blockers
    - Oral nicardipine 20–60 mg daily
- Withdraw other hypotensive agents (especially ACE inhibitors and diuretics) once good BP control is established.
- β-blockade is seldom necessary provided that good hydration is achieved

Assessment of fitness

- Controlled hypertension (170/90 mmHg)
- Postural hypertension present but not severe (blood pressure >90/60 mmHg on standing)
- Warm vasodilated peripheries
- Control of arrhythmias

Note: failure of maximum α-blockade to control symptoms may be an indication for urgent surgery.

Anaesthetic management

- Standard sedative premedication
- Monitoring
  - Standard anaesthetic monitoring
  - Direct arterial pressure monitoring
    - Central venous pressure (mainly for rapid drug access) after induction
  - Cardiac assessment
    - Pulmonary artery catheter no longer widely used
    - Transoesophageal echo may be very helpful, especially if cardiac dysfunction is present
    - Non-invasive cardiac output estimates may be helpful
      - Pulse contour analysis
      - Transoesophageal Doppler

Key clinical management points (continued)

Anaesthetic induction

- Propofol or thiopentone are suitable
- Vecuronium or rocuronium for muscle relaxation
- Volatiles: isoflurane or sevoflurane
- Blood pressure control
  - Magnesium sulphate
    - 2–4 g after induction if arterial blood pressure is high prior to intubation
    - 2 g/hour infusion
    - 2 g boluses as required for catecholamine surges
    - No defined upper dosage limit: up to 45 g has been given over a 5-hour period
  - Sodium nitroprusside
    - Continuous infusion
    - Less flexible than others
    - May cause venodilation and rapid swings in pressures
  - Calcium-channel blockers
    - Nicardipine infusion 2–6 µg/kg/min
- Following tumour removal, withdraw hypotensive agent
- Calcium chloride 1–3 g to reverse $MgSO_4$
- Phenylephrine infusion if necessary
- Aggressive fluid replacement
- Maintain haemoglobin 10–12 g/dL as viscosity is important for adequate blood pressure
- Check blood sugar

Post-operative care

- High-care unit admission
- Continuous blood pressure monitoring for 24 hours
- Vasoconstrictor therapy should not be necessary
- Monitor blood sugar hourly for first 24 hours

Follow-up

- All cases at high risk for recurrence should be reviewed annually for at least 5 years
  - Children, MEN syndromes, paraganglionomas, malignant tumours

References

1. Eisenhofer G, Kopin IJ, Goldstein DS (2004). Catecholamine metabolism: a contemporary view with implications for physiology and medicine. *Pharmacological Reviews*, **56**, 331–49.

2. Taupenot L, Harper KL, O'Connor DT (2003). The chromogranin–secretogranin family. *New England Journal of Medicine*, **348**,1134–49.

3. Drolet P, Girard M (1993). [The use of magnesium sulfate during surgery of pheochromocytoma: apropos of 2 cases] *Canadian Journal of Anaesthesia*, **40**, 521–5.

4. Eng C, Crossey PA, Milligan LM (1995). Mutations in the RET protooncogene and the von Hippel–Lindau disease tumour suppressor gene in sporadic and syndromic phaeochromocytomas. *Journal of Medical Genetics*, **32**, 934–7.

5. Neumann HP, Bausch B, McWhinney SR, *et al.* (2002). Germ-line mutations in nonsyndromic pheochromocytoma. *New England Journal of Medicine*, **346**, 1459–66.

6. Baysal BE, Ferrell RE, Willett-Brozick JE, *et al.* (2000). Mutations in SDHD, a mitochondrial complex II gene, in hereditary paraganglioma. *Science*, **287**, 848–51.

7. Dluhy RG (2002). Pheochromocytoma–death of an axiom. *New England Journal of Medicine*, **346**, 1486–8.

8. Eisenhofer G, Rivers G, Rosas AL, Quezado Z, Manger WM, Pacak K (2007). Adverse drug reactions in patients with phaeochromocytoma: incidence, prevention and management. *Drug Safety*, **30**, 1031–62.

9. Ishii C, lnoue K, Negishi K, Tane N, Awata T, Katayama S (2001). Diabetic ketoacidosis in a case of pheochromocytoma. *Diabetes Research and Clinical Practice*, **54**, 137–42.

10. Frankton S, Baithun S, Husain E, Davis K, Grossman AB (2009). Phaeochromocytoma crisis presenting with profound hypoglycaemia and subsequent hypertension. *Hormones*, **8**, 65–70.

11. Bravo EL, Tarazi RC, Fouad FM, Vidt DG, Gifford RWJ (1981). Clonidine-suppression test: a useful aid in the diagnosis of pheochromocytoma. *New England Journal of Medicine*, **305**, 623–6.

12. Lenz T, Ross A, Schumm-Draeger P, Schulte KL, Geiger H (1998). Clonidine suppression test revisited. *Blood Pressure*, **7**, 153–9.

13. Lenders JW, Pacak K, Eisenhofer G (2002). New advances in the biochemical diagnosis of pheochromocytoma: moving beyond catecholamines. *Annals of the New York Academy of Sciences*, **970**, 29–40.

14. Peaston RT, Ball S (2008). Biochemical detection of phaeochromocytoma: why are we continuing to ignore the evidence? *Annals of the Clinical Biochemistry*, **45**, 6–10.

15. Pacak K, Eisenhofer G, Ahlman H, *et al.* (2007). Pheochromocytoma: recommendations for clinical practice from the First International Symposium. October 2005. *Nature Clinical Practice. Endocrinology and Metabolism*, **3**, 92–102.

16. Mayo-Smith WW, Boland GW, Noto RB, Lee MJ (2001). State-of-the-art adrenal imaging. *Radiographics*, **21**, 995–1012.

17. Meunier JP, Tatou E, Bernard A, Brenot R, David M (2001). Cardiac pheochromocytoma. *Annals of Thoracic Surgery*, **71**, 712–13.

18. Pacak K, Goldstein DS, Doppman JL, Shulkin BL, Udelsman R, Eisenhofer G (2001). A 'pheo' lurks: novel approaches for locating occult pheochromocytoma. *Journal of Clinical Endocrinology and Metabolism*, **86**, 3641–6.

19. Hoegerle S, Nitzsche E, Altehoefer C, *et al.* (2002). Pheochromocytomas: detection with ^{18}F DOPA whole body PET: initial results. *Radiology*, **222**, 507–12.

20. O'Riordan JA (1997). Pheochromocytomas and anesthesia. *International Anesthesiology Clinics*, **35**, 99–127.

21. Boutros AR, Bravo EL, Zanettin G, Straffon RA (1990). Perioperative management of 63 patients with pheochromocytoma. *Cleveland Clinic Journal of Medicine*, **57**, 613–17.

22. Russell WJ, Metcalfe IR, Tonkin AL, Frewin DB (1998). The preoperative management of phaeochromocytoma. *Anaesthesia and Intensive Care*, **26**, 196–200.

23. Pacak K (2007). Preoperative management of the pheochromocytoma patient. *Journal of Clinical Endocrinology and Metabolism*, **92**, 4069–79.

24. Prys Roberts C (2000). Phaeochromocytoma: recent progress in its management. *British Journal of Anaesthesia*, **85**, 44–57.

25. Bravo EL (2002). Pheochromocytoma. An approach to anithypertensive management. *Annals of the New York Academy of Sciences*, **970**, 1–10

26. Desmonts JM, Marty J (1984). An anaesthetic management of patients with pheochromocytoma. *British Journal of Anaesthesia*, 56781–9

27. Oh TE, Turner CW, Ilett KF, Waterson JG, Paterson JW (1978). Mechanism of the hypertensive effect of droperidol in pheochromocytoma. *Anaesthesia and Intensive Care*, **6**, 322–7.

28. Breslin DS, Farling PA, Mirakhur RK (2003). The use of remifentanil in the anaesthetic management of patients undergoing adrenalectomy: a report of three cases. *Anaesthesia*, **58**, 358–62.

29. Bellingham GA, Dhir AK, Luke PP (2008). Case report: retroperitoneoscopic pheochromocytoma removal in an adult with Eisenmenger's syndrome. *Canadian Journal of Anaesthesia*, **55**, 295–301.

30. Matsuura T, Kashimoto S, Okuyama K, Oguchi T, Kumazawa T (1995). [Anesthesia with transesophageal echocardiography for removal of pheochromocytoma]. *Masui*, **44**, 1388–90.

31. Atallah F, Bastide-Heulin T, Soulie M, *et al.* (2001). Haemodynamic changes during retroperitoneoscopic adrenalectomy for phaeochromocytoma. *British Journal of Anaesthesia*, **86**, 731–3.

32. Joris JL, Hamoir EE, Hartstein GM, *et al.* (1999). Hemodynamic changes and catecholamine release during laparoscopic adrenalectomy for pheochromocytoma. *Anesthesia and Analgesia*, **88**, 16–21.

33. Beeton AG, Shipton EA, Katz BJ (1992). Unexplained hypertension during induction of a patient with phaeochromocytoma. *South African Journal of Surgery*, **30**, 165–7.

34. Bullough A, Karadia S, Watters M (2001). Phaeochromocytoma: an unusual cause of hypertension in pregnancy. *Anaesthesia*, **56**, 43–6.

35. Niruthisard S, Chatrkaw P, Laornual S, Sunthornyothin S, Prasertsri S (2002). Anesthesia for one-stage bilateral pheochromocytoma resection in a patient with MEN type IIa: attenuation of hypertensive crisis by magnesium sulfate. *Journal of the Medical Association of Thailand*, **85**, 125–30.

36. Pitt-Miller P, Primus E (2000). Use of magnesium sulphate as adjunctive therapy for resection of phaeochromocytoma. *West Indian Medical Journal*, **49**, 73–5.

37. Pivalizza EG (1995). Magnesium sulfate and epidural anesthesia in pheochromocytoma and severe coronary artery disease. *Anesthesia and Analgesia*, **81**, 414–16.

38. Poopalalingam R, Chin EY (2001). Rapid preparation of a patient with pheochromocytoma with labetolol and magnesium sulfate. *Canadian Journal of Anaesthesia*, **48**, 876–80.

39. Huddle KR, Mannell A, James MF, Plant ME (1991). Phaeochromocytoma. A report of 10 patients. *South African Medical Journal*, **79**, 217–20.

40. James MF (1985). The use of magnesium sulfate in the anesthetic management of pheochromocytoma. *Anesthesiology*, **62**, 188–90.

41. James MF (1989). Use of magnesium sulphate in the anaesthetic management of phaeochromocytoma: a review of 17 anaesthetics. *British Journal of Anaesthesia*, **62**, 616–23.

42. Brunt LM, Moley JF, Doherty GM, Lairmore TC, DeBenedetti MK, Quasebarth MA (2001). Outcomes analysis in patients undergoing laparoscopic adrenalectomy for hormonally active adrenal tumors. *Surgery*, **130**, 629–34.

43. Chiu M, Crosby ET, Yelle JD (2000). Anesthesia for laparoscopic adrenalectomy (pheochromocytoma) in an anemic adult Jehovah's Witness. *Canadian Journal of Anaesthesia*, **47**, 566–71.

44. Darvas K, Pinkola K, Borsodi M, Tarjanyi M, Winternitz T, Horanyi J (2000). General anaesthesia for laparascopic adrenalectomy. *Medical Science Monitor*, **6**, 560–3.

45. Gill IS (2001). The case for laparoscopic adrenalectomy. *Journal of Urology*, **166**, 429–36.

46. Guazzoni G, Cestari A, Montorsi F, *et al.* (2001). Eight-year experience with transperitoneal laparoscopic adrenal surgery. *Journal of Urology*, **166**, 820–4.

47. Janetschek G, Neumann HP (2001). Laparoscopic surgery for pheochromocytoma. *Urologic Clinics of North America*, **28**, 97–105.

48. Kazaryan AM, Mala T, Edwin B (2001). Does tumor size influence the outcome of laparoscopic adrenalectomy? *Journal of Laparoendoscopic and Advanced Surgical Techniques. Part A*, **11**, 1–4.

49. Salomon L, Rabii R, Soulie M, *et al.* (2001). Experience with retroperitoneal laparoscopic adrenalectomy for pheochromocytoma. *Journal of Urology*, **165**, 1871–4.

50. Toniato A, Piotto A, Pagetta C, Bernante P, Pelizzo MR (2001). Technique and results of laparoscopic adrenalectomy. *Langenbecks Archives of Surgery*, **386**, 200–3.

51. Tauzin-Fin P, Hilbert G, Krol-Houdek M, Gosse P, Maurette P (1999). Mydriasis and acute pulmonary oedema complicating laparoscopic removal of phaechromocytoma. *Anaesthesia and Intensive Care*, **27**, 646–9.

52. Sprung J, O'Hara JF, Gill IS, Abdelmalak B, Sarnaik A, Bravo EL (2000). Anesthetic aspects of laparoscopic and open adrenalectomy for pheochromocytoma. *Urology*, **55**, 339–43.

53. Sood J, Jayaraman L, Kumra VP, Chowbey PK (2006). Laparoscopic approach to pheochromocytoma: is a lower intraabdominal pressure helpful? *Anesthesia and Analgesia*, **102**, 637–41.

54. Davies MJ, McGlade DP, Banting SW (2004). A comparison of open and laparoscopic approaches to adrenalectomy in patients with phaeochromocytoma. *Anaesthesia and Intensive Care*, **32**, 224–9.

55. Levin H, Heifetz M (1990). Phaeochromocytoma and severe protracted postoperative hypoglycaemia. *Canadian Journal of Anaesthesia*, **37**, 477–8.

56. Kastelan D, Ravic KG, Cacic M, *et al.* (2007). Severe postoperative hypoglycemia in a patient with pheochromocytoma and preclinical Cushing's syndrome. *Medical Science Monitor*, **13**, CS34–7.

Chapter 9

Endocrine emergencies

PA Farling and JA Silversides

Introduction

Emergency situations involving the endocrine system are rare and may mimic other causes of life threatening cardiovascular collapse. However, if they are recognized and managed appropriately, the patient may survive without significant sequelae. The emergency management of pituitary apoplexy, thyroid storm, myxoedema coma, hyperparathyroid crisis, hypocalcaemia, adrenal insufficiency, phaeochromocytoma, hypoglycaemia, diabetic ketoacidosis, hyperglycaemic hyperosmolar state, and carcinoid are discussed in this chapter. These conditions have been mentioned in previous chapters, but collecting the principles of emergency management will simplify access to the information for clinicians involved in acute care. Successful management of endocrine emergencies requires a multidisciplinary approach including anaesthetists, endocrinologists, surgeons, accident and emergency specialists, and intensive care specialists.

Pituitary apoplexy

Overview

Apoplexy is an archaic term defined as unconsciousness or incapacity resulting from a stroke. Pituitary apoplexy is a rare clinical syndrome caused by sudden haemorrhage or infarction of the pituitary gland, generally within a pituitary adenoma.[1] Since an adenoma is invariably involved, the term *pituitary tumour apoplexy* is more correct.[2] The sudden increase in size of the contents of the sella turcica causes compression of surrounding structures, including the portal veins, giving rise to the classical signs and symptoms. There is significant morbidity and mortality and diagnosis may be delayed if the patient and clinicians are unaware of the underlying adenoma.

Simmonds' syndrome is the term for panhypopituitarism following trauma, vascular lesions, or tumour.[3] Clinical manifestations range from a relatively benign event to the catastrophic apoplectic situation.

Sheehan's syndrome, first described in 1937,[4] is a complication of pregnancy. It describes ischaemia of the anterior pituitary following major obstetric haemorrhage. Hypertrophy of lactotrophs during pregnancy results in enlargement of the pituitary. The anterior pituitary receives its blood supply via the portal venous system, which is a low-pressure system. Hence hypotension following haemorrhage causes ischaemia, necrosis, and reduced pituitary secretion.

Presentation

The classical presentation is a sudden severe headache, vomiting, visual impairment, and reduced function of the pituitary gland. Hypertension has been reported in 26% of cases,[5] and meningismus may be present. The visual disturbance comprises restriction of visual fields, deterioration of visual acuity, and weakness of ocular motility. These are due to displacement of the optic nerves and chiasma, and impingement upon the third, fourth, and sixth cranial nerves. There is often a rapid reduction in the level of consciousness that may complicate the diagnosis. This is due to either a mass effect of the expanded pituitary or to hydrocephalus. Signs of meningeal irritation due to extravasation of blood into the subarachnoid space are less common, but a case of pituitary apoplexy mimicking acute meningitis has been reported.[6]

Damage to the anterior pituitary leads to multiple acute hormonal deficiencies. Corticotrophic deficiency, leading to secondary adrenal failure, may be life threatening if untreated, and chronic deficiencies may result.

Pituitary apoplexy has been described following spinal anaesthesia,[7] angiography,[8] laparoscopic surgery,[9] pituitary function testing,[10] and liposuction.[11]

Diagnosis

The diagnosis is suspected by the typical clinical presentation, and confirmed by ophthalmic examination, imaging, and measurement of pituitary hormones. Computed tomography (CT) and magnetic resonance imaging (MRI) will show a pituitary tumour with haemorrhagic or necrotic components. CT is most useful in the acute setting, while MRI is useful for identifying blood components in the sub-acute setting (4 days to 1 month).[1] MRI correctly identified pituitary haemorrhage more often than CT and therefore is felt to be the imaging method of choice.[5] Catheter or MR angiography may be required to exclude an aneurysm.

Tests of hypothalamic and pituitary dysfunction will include thyroid-stimulating hormone (TSH), thyroxine (T_4), the insulin tolerance test for adrenocorticotrophic hormone, etc., and are best supervised by endocrinologists.

Management

Initial management of patients with pituitary tumour apoplexy includes administration of intravenous fluids and corticosteroids. Hydrocortisone treatment must always be initiated immediately at a dose of 50 mg every 6 hours. Subsequent management is controversial, as some authors advocate early trans-sphenoidal surgical decompression for all patients. Others chose to withhold surgery from patients with normal levels of consciousness and without visual field defects. The small number of patients makes it difficult to compare surgical and conservative management. Patient selection is critical, as urgent surgical decompression may save life and vision and will optimize the chance of regaining or maintaining pituitary function. Removal of the tumour will prevent any recurrence of apoplectic symptoms.

Outcome

Mortality from pituitary apoplexy reduced from 83% in 1950 to 6.7% in 1984 following the introduction of surgical intervention and improved medical care.[12] All patients presenting with pituitary apoplexy will require long-term follow-up to treat any residual tumour or pituitary dysfunction. Long-term replacement of corticosteroids, thyroxine, testosterone, and desmopressin may be required. Those patients who underwent transsphenoidal surgery within 8 days had complete restoration of visual acuity.[13,14]

Thyroid crisis (see also Chapter 4)

Overview

Thyrotoxic crisis, also known as thyroid storm, is a rare but life-threatening condition requiring immediate treatment, preferably in an intensive care unit. Thyroid storm is frequently mentioned in textbooks of anaesthesia, but is rarely seen now because of the widespread use of anti-thyroid drugs, such as carbimazole, and β-blockers. Its incidence is about 1–2% among patients with overt hyperthyroidism. A thyrotoxic crisis occurs predominantly in the elderly, and is three to five times more common in women than in men. The overall mortality is 10–20%.[15]

Presentation

The pathogenesis is not fully understood, but an increased sensitivity to catecholamines appears to be an important mechanism, and a number of endogenous and exogenous stress factors can provoke the onset of a thyrotoxic storm. It occurs in uncontrolled hyperthyroid patients as a result of a trigger such as surgery, infection, or trauma. Cases have been described following Caesarean section[16] and in a severely burned patient.[17]

Diagnosis

The diagnosis of a thyrotoxic crisis is made entirely on the clinical findings. It should be remembered that here is no difference in thyroid hormone levels between patients with uncomplicated thyrotoxicosis and those undergoing a thyroid storm.

Management

Medical treatment is based on three principles:

- counteracting the peripheral effects of thyroid hormones
- inhibition of thyroid hormone synthesis
- treating systemic complications.

These measures should bring about clinical improvement within 12–24 hours. Supportive management of thyroid crisis includes hydration, cooling, and inotropes. β-blockade (usually with propranolol) together with anti-thyroid drugs forms the first line of treatment. However, esmolol was successful in treating a child of 14 months who developed a thyroid crisis 3 hours after thyroidectomy.[18] An 85-year-old patient with multinodular goitre and severe thyrotoxicosis was also managed with esmolol.[19] However, it should be noted that a thyroid crisis has been reported during β-blockade.[20]

The administration of thionamides depends on the circumstances. As only oral forms are available, it may be difficult to administer these drugs in a disorientated and uncooperative patient and the placement of a nasogastric tube may be considered. However, many patients exhibiting a thyroid storm may already have lost their source of hormone (following thyroidectomy) or the source of excess TSH (e.g. following removal of the placenta in a pregnant patient). In such circumstances, thionamides would be of no value. Iodides may help in limiting thyroid hormone release, and intravenous contrast agents have been suggested as a valuable and reasonably safe source of intravenous iodine. Contrast agents have been described as causing thyroid crisis and are probably best given once anti-thyroid drugs have been administered. However, as the hormones have a relatively long half-life, the influence of any anti-thyroid medication will be significantly delayed, probably for several hours.

Sedation is frequently required, and intravenous chlorpromazine 5 mg is the drug of choice as it has good antipyretic and α-antagonistic actions in addition to excellent sedation.

An acute thyroid crisis on induction of anaesthesia, which was mistakenly diagnosed as malignant hyperthermia, was successfully treated with 1 mg/kg boluses of dantrolene.[21] Christensen and Nissen[22] reported the successful use of dantrolene to treat thyroid crisis in a child who had not responded to conventional measures. However, while dantrolene will effectively reduce temperature, it will not necessarily improve haemodynamic disturbances.

In situations of prolonged severe hyperthyroid crisis, plasmapheresis has been used to remove thyroid-binding globulins,[23] and cholestyramine can be administered orally as it binds thyroid hormone within the gastrointestinal tract.

Since thyroid hormones sensitize the adrenergic receptors to endogenous catecholamines, magnesium sulphate would seem to be, theoretically, a useful drug. Magnesium reduces the incidence and severity of dysrrhythmias due to catecholamines.

Malignant hyperthermia has occurred in a patient with Graves' disease during subtotal thyroidectomy.[24]

Outcome

Any delay in therapy (e.g. by awaiting additional laboratory results) must be strictly avoided because the mortality rate may rise to 75%. Thus early thyroidectomy should be considered as the treatment of choice if medical treatment fails to result in clinical improvement.

If death occurs following thyroid storm, it is most likely to be cardiopulmonary failure, particularly in the elderly.[15]

Myxoedema coma

Overview

Myxoedema coma is rare, appearing in 0.1% of cases of hypothyroidism.[25] It is a life-threatening clinical condition which can occur in a fully treated or a neglected hypothyroid patient. The incidence is greater in females than males (F:M ratio of 5–10:1) and mortality rates of up to 80% have been reported in the past. Patients exhibit disorientation, lethargy, and psychosis that may proceed to coma. It may be precipitated by infection, environmental exposure, trauma, other metabolic stresses, or certain drugs, particularly diuretics, sedatives and tranquillisers.

Diagnosis

The classical features include hypothermia, respiratory depression, and unconsciousness in a patient with known, or clinical evidence of, hypothyroidism. Thyroid function tests will show elevated TSH in primary hypothyroidism, but TSH may be normal or low if the hypothyroidism is secondary to pituitary failure. Free T_4 will be low and T_3 resin uptake will be increased, but these hormones only need to be measured if the diagnosis is in doubt. Hyponatraemia is common because of elevated levels of antidiuretic hormone. Blood glucose levels range from normal to low because of decreased gluconeogenesis and reduced insulin clearance. Hypoventilation will cause hypoxia and hypercapnia. A chest X-ray will be required, as chest infections and pericardial effusions may complicate myxoedema coma. Abdominal radiographic series may show an associated ileus. CT will rule out other causes of coma, including intracerebral haemorrhage.

Core temperature is likely to be reduced and ECG confirms bradycardia, low voltage, prolonged PR interval, T-wave abnormalities, and electrical alteration if an effusion is present.

Management

Treatment is contemporaneous with evaluation of other potential causes of coma. Intensive care admission will be required when mechanical ventilation is necessary. Passive rewarming, cautious plasma volume expansion, and correction of hypoglycaemia should be initiated. Aggressive rewarming may lead to vasodilatation and hypotension.

There is no consensus on the most appropriate form of thyroid hormone supplementation. Aggressive replacement with T_3 will result in abrupt increases in metabolism that may precipitate myocardial ischaemia,[26] but too conservative an approach is also associated with poor outcome. A starting dose of thyroxine 300–500 µg followed by 50–100 µg intravenously daily until the patient can take oral medication is currently recommended. If the response is poor, 10 µg of T_3 may be given intravenously every 4 hours with careful and continuous ECG monitoring until an adequate response is obtained.

Severe hyponatraemia will require hypertonic saline therapy—initially 200 mL of 2.7% saline as an intravenous bolus. The serum sodium should not increase by more than 12 mmol/L in a 24 hour period.

Blood glucose must be monitored frequently in these patients and intravenous dextrose given as required.

Adrenal insufficiency is commonly associated with thyroid failure, so patients with myxoedema coma should be treated with hydrocortisone 100 mg every 8 hours. The hydrocortisone dose is reduced as the patient's condition improves.

Sedatives and narcotics should be avoided, as reduced metabolism will lead to prolongation of their effects.

Outcome

Historically, the mortality from myxoedema coma had been as high as 80%, but early recognition and improved management has reduced it to 20–40%.[27] Predictors of outcome include increased age, cardiovascular compromise, and reduced consciousness.[28]

Follow-up is required to assess the recovery of thyroid and pituitary–adrenal function. Most patients will require lifelong thyroid hormone supplementation.

Parathyroid crisis (see also Chapter 5)

Overview

Parathyroid crisis (also known as acute hyperparathyroidism, parathyroid storm, and parathyrotoxicosis) is an uncommon endocrine emergency and represents an extreme manifestation of primary hyperparathyroidism with resultant severe and symptomatic hypercalcaemia. The anaesthetist may be involved in the management of these patients presenting for parathyroidectomy or other surgery, in the peripartum period, or in the intensive care unit.

Presentation

Although no consensus definition exists, parathyroid crisis is generally accepted as comprising the acute onset of signs and symptoms attributable to severe hypercalcaemia (usually >3.5 mmol/L) in association with biochemical evidence of hyperparathyroidism. It accounts for 1–6% of patients requiring parathyroidectomy, and is the most common cause of hypercalcaemic crisis.[29]

Signs and symptoms affect the nervous, gastrointestinal, renal, and cardiovascular systems, and are thought to arise from a combination of interference with cell signalling, abnormal calcium deposition, and dehydration. The majority of patients have some form of neurological disturbance, ranging from mild lethargy to coma and seizures. Generalized neuromuscular weakness is present in some cases. Accompanying this are gastrointestinal symptoms (usually nausea), anorexia, and dyspepsia, progressing to constipation, vomiting, and sometimes abdominal pain. Polyuria and polydypsia result from stimulation of the calcium-sensing receptor in the thick ascending limb of the loop of Henle, leading to inhibition of calcium, magnesium, sodium, and water reabsorption.[30] This results in severe dehydration and a fall in glomerular filtration rate (GFR) when thirst mechanisms fail, such as with decreased conscious level. Acute renal failure may also result from renal arterial vasoconstriction and from nephrolithiasis and nephrocalcinosis. When the GFR falls, calcium elimination is further reduced, leading to further rises in serum calcium. Severe dehydration is invariably present, although this may be masked by profound vaso-constriction, and indeed hypertension is common. Various electrocardiographic abnormalities have been described, including shortened QT interval and ST elevation mimicking myocardial infarction. Tachyarrhythmias, conduction defects, bradyarrhythmias, and asystole can all occur, and have been reported at induction of anaesthesia,[29] and the potential for cardiac glycoside toxicity is increased.

Patients with hypercalcaemia due to hyperparathyroidism are said to exist in a state of 'equilibrium hypercalcaemia' until there is a surge in parathyroid hormone (PTH) secretion or a fall in calcium excretion. Histological examination of excised parathyroid glands in patients with severe hypercalcaemia frequently reveals areas of recent haemorrhage or cystic changes, in keeping with an acute pathological event resulting in the release of large amounts of PTH. Extra-glandular conditions that have been implicated in the precipitation of parathyroid crises include vomiting and diarrhoea, acute renal failure (through the mechanisms described above), acute pancreatitis, thyrotoxicosis, malignancy, and commencement of thiazide diuretics.

The relationship between parathyroid crisis and acute pancreatitis is noteworthy. Several case series have confirmed a 25–34% incidence of pancreatitis in patients with parathyroid crisis,[31] although this remains a rare cause of pancreatitis. Possible mechanisms for the association include pancreatic duct obstruction due to deposition of calcium and excessive calcium-mediated trypsinogen activation. The resultant systemic inflammatory response with reduced GFR may result in reduced calcium elimination and thus an acute worsening of hypercalcaemic symptoms.

Although pregnancy confers protection against maternal parathyroid crisis due to active transport of calcium across the placenta, patients may develop hypercalcaemia due to hyperemesis gravidarum, or may present post-partum when this protective mechanism is lost.

Diagnosis and management

Emergency treatment of hypercalcaemia and life-threatening complications such as hypovolaemia must not be delayed by a search for the cause. Nevertheless, parathyroid crisis must be differentiated from other causes of severe hypercalcaemia (Table 9.1), most of which are associated with reduced levels of PTH. Severe hypercalcaemia (corrected for serum albumin concentration and preferably confirmed by measuring ionised calcium) is often associated with mild hypophosphataemia, hyperchloraemia and elevated alkaline phosphatase (ALP). The key investigation, however, is serum PTH level, which, if not suppressed in the presence of hypercalcaemia, is diagnostic of PTH-dependent hypercalcaemia.

Table 9.1 Causes of hypercalcaemia

PTH normal or elevated
Primary or tertiary hyperparathyroidism
Lithium-induced hyperparathyroidism
Familial hypocalciuric hypercalcaemia
PTH suppressed
Malignancy
Bony metastases
Multiple myeloma
Secretion of PTH-related peptide
Prolonged immobilization
Post-hypocalcaemic hypercalcaemia
Vitamin D excess
Intoxication
Granulomatous disease
Excess calcium intake
Iatrogenic (e.g. total parenteral nutrition))
Milk-alkali syndrome
Endocrine disorders
Adrenal insufficiency
Thyrotoxicosis
Acromegaly
Phaeochromocytoma

Familial hypocalciuric hypercalcaemia, although an important differential diagnosis in the asymptomatic or mildly symptomatic patient, is not associated with hypercalcaemic crisis. However, lithium-induced hyperparathyroidism may present acutely with parathyroid crisis, and usually resolves with cessation of lithium therapy and medical management of hypercalcaemia.

Causes of hyperparathyroidism in patients with parathyroid crisis are similar to those in patients with less severe hyperparathyroidism: benign hyperplasia, adenoma (which may be ectopic), parathyroid cyst, and carcinoma.

The principles of management are correction of volume depletion, increasing elimination of calcium, and surgical excision of diseased parathyroid glands. Large volumes of 0.9% saline should be given for rehydration, dilution of serum calcium, and calciuresis that is natriuresis dependent. Careful monitoring of volume status is required, and invasive monitoring may assist with fluid management. Once normal volume has been restored, the addition of a loop diuretic such as furosemide may promote further calciuresis by inhibiting sodium absorption (and thus passive calcium absorption) in the thick ascending limb of the loop of Henle. However, excessive use of furosemide, leading to hypovolaemia, may exacerbate calcium retention and must be avoided. Rehydration and promotion of calciuresis in this way may be expected to lower serum calcium by approximately 0.5 mmol/L over 24–48 hours. In contrast with loop diuretics, thiazides, amiloride, and carbonic anhydrase inhibitors all promote calcium absorption and must be discontinued in parathyroid crisis.

In the event of oliguric renal failure unresponsive to volume replacement, intermittent haemodialysis with a calcium-free dialysate can be used to lower calcium levels effectively. It must be noted that even in the absence of a low-calcium or calcium-free dialysate, the calcium concentration in standard dialysate fluid is lower than the serum concentration in parathyroid crisis and thus will tend to reduce serum calcium. Rebound hypercalcaemia between haemodialysis episodes is well known, and continuous venovenous haemodiafiltration with citrate anticoagulation to chelate calcium has been used successfully for control of calcium in this setting.

Bisphosphonates are a group of drugs that inhibit osteoclast function, thereby decreasing calcium mobilization due to bone resorption. Although most studies of bisphosphonate use for hypercalcaemia have been in the context of malignancy, they are widely accepted as being effective calcium-lowering agents in parathyroid crisis.[32] The most widely used regimen is intravenous pamidronate 60–90 mg infused over 2–4 hours, which can be expected to decrease serum calcium within 24 hours, although the newer drug zoledronate (4–8 mg infused over 5 minutes) may be more effective. Common side-effects of bisphosphonates include fever, anaemia, constipation, and dyspnoea. Renal failure can occur.

Calcitonin (given subcutaneously in a dose of 4 IU every 12 hours) is a less potent inhibitor of osteoclast function than the bisphosphonates; however, it has the advantage of a faster onset (12–24 hours), and in the emergency setting combination therapy is to be recommended.

The novel calcimimetic agent cinacalcet binds to the CaR, increasing sensitivity to circulating calcium and reducing PTH and calcium levels in patients with primary hyperparathyroidism. While neither studied specifically nor currently licensed in the UK for the emergency treatment of parathyroid crisis, cinacalcet has been demonstrated to produce a significant fall in serum calcium within 12–24 hours of the first dose (typically 30–90 mg every 12 hours) with an acceptable incidence of side-effects.[33]

Mithramycin, a chemotherapeutic drug with calcium-lowering effects which was at one time the mainstay of therapy, is no longer in common use because of its side-effect profile. The usefulness of gallium nitrate is limited by an unacceptably high incidence of renal failure. Intravenous phosphate infusions, while lowering serum calcium, are associated with precipitation of calcium phosphate complexes and organ damage, and should be used only for treatment of significant hypophosphataemia.

Patients should undergo continuous cardiac monitoring in view of the risk of sudden arrhythmias, and coexisting hypokalaemia should be corrected. The optimum pharmacological management of hypercalcaemia-associated tachyarrhythmias has not been determined, although verapamil has been used successfully in one small animal study, whereas amiodarone was associated with deterioration in one patient with coexisting cardiomyopathy. Bradyarrhythmias may not respond to atropine and pacing may be required, while successful defibrillation of hypercalcaemia-associated tachyarrhythmias has been reported.

With effective medical therapy now readily available, the need for emergency parathyroidectomy with associated high mortality rate is no longer present. Therefore parathyroidectomy should be delayed until dehydration has been treated and hypercalcaemia at least partially controlled. While bilateral neck exploration with intra-operative localization of parathyroid tissue remains normal practice, pre-operative localization of abnormal parathyroid tissue using a combination of ultrasound and scintigraphy may allow a less invasive unilateral approach.

Outcome

With recent developments in medical therapy, the mortality from this condition has fallen dramatically and death from parathyroid crisis is now rare. Surgical management provides long-term control of hyperparathyroidism and long-term survival can be expected.

Acute hypocalcaemia

Overview

Unlike chronic mild hypocalcaemia, acute symptomatic hypocalcaemia is unusual, but anaesthetists may encounter this emergency following parathyroidectomy, and in critical care units in the context of septic shock or severe pancreatitis.

Pathophysiology

Only a small proportion of the body's calcium stores is available as free ionized calcium. The majority is stored in bone, and even most of that transported in the blood is protein bound in a pH-dependent manner. Calcium levels are regulated by PTH and vitamin D. These normally respond to hypocalcaemia by increasing calcium absorption in renal and gastrointestinal tracts and stimulating osteoclast-mediated bone reabsorption.

Total calcium levels dependon albumin. Therefore serum calcium should be corrected for hypoalbuminaemia using the formula

$$[Ca]_{corr} = [Ca] + 0.02 \times (40\text{-albumin } [g/L]).$$

Ionized calcium falls when protein binding is increased, such as with respiratory alkalosis, catecholamines, glucagon, and growth hormone. Hypocalcaemia may also occur when levels of calcium-chelating agents increase. Examples of this are in hyperphosphataemia (renal failure, rhabdomyolysis, and tumour lysis syndrome), rapid phosphate supplementation, citrate administration in massive blood transfusion or as anticoagulation in continuous renal replacement therapy; or in severe acute pancreatitis and other critical illness, where free fatty acids form calcium complexes. Other causes of hypocalcaemia include vitamin D deficiency; hypomagnesaemia, leading to impaired PTH secretion and activity; and antiretroviral and antineoplastic drugs.

Peri-operatively, hypocalcaemia commonly occurs following parathyroidectomy and occasionally as a complication of thyroidectomy. Patients most at risk are those with chronic renal failure and secondary or tertiary hyperparathyroidism, and those with generalized parathyroid hyperplasia rather than adenoma, most likely reflecting the surgical procedure performed, as subtotal parathyroidectomy is used more commonly than localized resection in these groups. The mechanisms of hypocalcaemia are inadvertent removal, or damage to, all functional parathyroid tissue. Suppression of remaining normal glands may occur after removal of autonomous adenoma. The 'hungry bone syndrome' whereby bone, demineralized following long-term exposure to high levels of PTH, sequesters large amounts of calcium when the PTH level falls rapidly post-operatively. It has also been described following surgical or radio-iodine treatment of Graves' disease. A similar entity, 'hungry tumour syndrome', may occur due to osteoblastic metastases in prostate or breast carcinoma or chondrosarcoma.[34]

Presentation and investigation

The majority of symptoms and signs of severe hypocalcaemia relate to increased neuronal excitability. Peri-oral paraesthesiae, muscle cramps and hyper-reflexia may progress to muscle spasms, altered conscious level, seizures, and laryngeal spasm. Impaired myocardial contractility can lead to cardiac failure and hypotension; and conduction defects including prolongation of the QT interval may occur. Physical signs include Chvostek's sign (facial twitching in response to tapping over the facial nerve) and Trousseau's sign (carpal spasm in response to inflation of a blood pressure cuff for 3–5 minutes).

Investigation should include urgent serum calcium, phosphate, and albumin, ionized calcium, and alkaline phosphatase (ALP) and PTH levels. Depending on the clinical setting, magnesium, amylase, creatine kinase, urea, creatinine, and vitamin D levels may be helpful in identifying the cause of hypocalcaemia.

Post-operatively, hypoparathyroidism is associated with normal ALP and elevated serum phosphate levels, while hungry bone syndrome tends to cause low serum phosphate and elevated ALP levels.

Management

Treatment of hypocalcaemia will vary according to clinical and biochemical severity, with an ionized calcium level <0.8 mmol/L considered an indication for intravenous therapy even in the absence of symptoms. Where life-threatening complications are present, a bolus of 0.11 mmol/kg (children) or 2.25–4.5 mmol (adults) of 10% calcium gluconate or 10% calcium chloride may be given over 5–10 minutes and repeated as necessary, with ECG monitoring. The chloride solution contains approximately three times as much calcium per gram as the gluconate and thus is more immediately effective, but it should be given through a central vein as it may cause tissue necrosis if extravasation occurs.

Following the initial bolus, an infusion of intravenous calcium solution at 0.1–0.5 mmol/kg/hour should be titrated, ideally to the ionized calcium level. Sodium bicarbonate should not be given in the same line as precipitation will occur.

Most post-operative hypocalcaemia is mild, and treatment is with oral calcium salts. In some centres, oral calcium therapy is given routinely in the post-operative period.

Outcome

Post-operative hypocalcaemia is usually transient, lasting for 24–48 hours, although a minority of patients will require long-term therapy with calcium salts, vitamin D, and occasionally thiazide diuretics to promote calcium reabsorption.

Adrenal insufficiency (see also Chapter 7)

Overview

Adrenal insufficiency, also known as Addisonian crisis, is a rare disorder, but its prevalence is increasing.[35] The most frequent cause of primary adrenal insufficiency in Western countries is autoimmune adrenalitis. Other causes include tuberculosis, septicaemia, AIDS, haemorrhage, and tumours. Primary insufficiency involves a decrease in both glucocorticoid and mineralocorticoid activity. Secondary adrenal insufficiency is due to a lack of adrenocorticotrophic hormone because of suppression by exogenous steroids, hypopituitarism, or pituitary tumours, or following hypophysectomy.

Most crises occur in undiagnosed Addison's disease and failure to increase the steroid dose following infection or stress in patients on steroid replacement therapy. Occasionally, an acute adrenal insufficiency crisis can become a life-threatening condition because of acute interruption of a normal or hyperfunctioning adrenal or pituitary gland or a sudden interruption of adrenal replacement therapy (see Chapter 1).

Presentation

The clinical features of chronic adrenal insufficiency include weakness, fatigue, postural hypotension, nausea, vomiting, diarrhoea, weight loss, and hyperpigmentation. Hyperpigmentation occurs in areas of the skin not exposed to the sun because melanocyte-stimulating hormone shares the same precursor as adrenocorticotrophic hormone (ACTH). Classically, an Addisonian crisis presents as hypotension, hypoglycaemia, hyponatraemia, and hyperkalaemia in a patient with abdominal, leg, or back pain. Reduced production of aldosterone causes the hyponatraemia and hyperkalaemia and results in a metabolic acidosis as sodium reabsorption in the distal tubule of the kidney is linked with H^+ secretion.

Autoimmune adrenal disease may be associated with hypothyroidism and diabetes. Treatment with thyroxine may precipitate an adrenal crisis because hypothyroidism reduces cortisol clearance but thyroxine will stimulate metabolism and increase cortisol requirements.

The differential diagnoses include hypovolaemic shock and septic shock.

Diagnosis

Routine blood tests will show low sodium, high potassium, high calcium, and low blood glucose. Eosinophilia is reported in 20% of cases. Random cortisol levels will be low. In primary adrenal insufficiency ACTH levels will be high. In secondary adrenal insufficiency ACTH levels will be low. Aldosterone and renin levels may also be helpful. Ultrasound, CT, and MRI will be required depending on the cause of the adrenal problem.

Management

The initial treatment involves fluid replacement with 2–3 L of 0.9% saline and glucocorticoid replacement. Hydrocortisone 100 mg intravenously every 6 hours should commence immediately without waiting for synacthen testing.

   The chronic replacement dosage for patients with adrenal insufficiency should be as low as possible, with clear instructions for dosage adjustments in case of stress or acute emergencies.[36] Chronic glucocorticoid replacement consists of hydrocortisone 15–25 mg/day in divided doses and dose monitoring is largely based on clinical judgement. Fludrocortisone 0.05–0.2 mg/day is given for substitution in mineralocorticoid deficiency, aiming at normotension, normokalaemia, and a plasma renin activity in the upper normal range. It has recently been shown that, despite adequate glucocorticoid and mineralocorticoid replacement, well-being in patients with adrenal insufficiency is still impaired. Several studies have demonstrated that oral dehydroepiandosterone 25–50 mg/day may improve mood, fatigue, well-being, and, in women, sexuality, suggesting that dehydroepiandosterone should become part of the standard treatment regime. However, large phase III trials of dehydroepiandosterone for adrenal insufficiency are still lacking and it has not yet been approved for the treatment of this disease.

   Careful and repeated education of patients and their partners is the best strategy for avoiding adrenal crises. Patients with known adrenal insufficiency should carry steroid cards or MedicAlert® bracelets. Patients, and their relatives and general practitioners, should repeatedly receive verbal and written instructions on how to deal with physical and severe psychic stress. Early dose adjustments are required to cover the increased glucocorticoid demand in stress. For example, in minor illnesses the steroid dose should be doubled until the patient recovers and then the dose should be gradually reduced. Patients and their relatives can be taught how to use an emergency intramuscular injection of hydrocortisone.[37]

Phaeochromocytoma (see also Chapter 8)

Overview

Phaeochromocytoma is an example of a tumour of the amine precursor uptake and decarboxylation (APUD) cells. A hypertensive crisis in a patient with a phaeochromocytoma may present with a severe pounding headache, sweating, pallor, palpitations, and numbness or tingling. The onset may be sudden and can be precipitated by straining, exercise, pressure on the abdomen, angiography (particularly with older ionic contrast agents), and drugs such as anaesthetic agents. An episode can last from a few minutes to several hours, and may occur at various intervals from several times a day to less than once a month. It has been mistaken for malignant hyperthermia, as pyrexia and increased metabolic rate may form part of the syndrome.[38] Severe end-organ damage may occur, leading to multiple organ failure and death in a high proportion of cases, if diagnosis is delayed.[39–41]

Diagnosis

The differentiation of causes of hypertensive crises is difficult, but suspicion of secondary hypertension should always be raised if a hypertensive crisis occurs in a young person. Other endocrine causes include excesses of glucocorticoids, aldosterone, and renin. Non-endocrine causes include subarachnoid haemorrhage, acute glomerulonephritis, and eclampsia, and these require detailed clinical, biochemical, and radiological assessment. Severe hypertension has the potential to cause cerebrovascular, cardiovascular, renal, and eye damage.

Management

Urgent treatment is required to reduce the blood pressure in a progressive but controlled manner. The choice will depend upon the experience of the individual clinician. Endocrinologists may be more familiar with the use of intravenous α-blockers such as phenoxybenzamine 1 mg/kg infusion over 2 hours or phentolamine 1–5 mg increments. β-blockers may also be used, but must always be given after the α-blocker to prevent unopposed α-mediated vasoconstriction which may worsen the hypertension. Anaesthetists may prefer to use an infusion of sodium nitroprusside or nitroglycerin. These require intra-arterial monitoring of blood pressure to avoid rebound hypotension, and cyanide toxicity is an extremely rare complication of sodium nitroprusside. The use of magnesium has been discussed in Chapter 7 and it has proved valuable where other vasodilators have failed to control the hypertension.[42] It should probably be regarded as the first-line treatment for hypertensive crisis in obstetrics, as its safety for both mother and fetus is well established and it is an ideal first agent for most cases.

Following control of the hypertensive crisis, the patient will require referral for surgical excision of the phaeochromocytoma.

Hypoglycaemia

Overview

Normal blood glucose levels are between 4 and 10 mmol/L. Hence hypoglycaemia may be considered at a blood glucose of <3.9 mmol/L. Commonly, this occurs following an imbalance of insulin therapy in patients with diabetes mellitus or following the use of sulphonylurea. Rarer causes include insulinoma, breast and adrenal carcinoma, early pregnancy, prolonged fasting, and long periods of strenuous exercise, particularly when on β-blockers. Aspirin can induce hypoglycaemia in some children, and it occurs in chronic alcoholics and binge drinkers. Unripe ackee fruit from Jamaica produce hypogly-cin toxins.

Presentation

Symptoms of hypoglycaemia are caused by an autonomic disturbance or neuroglycope-nia. The autonomic symptoms tend to occur at a blood glucose level of around 3.3–3.6 mmol/L and neuroglycopenia at 2.6 mmol/L. Classical features include tachycar-dia, sweating, pallor, nausea, and light-headedness which may progress to confusion, altered behaviour, restlessness, loss of coordination, seizures, coma, and eventually death.

Many diabetic patients, particularly those with autonomic neuropathy, may develop a failure to recognize hypoglycaemic symptoms.

Management

Patients or their relatives manage most hypoglycaemic episodes by recognizing the early symptoms and taking appropriate action. Glucose tablets or gel may be used or the patient may ingest other sources of carbohydrate. Close monitoring of blood glucose and educa-tion are obviously important preventative measures. Patients who are unconscious should receive 50 mL of 50% dextrose intravenously. Response is often rapid; however, 50% dextrose is an irritant to peripheral veins. Glucagon 1 mg may be used followed by an infusion of 10% dextrose.

Insulinoma is a rare APUD tumour of the β-cells of the pancreas that secret insulin. Patients are often overweight, as they attempt to compensate for the hypoglycaemia. The diagnosis is made by a low fasting blood sugar (<2.2 mmol/L), increased insulin levels, increased C-peptide, and absence of sulphonylurea in the plasma. Medical man-agement includes the use of diazoxide, a benzothiazide that inhibits the release if insulin. Tumours are usually benign and intra-operative ultrasound may be required to localize them in the pancreas. Blood glucose is monitored peri-operatively and levels of C-peptide may be used to indicate complete resection.

Diabetic ketoacidosis

Overview

Diabetic ketoacidosis (DKA) is a common life-threatening emergency which may occur in the peri-operative period and/or necessitate treatment in a critical care unit. DKA is characterized by hyperglycaemia, ketosis, and metabolic acidosis with severe dehydra-tion. The rate of hospital admission for DKA continues to rise despite advances in diabetes care, largely because of the increasing prevalence of diabetes.[43]

Pathophysiology

Insulin is essential for the uptake and utilization of carbohydrate, fat, and protein in liver, muscle and adipose tissue. Absolute or relative deficiency, together with an excess of insulin counter-regulatory hormones (ICRHs) such as catecholamines, glucagon, growth hormone and cortisol, leads to a profoundly catabolic state similar to that occurring in starvation. Glucagon stimulates hepatic glycogenolysis and gluconeogenesis, causing hyperglycaemia which is exacerbated by failure of uptake and utilization of glucose by peripheral tissues due to insulin deficiency.[44]

In the liver and adipose tissue, catecholamine-mediated lipolysis liberates free fatty acids (FFAs) and glycerol and provides substrate for oxidation and further gluconeogenesis, respectively. This process also results in the formation of very-low-density lipoprotein, manifesting as hypertriglyceridaemia. Oxidation of accumulated FFAs produces acetyl coenzyme A (acetyl CoA), which, instead of entering the citric acid cycle or being converted to malonyl CoA (the first step in lipogenesis), is diverted to form the ketone bodies aceto-acetyl CoA, β-hydroxybutyrate, and acetoacetone. These are weak acids which dissociate at physiological pH, leading to a raised hydrogen ion load and a high anion gap metabolic acidosis.

Protein metabolism is also altered as part of the decreased insulin-to-glucagon ratio, with proteolysis occurring in muscle cells to release free amino acids which act as the major substrate for gluconeogenesis.

Lipolysis is associated with production of vasodilatory prostaglandins, which have been linked to the nausea, vomiting, and abdominal pain which are frequent symptoms of DKA.

A number of mechanisms contribute to the severe dehydration present in DKA. The renal transfer maximum for glucose is approximately 11 mmol/L. When plasma glucose concentration exceeds this threshold, reabsorption is inadequate to prevent glycosuria, leading to an osmotic diuresis and natriuresis. Ketone bodies are also osmotically active, and their concentration in DKA exceeds the tubular capacity for reabsorption, contributing to osmotic diuresis. Insulin deficiency itself further reduces tubular reabsorption of water, sodium, and potassium.

Because of the reduced ability of glucose to enter cells, together with increased gluconeogenesis, the extracellular compartment becomes hypertonic, driving water from the intracellular compartment, so that dehydration is both intra- and extracellular. This is one reason for the paradoxical occurrence of hyponatraemia despite large-volume free water loss; the other reasons is severe hyperlipidaemia and 'pseudo-hyponatraemia'.

Urinary sodium excretion is low relative to water excretion, in part because of secondary hyperaldosteronism, which also contributes to excessive urinary potassium loss. The typical potassium deficit has been reported to be in the range 5–10 mmol/kg body weight. Despite this, serum potassium concentration may be elevated because of movement of potassium from intracellular to extracellular compartments. Contributory factors to this potassium shift include acidosis and insulin deficiency.

In summary, deficiency of insulin together with increased levels of ICRHs lead to a state of hyperglycaemia, ketosis, and metabolic acidosis, together with intracellular and extracellular dehydration and electrolyte depletion (Table 9.2).

Table 9.2 Typical body deficits in diabetic ketoacidosis and hyperglycaemic hyperosmolar state

	DKA	HHS
Total water (L)	6	9
Water (mL/kg)	100	100–200
Na^+ (mmol/kg)	7–10	5–13
Cl^- (mmol/kg)	3–5	5–15
K^+ (mmol/kg)	3–5	4–6
PO_4 (mmol/kg)	5–7	3–7
Mg^{2+} (mmol/kg)	2–4	2–4
Ca^{2+} (mmol/kg)	2–4	2–4

© 2004 American Diabetes Association. From *Diabetes Care*, Vol. **27**, 2004; S94–S102. Reprinted with permission from The American Diabetes Association.

Presentation

DKA may occur as the first manifestation of type 1 diabetes mellitus (DM), but more commonly its occurrence is precipitated in known diabetic patients by omission or inadequate use of insulin, or by a physiological stressor such as infection. It may also occur in type 2 DM, although this is relatively unusual. Euglycaemic DKA is a rare entity and appears to occur in the setting of prolonged deficiency of carbohydrate intake and depletion of hepatic glycogen stores.[45]

Infection is the most common precipitant of DKA, with respiratory and urinary tracts the most common sites. Seemingly minor skin and peri-anal infections, to which diabetic patients are prone, and intra-abdominal pathology, such as appendicitis, may also precipitate DKA. Other precipitants include myocardial infarction, trauma, pregnancy, acute pancreatitis, surgery, catecholamine excess, and drugs with a hyperglycaemic effect, such as glucocorticoids and thiazides.[46]

Symptoms of DKA typically develop over hours or days and are those of diabetes mellitus: polyuria, polydipsia, and lethargy, together with those of the precipitating event. Gastrointestinal symptoms are usually limited to nausea and vomiting, but abdominal pain and distension, reflecting paralytic ileus, may occur. On examination, patients are clinically dehydrated, may be haemodynamically unstable, and may exhibit abnormal neurological signs including headache, abnormal tendon reflexes, and cranial nerve deficits, drowsiness, or coma. Decreased conscious level correlates with elevated serum osmolality and lower pH,[47] but may also reflect the presence of cerebral oedema. Abnormal respiratory patterns are common and range from rapid shallow breathing to the classical deep slow ventilatory pattern (Kussmaul's respiration) associated with partial respiratory compensation for metabolic acidosis. A distinctive odour of acetone may be detectable.

Investigations and diagnosis

Investigations should be aimed at establishing the diagnosis and identifying an underlying cause. The diagnosis can usually be made with point-of-care testing of capillary blood

Table 9.3 Diagnostic criteria for diabetic ketoacidosis and hyperglycaemic hyperosmolar state

	DKA			HHS
	Mild	**Moderate**	**Severe**	
Plasma glucose (mmol/L)	>14	>14	>14	>33
Arterial pH	7.25–7.30	7.0–7.24	<7.0	>7.3
Serum bicarbonate (mmol/L)	15–18	10–15	<10	>15
Urinary ketones	Positive	Positive	Positive	Small
Serum ketones	Positive	Positive	Positive	Small
Effective serum osmolality (mOsm/kg)	Variable	Variable	Variable	>320
Anion gap	>10	>12	>12	Variable
Alteration in mental status	Alert	Alert/drowsy	Stupor/coma	Stupor/coma

(c) 2004 American Diabetes Association. From *Diabetes Care*, Vol. **27**, 2004; S94–S102. Reprinted with permission from The American Diabetes Association.

glucose, arterial blood gas analysis, and dipstick urinalysis to confirm the presence of hyperglycaemia (blood glucose typically >17 mmol/L), metabolic acidosis (pH <7.3), and ketonuria (++ or more). The diagnostic criteria given in Table 9.3 are widely used.[48] The principle differential diagnoses are starvation ketosis, which results from prolonged deficiency of carbohydrate intake, and alcoholic ketoacidosis which is associated with vomiting after a recent ethanol binge on a background of poor carbohydrate intake.[49] Blood glucose is usually low or normal in both these conditions. Laboratory investigations should include urea, creatinine and electrolyte concentrations; haematocrit; leucocyte count and differential cell count; laboratory blood glucose; and serum osmolality. Other investigations should focus on a search for infection or other precipitant, and may include cultures of blood, sputum, urine, or other specimens, other microbiological tests, electrocardiography, troponin, and chest radiograph or other imaging as dictated by the clinical picture.

In addition to the criteria for diagnosis, other common laboratory abnormalities include leucocytosis, which is common even in the absence of infection, hyperamylasaemia, which rarely results from pancreatitis in this setting, hypophosphataemia, hypomagnesaemia, hyperlipidaemia, and hyponatraemia, as discussed above. Sodium concentration should be corrected for the degree of hyperglycaemia using the formula

$$[Na]_{corr} = [Na] + \{0.44 \times ([Glu] - 5.5)\}.$$

The detection of ketone bodies in urine relies on the reaction of ketones with nitroprusside, which gives a positive result with acetoacetate and acetone, but does not react with β-hydroxybutyrate, the predominant ketoacid in DKA. Point-of-care testing of capillary β-hydroxybutyrate levels has been developed, with levels >3 mmol/L strongly correlated with acidosis, and this appears to be a more useful test for following the response to therapy.

Cerebral oedema in DKA

The most feared complication of DKA is cerebral oedema which occurs in <1% of children treated for DKA and even more rarely in adults, and has a mortality rate of 20–50%.[50] Although uncommon, it is noteworthy for being widely regarded as a consequence of therapy, and fear of precipitating cerebral oedema has been a major consideration in the development of treatment guidelines.[48]

The pathophysiology is poorly understood. It is hypothesized that insulin therapy, together with infusion of large volumes of hypotonic fluid, results in a rapid increase in brain cell volume manifesting as cerebral oedema and eventual brain herniation. The evidence for this relies largely on observed associations between cerebral oedema and an attenuated rise in plasma sodium concentrations with rehydration, thought by some to result from excess free water load. While these associations appear fairly consistent, no consistent association with the rate or type of fluid administered has been demonstrated.[50] The largest study to date (61 cases of cerebral oedema in 6977 cases of DKA) identified the following risk factors for cerebral oedema:[51]

- higher blood urea nitrogen concentration, reflecting a greater degree of dehydration
- lower partial pressure of carbon dioxide, reflecting hyperventilation in response to metabolic acidosis
- lower rate of increase in plasma sodium concentration
- use of bicarbonate therapy for acidosis.

The significance of the association between lack of increase in plasma sodium concentration and cerebral oedema is not easy to determine. It has been suggested that, rather than being a function of administered fluid, this may reflect excess endogenous antidiuretic hormone activity or cerebral salt-wasting in patients with cerebral oedema, and remains an association rather than a proven causative factor.

Evidence against the influence of fluid administration in precipitating DKA includes radiological evidence of subclinical cerebral oedema in many DKA patients before commencement of therapy. There is also evidence of cerebral vasoconstriction in association with hypocapnia and reduced cerebral blood flow with brain ischaemia and subsequent reperfusion injury leading to cytotoxic oedema.

Overall, current evidence points to the most severe DKA patients being at highest risk of cerebral oedema, with a fall in or lower rate of rise in plasma sodium as an association, and the use of bicarbonate as a possible risk factor. While the mechanisms are unclear, current consensus is to minimize fluid shifts by controlled rehydration and fall in effective serum osmolality.

Management

The key aspects of management are fluid resuscitation and rehydration, insulin therapy, replacement of electrolyte losses, and treatment of any precipitating infection.

The optimal rate and type of fluid for rehydration in DKA remains controversial, with persistent concerns that cerebral, pulmonary, and interstitial oedema may be precipitated by use of the 'wrong' fluid or by an overly rapid rate of administration and decline in effective serum osmolality.[47] As discussed, the fluid loss is both intra- and extracellular, and the majority of patients with DKA present with only mild hypoperfusion. The most obvious solution is to choose the fluid which most closely approximates the deficit—this is 0.45% saline. However, this is inefficient for expansion of the intravascular compartment and restoration of tissue perfusion, and enough concern persists with regard to hypotonic fluids and cerebral oedema that its use is usually reserved for replacement of total deficit once perfusion has been restored. For resuscitation purposes, 0.9% saline is the most widely used fluid, with colloids and Hartmann's solution as possible alternatives. There is no evidence in favour of one fluid or the other; proponents of colloids argue that the lower volume required lowers the risk of oedema, while Hartmann's solution carries less risk of the hyperchloraemic acidosis which frequently complicates fluid resuscitation.[52] Following restoration of tissue perfusion, which usually requires only 10–20 mL/kg (1–2 L in the typical adult), a more gradual replacement of the total deficit, typically 5–10 L in adults or 7–10% body weight in children, is required, usually over 24–48 hours. The fluid used for this will depend on measurement of serum electrolytes, but 0.9% saline and 0.45% saline are frequently used, guided by the plasma sodium concentration.[48] Osmotic diuresis will continue until hyperglycaemia resolves, so ongoing fluid losses must be taken into account when determining the rate of fluid administration.

Once blood glucose levels are below 12 mmol/L, it is usual to switch to 5% dextrose (in adults) or 0.45% saline with 5% dextrose (in children) as the rehydration fluid, both to lessen the risk of hypoglycaemia and to reduce the rate of fall in effective serum osmolality and associated theoretical risk of cerebral oedema.[48]

Intravenous insulin replacement is required for treatment of hyperglycaemia and clearance of ketones. Typically, an infusion of short-acting insulin is commenced at 0.1 IU/kg/hour and adjusted according to the rate of change in plasma glucose concentrations, aiming for a fall of 2.5–4 mmol/L/hour. There appears to be no advantage in an initial bolus of insulin provided that an infusion can be started without excessive delay.[53] Intravenous insulin by infusion should normally be continued until ketoacidosis is resolved and the patient is able to eat and drink normally, at which point the patient's regular regime may be restarted or a suitable regime commenced. However, in the peri-operative or critical care setting, it may be necessary to continue until after surgery and/or recovery of gut function. Subcutaneous or intramuscular administration of short-acting insulin, titrated against hourly measurements of blood glucose, is an alternative option, although it is not recommended where perfusion is compromised and absorption is unpredictable.

Replacement of the potassium deficit will be necessary, although the timing may vary. The initial potassium concentration may be high, normal, or low, but will always fall with correction of acidosis and administration of insulin. For this reason, if hypokalaemia is present initially, replacement should commence prior to administration of insulin. If hyperkalaemia is present, replacement should be delayed until a downward trend has been observed. A typical regime is to add 20–40 mmol of potassium to each litre of fluid, depending on the serum potassium concentration.

Replacement of other electrolytes, specifically phosphate and magnesium, is more controversial. While phosphate deficiency is invariably present, and is frequently associated with depletion of 2,3-diphosphoglycerate and left shift of the oxyhaemoglobin dissociation curve, routine replacement has not been associated with clinical benefit. Therefore replacement is usually undertaken only when hypophosphataemia is moderate to severe (<0.3–0.5 mmol/L) or in the presence of impending or actual cardiac or respiratory failure.[48] If needed, 10–20 mmol of phosphate in the form of dipotassium hydrogen phosphate may be added to intravenous fluids or given as an infusion through a central venous catheter over several hours; alternatively, enteral supplementation may be used. Similarly, routine magnesium replacement has not been demonstrated to be of benefit, but may be worthwhile if deficiency is severe or arrhythmias are present.

The use of bicarbonate for treatment of severe acidosis is controversial, as it is associated with hypokalaemia and overshoot alkalosis, and routine use at pH 6.9–7.1 has shown no benefit. The rationale for the use of bicarbonate is that low pH is associated with inhibition of the enzyme phosphofructokinase, which is essential for glycolysis and glucose utilization, and impairment of myocardial contractility. However, both these assertions have been challenged, and even if they are correct, there is no evidence that bicarbonate therapy is effective in reversing them.[52] Indeed, bicarbonate has been demonstrated to worsen intracellular acidosis in some settings. The routine use of bicarbonate cannot be recommended, but many clinicians still consider its use at pH <6.9, particularly if haemodynamic instability is present.

Most patients with DKA do not require critical care; those who do are the most severely affected and those with complex precipitating factors. Therefore invasive haemodynamic monitoring is not needed routinely, although it may be useful for regular blood sampling. Electrocardiographic monitoring may be useful in severe hyper- or hypokalaemia, and continuous pulse oximetry should be used if respiratory infection or pulmonary oedema is present. The most critical aspects of monitoring are regular clinical assessment and blood sampling for glucose, electrolytes, and venous or arterial blood gases.

Mechanical ventilation in DKA, although rarely required, poses a difficult question. What level of carbon dioxide should be targeted—normocarbia or compensatory hypocarbia for metabolic acidosis? There is little evidence on which to base an answer, although it is argued that aiming for partially compensatory hypocarbia and allowing the carbon dioxide level to rise slowly, with correction of the metabolic acidosis, is physiologically sound. This will also avoid the risk of reactive hyperaemia associated with sudden correction of CO_2-mediated cerebral vasoconstriction.

Where surgery is required in the setting of DKA, the correct timing is important. While surgical treatment of infection may be required for longer-term glucose control, it is preferable to ensure fluid resuscitation and correction of acidosis prior to surgery if possible.

Outcome

Complications of DKA are rare and mortality is now <5%.[43] As discussed above, cerebral oedema is the most serious complication and requires prompt treatment with mechanical ventilation for carbon dioxide control and osmotherapy with mannitol and/or hypertonic saline. Other complications include hyperchloraemia, which results from large-volume infusions of saline and may account for slow resolution of metabolic acidosis, gastrointestinal haemorrhage, rhabdomyolysis, and venous thromboembolism. Treatment for these is along conventional lines.

Hyperglycaemic hyperosmolar state

Hyperglycaemic hyperosmolar state (HHS), previously known as hyperosmolar non-ketotic coma (HONK), is much less common than diabetic ketoacidosis, but it carries a higher mortality and, like DKA, may present in the peri-operative period or require treatment in a critical care unit.

Pathophysiology

As with DKA, the development of HHS is the result of insulin deficiency and increase in ICRHs, usually in the context of an acute precipitant such as infection.

However, in contrast with DKA, insulin deficiency in HHS is relative and not absolute, in keeping with the insulin resistance encountered in type 2 DM. The minimal persisting effect of insulin, while insufficient to prevent glycogenolysis, gluconeogenesis, and therefore hyperglycaemia, appears to be sufficient to prevent lipolysis and production of ketoacids. There is also evidence that ICRH levels, although elevated, are not as high as in DKA, and that the hyperosmolar state produced by hyperglycaemia and water loss through osmotic diuresis inhibits lipolysis and ketoacid generation. Renal impairment is an important factor, since the markedly elevated glucose levels seen in HHS (up to 100 mmol/L) do not occur unless renal perfusion declines and the 'safety valve' of urinary glucose loss fails.

Therefore the predominant pathological features of HHS relate to hyperglycaemia, osmotic diuresis, and resultant electrolyte depletion, often exacerbated by inability to drink enough free water to replace urinary losses.

Presentation

Patients with HHS are predominantly elderly, usually with known type 2 diabetes, and often limited in their ability to drink sufficient water to replace urinary losses, leading to a slow increase in osmolality and decline in neurological status. For this reason, patients in nursing homes and those hospitalized and kept fasting peri-operatively are at particular risk. However, the increasing prevalence of type 2 diabetes in children and adolescents has led to reports of HHS as the presenting feature of childhood DM, and it may also occur in association with type 1 diabetes mellitus.

The list of reported precipitants for HHS is extensive, but poor compliance with insulin therapy, or essentially any physiological stressor, may increase levels of stress hormones and precipitate hyperglycaemia in a patient with insulin resistance, resulting in HHS. Examples include infection, surgery, trauma, dialysis, and stroke. Similarly, many drugs have been associated with HHS, mainly hyperglycaemic agents and diuretics; they include glucocorticoids, thiazides, β-blockers, immunosuppressants, lithium, and neuroleptics.[49]

Dehydration develops slowly, usually over days or even weeks, with a history of increasing polyuria and polydipsia, often with symptoms of a precipitating event such as respiratory or urinary tract infection. Examination reveals profound dehydration, although usually without major haemodynamic instability. Tachycardia and low-grade pyrexia may be present, but the hyperventilation of DKA is absent. By the time of presentation, glomerular filtration may have fallen sufficiently that urinary output is minimal.

Neurological deficits are common, with alterations in conscious level ranging from mild drowsiness to coma, closely related to serum osmolality.[54] Seizures, motor deficits, abnormal reflexes, sensory defects, and behavioural disturbances may all occur and are closely related to serum osmolality. Gastroparesis commonly results in nausea and vomiting, but the presence of abdominal pain should prompt a search for intercurrent pathology.

Investigations and diagnosis

Laboratory findings are those of hyperglycaemia, typically with blood glucose levels <35 mmol/L and occasionally up to 100 mmol/L. There is elevated serum osmolality, greater than 320 mOsm/kg and occasionally as high as 400 mOsm/kg, reflecting hyperglycaemia and a water deficit of up to 25% (8–12 L in a 70-kg adult). Measured serum sodium is usually high, despite a low total body sodium. This is attributable mainly to movement of water from intra- to extracellular compartments and dilution of sodium in extracellular fluid. Various formulae attempt to produce a corrected sodium level for the degree of hyperglycaemia: one such formula adds 1 mmol/L sodium to the measured value for each 2.3 mmol/L elevation in glucose above normal.[55]

Although a mild ketosis or hypoperfusion-related lactic acidosis may exist, the severe metabolic acidosis that is characteristic of DKA is notably absent.

Plasma potassium concentration may be low, normal, or high, but again there is invariably a large intracellular deficit and levels will fall with insulin therapy. Similarly, phosphate and magnesium levels are usually decreased and fall further with insulin administration. Urea and creatinine are invariably elevated, in keeping with pre-renal or renal insufficiency with an increased urea-to-creatinine ratio.

Other laboratory abnormalities include hyperlipidaemia, which may contribute to pseudo-hyponatraemia, hyperamylasaemia, and falsely elevated protein, haematocrit, and bilirubin levels due to a concentration effect. As in DKA, leucocytosis is common and not specific for the presence of infection. Further investigations such as ECG and imaging may be necessary to uncover a precipitating cause of HHS.

Management

The main aspects of management are fluid resuscitation and rehydration, insulin therapy, and replacement of electrolyte deficits.

Resuscitation is likely to include administration of rapid fluid boluses, initially for the restoration of tissue perfusion. A need for critical care in patients with HHS is unusual, but aspects of supportive care may occasionally include intubation and ventilation in the comatose patient. Arterial, and occasionally central venous, access for monitoring of fluid therapy may be required. There may be a need for renal replacement therapy if volume replacement is insufficient to restore adequate renal function.

Boluses of 0.9% saline are generally used for resuscitation purposes, remembering that this is hypotonic relative to plasma. Once adequate intravascular volume has been restored, usually after 10–20 mL/kg (1–2 L in an average adult), attention should be paid to careful correction of the intra- and extracellular fluid deficit, sodium concentration, and serum osmolality. The general consensus is that the deficit should be replaced over 36–48 hours.[48] This balances the need for rehydration with the risks of cerebral oedema (in younger, mainly paediatric, patients), pulmonary oedema, and central pontine myelinolysis attributed to rapid fluid and sodium flux.

The optimum fluid replacement strategy beyond the fluid resuscitation stage is controversial. The perceived advantage of 0.9% saline is a more gradual fall in sodium levels and effective serum osmolality, while 0.45% saline more closely approximates the fluid and electrolyte deficit, and is less closely associated with hypernatraemia and hyperchloraemic acidosis. Hartmann's solution may represent a useful compromise. American Diabetes Association guidelines recommend the use of 0.9% saline for resuscitation, followed by 0.45% saline if corrected plasma sodium is normal or high, or continued use of 0.9% saline if corrected plasma sodium is low.[48] Regardless of the fluid used, frequent clinical and laboratory evaluation with adjustment to prevent overly rapid changes in sodium concentration and effective serum osmolality (measured serum osmolality minus urea concentration) is crucial to minimize the risk of iatrogenic complications. A rate of decline in effective serum osmolality no greater than 3 mOsm/kg/hour has been suggested as a target.[48] The rate of fluid administration required is typically 4–14 mL/kg/hour, and should be adjusted according to clinical and haemodynamic parameters.

Potassium should be added to intravenous fluids once renal function is established and serum concentrations are known. Typically 20–40 mmol potassium, in the form of KCl or K_2HPO_4, per 1000 mL fluid is required as serum levels fall with insulin administration.

Insulin therapy should be commenced only when rehydration is under way and serum potassium is within or above normal limits, because of the potential for water and potassium movement into cells, resulting in further intravascular depletion and worsening hypokalaemia, respectively. Typically, an intravenous insulin infusion of 0.1 IU/kg/hour will lower plasma glucose by 2.5–4 mmol/L/hour, which is an acceptable rate of decline.[56] Failure of insulin levels to fall at this rate should prompt reassessment of insulin delivery and adequacy of hydration, since restoration of adequate renal perfusion will usually increase urinary glucose loss and produce a fall in serum glucose even before insulin has commenced. Once serum glucose has fallen to around 15 mmol/L, the infusion rate may be halved to 0.05 IU/kg/hour and 5% dextrose added to intravenous fluids to allow a more gradual decline in serum glucose, and thus osmolality, and to prevent hypoglycaemia.

There are no studies on management of the hypophosphataemia that invariably accompanies HHS. Extrapolation from studies of DKA suggest that routine replacement is not associated with detectable clinical benefit. However, most authorities suggest phosphate replacement in moderately severe hypophosphataemia if cardiac or respiratory failure is present or in the presence of muscular weakness. Similarly, magnesium concentrations should be checked and magnesium replaced if severe hypomagnesaemia is present or in the setting of cardiac arrhythmias.

Treatment of any precipitant is essential. Most commonly this takes the form of treating infection with antibiotics, but occasionally surgical intervention is required. Surgery for any reason should ideally be delayed until hypovolaemia has been treated and hyperglycaemia and hyperosmolarity have resolved.

Because of the hyperosmolar state and increased blood viscosity and thrombotic risk, prophylactic low molecular weight heparin should be given early in the course of treatment.

Complications and outcome

Complications of HHS include venous and arterial thrombosis, leading to stroke, myocardial infarction, mesenteric infarction, and deep venous thrombosis. Rhabdomyolysis is a recognized complication, and a malignant-hyperthermia-like syndrome of pyrexia, rhabdomyolysis, and cardiovascular instability has been reported in several patients. Dantrolene may be of benefit in this extremely rare situation. Acute renal failure, cerebral oedema, non-cardiogenic pulmonary oedema, and multi-organ failure may occur. Hypoglycaemia and central pontine myelinolysis are related to treatment and are largely preventable with careful monitoring of clinical and laboratory parameters.

Overall mortality for HHS is of the order of 15%, considerably higher than that for DKA, reflecting the higher average age and increased comorbidities of those affected. However, the majority of patients will recover with no sequelae.

Carcinoid crisis (see also Chapter 6)

Overview

Carcinoid is an APUD tumour derived from argentaffin cells. Vasoactive peptides, including serotonin, bradykinin histamine, and prostaglandins, are produced which have dramatic effects when secreted into the systemic circulation. A carcinoid crisis is the result of a massive outpouring of these vasoactive peptides.

Carcinoids are usually found in the gastrointestinal tract, and hence hepatic metastases or a primary in an area not drained by the portal venous system are required to produce the carcinoid syndrome and crisis.

Presentation

Flushing, diarrhoea, and bronchospasm are classical features, and hypotension, hypertension, tachycardia, and hyperglycaemia may occur. A crisis is distinguished from a severe episode of the carcinoid syndrome by the sudden and violent onset of different symptoms at once. Crises are precipitated by endogenous or exogenous catecholamines, so anxiety and various forms of stress have been implicated. Mechanical stimulation of the tumour, hypotension, hypertension, hypercapnia, and hypothermia have all been reported as triggers of a crisis. Histamine-releasing drugs such as morphine should be avoided. A catecholamine tracer ($[^{18}F]$DOPA) used in PET scanning precipitated a crisis in a patient with metastatic carcinoid tumour.[57] A crisis following administration of a drug can be mistaken for an anaphylactic reaction.

Diagnosis

Serotonin and its metabolites (5-hydroxy-indole acetic acid 5-HIAA)) are raised, while tryptophan is reduced.

Management

Octreotide prevents the release of mediators and is used for long-term maintenance therapy. It should also be administered as premedication and may be given at induction of anaesthesia; increments of 100–500 µg should be used for intra-operative episodes of hypotension.

Ketanserin (10 mg bolus intravenously) blocks the actions of mediators and decreases central sympathetic outflow.[58]

Labetalol and esmolol may be used to control hypertension.

The use of inotropes, containing catecholamines, to manage episodes of hypotension may be counter-productive as they stimulate further serotonin secretion. A death occurred following fine-needle biopsy of hepatic metastases when adrenaline and dopamine were used to resuscitate a patient who had a carcinoid crisis.[59] However, there have been no reports of this occurring following the use of octreotide, and the risk is probably justified in patients where catecholamines are thought necessary to control resistant hypotension or bronchospasm. Nevertheless, volume replacement and octreotide should be the first line of treatment of hypotension.

Patients undergoing cardiac surgery for carcinoid valve disease have been given adrenaline to wean them from bypass when myocardial function was poor, but this is done in the presence of an octreotide infusion.[60]

Summary

Endocrine emergencies are rare, but increased awareness and understanding of pathophysiology combined with improved diagnosis and management have decreased the mortality associated with these conditions.

Key clinical management points

Pituitary apoplexy

Diagnosis

- ◆ Clinical presentation
  - Sudden onset of headache with hypertension and meningismus

Key clinical management points (continued)

- Fundoscopy
- CT/MRI for pituitary haemorrhage

Management

- Fluid resuscitation and corticosteroids
  - Hydrocortisone initiated immediately at a dose of 50 mg every 6 hours
- Consider surgical decompression

Thyroid crisis

Diagnosis

- Suspect thyroid crisis on clinical grounds in a patient with a history of previous thyroid disease

Diagnostic tests (do not delay treatment while waiting for results)

- TSH (should be low)
- T_4 and T_3 for confirmation only

Immediate management

- Oxygen
- β-blockade
  - Propranolol 100 mg by slow intravenous injection
  - Esmolol 1–2 mg/kg intravenously followed by an infusion titrated against symptoms
- Anti-thyroid drugs (not to be used if source of hormone is removed)
  - Propylthiouracil 200 mg orally
  - Carbimazole 30 mg orally
- Intravenous fluid
  - Establish good intravenous access
    - Cold Ringer's lactate 1 L rapidly; further fluids in response to clinical signs
    - Consider added dextrose if blood sugar falls
- Sedation
  - Chlorpromazine 5 mg intravenously repeated as necessary to maximum of 50 mg
- Surface cooling
- Supportive therapy as indicated
- Further management

Key clinical management points (continued)

- Intravenous iodine
  - Iopanoic acid 500 mg four times a day
  - Potassium iodide solution
- Removal of hormone
  - Cholestyramine orally
  - Plasmapheresis
- Plan thyroidectomy where appropriate

Myxoedema coma

Diagnosis

Suspect myxoedema on clinical grounds in older patients especially where there is a prior history of treated hyperthyroidism.

Diagnostic tests (do not delay treatment while waiting for results):

- TSH (should be high, unless pituitary failure)
- ECG and chest X-ray

Immediate management

- Symptomatic
  - Passive rewarming
  - Measure and treat blood glucose appropriately
- Ventilatory support if necessary
- Intravenous fluid
  - Establish good intravenous access
    - Warmed Ringer's lactate 1 L carefully (consider added glucose)
- Thyroid hormone
  - Thyroxine (T_4) 300–500 µg followed by 50–100 µg thyroxine intravenously daily
  - T_3 10 µg every 4 hours if response to T_4 is poor. Continuous ECG monitoring

Supportive therapy as indicated

- Consider steroids

Parathyroid crisis

Diagnosis

- Clinical suspicion
- Measure corrected serum calcium: $[Ca]_{corr} = [Ca] + 0.02 \times (40 - albumin [g/L])$

Key clinical management points (continued)

Management

- Supportive therapy for arrhythmias, coma, acute renal failure
- Withhold thiazide diuretics
- Rehydration with 0.9% saline
- Loop diuretics (e.g. furosemide) once fluid replete
- Bisphosphonate (e.g. pamidronate 60–90 mg or zoldronate 4–8 mg)
- Calcitonin 4 IU every 12 hours
- Cinacalcet 30–90 mg every 12 hours
- Parathyroidectomy when stable and calcium level <3 mmol/L

Acute hypocalcaemia

Diagnosis

- Check ionized calcium, serum calcium, albumin, ALP, and phosphate

Management

- Correct serum calcium for albumin concentration:

  $[Ca]_{corr} = [Ca] + 0.02 \times (40 - \text{albumin } [g/L])$

- Emergency intravenous calcium therapy if severe symptoms or ionized calcium <0.8 mmol/L
  - 0.11 mmol/kg (children) or 2.25–4.5 mmol (adults) over 5–10 minutes
- ECG monitoring
- Follow up infusion of 0.1–0.5 mmol/kg/hour titrated to relief of symptoms and ionized calcium >1.0 mmol/L
- Consider switch to oral calcium salts when levels are stable

Adrenal insufficiency

Diagnosis

- Clinical presentation
  - Hypotension, hypoglycaemia, hyponatraemia, and hyperkalaemia in a patient with abdominal, leg, or back pain
  - Shock with low peripheral resistance resembling septic shock
  - Low sodium, high potassium, high calcium, and low blood glucose
  - Random cortisol levels low
  - Primary adrenal insufficiency
    - ACTH levels high
  - Secondary adrenal insufficiency
    - ACTH levels low

Key clinical management points (continued)

Management

- ◆ Fluid resuscitation and corticosteroids
  - Hydrocortisone initiated immediately at a dose of 100 mg every 6 hours
  - Chronic glucocorticoid therapy
    - Hydrocortisone 15–25 mg/day in divided doses
    - Fludrocortisone 0.05–0.2 mg/day for in mineralocorticoid deficiency

Phaeochromocytoma

Diagnosis

Suspect the diagnosis in young patients with atypical hypertension. It frequently presents as a hypertensive crisis during an intervention (pregnancy, especially at or immediately after delivery, surgery, interventional radiology, biopsy, etc). It may present with various complications.

- ◆ Severe left ventricular failure
  - ECG may show acute left ventricular strain
  - Echocardiography may reveal LVH, LAH and decreased ejection fraction
- ◆ Peripheral ischaemia
- ◆ Stroke
- ◆ Convulsions
- ◆ Pre-renal renal dysfunction (elevated urea/creatinine ratio)

Acute management

Once the diagnosis is suspected.

- ◆ During surgery
  - Manage the emergency (see below)
  - Is tumour resection likely to be simple?
    - Proceed to tumour excision once haemodynamic stability is established
    - Expect severe hypotension after tumour excision
    - May require aggressive fluid replacement and vasopressor management
    - Monitor haematocrit (see below)
  - Is tumour excision likely to be difficult/lengthy
    - Establish haemodynamic control
    - Abandon surgery
    - Manage emergency as below
    - Establish standard control
    - Schedule elective excision

Key clinical management points (continued)

- Admit to high care unit
- Establish monitoring
  - ECG
  - Arterial line
  - Central venous pressure
  - ??Pulmonary artery catheter
- Vasodilator therapy
  - Magnesium sulphate 4 g intravenous bolus followed by an infusion at 2 g/hour
  - Calcium-channel blockers
  - Phentolamine 1–5 mg intravenously repeated as required
  - Phenoxybenzamine 1 mg/kg infusion over 2 hours
  - Sodium nitroprusside
- ***Do not*** administer β-blockers until vasodilator therapy is well established; only use β-blockade for tachycardia with ischaemia (not strain)
- Careful fluid loading
  - Patients usually fluid depleted
  - Large volumes may be required
  - Administer fluids as a mix of crystalloids and colloids
  - Monitor haematocrit as marked falls in haemoglobin concentration may occur
- Confirm the diagnosis

Diabetic ketoacidosis and hyperglycaemic hyperosmolar state

- Assess need for oxygen, airway protection, ventilatory support, and fluid resuscitation
- Investigations
  - Full blood count, urea, creatinine, electrolytes, serum osmolality, glucose, venous or arterial blood gas, urinalysis, capillary β-hydroxybutyrate
  - Consider blood and other cultures, chest X-ray, ECG
- Calculate corrected serum sodium: $[Na]_{corr} = [Na] + \{0.44 \times ([Glu] - 5.5)\}$
- Calculate effective serum osmolality: serum osmolality – [urea]
- Estimate fluid deficit to be replaced over 48 hours
- Fluids
  - Bolus(es) of 10–20 mL/kg (1–2 L) isotonic crystalloid (Hartmann's solution, 0.9% saline) or colloid
  - When haemodynamically stable, rehydration therapy guided by clinical condition and investigations

Key clinical management points (continued)

- Typical requirements 4–14 mL/kg/hour
- Hartmann's solution, 0.9% saline, or 0.45% saline depending on corrected serum sodium and effective serum osmolality (if $[Na]_{corr}$ >155 mmol/L use 0.45% saline)
- Aim for ≤3 mOsm/L/hour fall in effective serum osmolality
- When serum glucose <12 mmol/L, switch to 0.45% saline + 5% dextrose

- Insulin
  - Commence short-acting insulin (e.g. Actrapid®) infusion 50 IU in 50 mL 0.9% saline at 0.1 IU/kg/hour
  - Adjust infusion rate hourly to obtain a fall in serum glucose of 2.5–4 mmol/L/hour
  - **DKA**: usual insulin regime can be restarted when β-hydroxybutyrate <1 mmol/L if clinically appropriate
  - **HHS**: no requirement for extended insulin regime

- Potassium
  - Add 20 mmol KCl per 500 mL fluid after initial fluid bolus and adjust according to serum potassium

- Monitoring
  - Vital signs including neurological status as clinically appropriate (minimum hourly)
  - Hourly capillary blood glucose and β-hydroxybutyrate
  - Recheck electrolytes, osmolality, and venous or arterial blood gas after 2 hours, then every 4 hours

- Other measures
  - Correct severe or symptomatic hypophosphataemia and hypomagnesaemia
  - Consider bicarbonate therapy if pH <6.9

Carcinoid crisis

Diagnosis

- Clinical presentation
  - Sudden onset of severe symptoms
    - Flushing, diarrhoea, and bronchospasm
    - Hypotension, hypertension, tachycardia, and hyperglycaemia.
  - Precipitated by stress or drugs
    - Histamine-releasing agents
    - Catecholamines
  - Elevated 5-HIAA levels

Key clinical management points (continued)

Management

- ◆ Octreotide 100–500 µg
- ◆ Volume therapy
- ◆ Avoid catecholamines unless essential for resuscitation

References

1. Chanson P, Lepeintre JF, Ducreux D (2004). Management of pituitary apoplexy. *Expert Opinion on Pharmacotherapy*, **5**, 1287–98.

2. Nawar RN, AbdelMannan D, Selman WR, Arafah BM (2008). Pituitary tumor apoplexy: a review. *Journal of Intensive Care Medicine*, **23**, 75–90.

3. Simmonds M (1914). Über hypophysisschwund mit todlichem ausgang. *Deutsche medizinische Wochenschrift*, **40**, 322–3.

4. Sheehan HL (1937). Postpartum necrosis of the anterior pituitary. *Journal of Pathology and Bacteriology*, **45**, 189–214.

5. Randeva HS, Schoebel J, Byrne J, Esiri M, Adams CB, Wass JA (1999). Classical pituitary apoplexy: clinical features, management and outcome. *Clinical Endocrinology*, **51**, 181–8.

6. Chibbaro S, Benvenuti L, Carnesecchi S, Faggionato F, Gagliardi R (2007). An interesting case of a pituitary adenoma apoplexy mimicking an acute meningitis. Case report. *Journal of Neurosurgical Sciences*, **51**, 65–9.

7. Lennon M, Seigne P, Cunningham AJ (1998). Pituitary apoplexy after spinal anaesthesia. *British Journal of Anaesthesia*, **81**, 616–18.

8. Suga T, Kagawa S, Goto H, Yoshioka K, Hosoya T (1996). [A case of pituitary adenoma progressing to pituitary apoplexy on the occasion of cerebral angiography]. *No Shinkei Geka*, **24**, 475–9.

9. Liu JK, Nwagwu C, Pikus HJ, Couldwell WT (2001). Laparoscopic anterior lumbar interbody fusion precipitating pituitary apoplexy. *Acta Neurochirurgica*, **143**, 303–6.

10. Masago A, Ueda Y, Kanai H, Nagai H, Umemura S (1995). Pituitary apoplexy after pituitary function test: a report of two cases and review of the literature. *Surgical Neurology*, **43**, 158–64.

11. Cohen A, Kishore K, Wolansky L, Frohman L (2004). Pituitary apoplexy occurring during large volume liposuction surgery. *Journal of Neuroophthalmology*, **24**, 31–3.

12. Cardoso ER, Peterson EW (1984). Pituitary apoplexy: a review. *Neurosurgery*, **14**, 363–73.

13. Agrawal D, Mahapatra AK (2005). Visual outcome of blind eyes in pituitary apoplexy after transsphenoidal surgery: a series of 14 eyes. *Surgical Neurology*, **63**, 42–6.

14. Abbott J, Kirkby GR (2004). Acute visual loss and pituitary apoplexy after surgery. *British Medical Journal*, **329**, 218–19.

15. Karger S, Fuhrer D (2008). [Thyroid storm–thyrotoxic crisis: an update]. *Deutsche medizinische Wochenschrift*, **133**, 479–84.

16. Pugh S, Lalwani K, Awal A (1994). Thyroid storm as a cause of loss of consciousness following anaesthesia for emergency Caesarean section. *Anaesthesia*, **49**, 35–7.

17. Naito Y, Sone T, Kataoka K, Sawada M, Yamazaki K (1997). Thyroid storm due to functioning metastatic thyroid carcinoma in a burn patient. *Anesthesiology*, **87**, 433–5.

18. Knighton JD, Crosse MM (1997). Anaesthetic management of childhood thyrotoxicosis and the use of esmolol. *Anaesthesia*, **52**, 67–70.

19. Vijayakumar HR, Thomas WO, Ferrara JJ (1989). Peri-operative management of severe thyrotoxicosis with esmolol. *Anaesthesia*, **44**, 406–8.

20. Strube PJ (1984). Thyroid storm during beta blockade. *Anaesthesia*, **39**, 343–6.

21. Bennett MH, Wainwright AP (1989). Acute thyroid crisis on induction of anaesthesia. *Anaesthesia*, **44**, 28–30.

22. Christensen PA, Nissen LR (1987). Treatment of thyroid storm in a child with dantrolene. *British Journal of Anaesthesia*, **59**, 523.

23. Adali E, Yildizhan R, Kolusari A, Kurdoglu M, Turan N (2008). The use of plasmapheresis for rapid hormonal control in severe hyperthyroidism caused by a partial molar pregnancy. *Archives of Gynecology and Obstetrics*, **279**, 569–71.

24. Nishiyama K, Kitahara A, Natsume H, *et al* (2001). Malignant hyperthermia in a patient with Graves' disease during subtotal thyroidectomy. *Endocrine Journal*, **48**, 227–32.

25. Schraga,E.D. Hypothyroidism and myxedema coma. Available online at: http://emedicine. medscape.com/article/768053-overview (accessed 20 January 2009).

26. McCulloch W, Price P, Hinds CJ, Wass JA (1985). Effects of low dose oral triiodothyronine in myxoedema coma. *Intensive Care Medicine*, **11**, 259–62.

27. Wartofsky L (2006). Myxedema coma. *Endocrinology and Metabolism Clinics of North America*, **35**, 687–98.

28. Beynon J, Akhtar S, Kearney T (2008). Predictors of outcome in myxoedema coma. *Critical Care*, **12**, 111.

29. Ziegler R (2001). Hypercalcemic crisis. *Journal of the American Society of Nephrology*, **12** (Suppl 17), S3–9.

30. Hebert SC (1996). Extracellular calcium-sensing receptor: implications for calcium and magnesium handling in the kidney. *Kidney International*, **50**, 2129–39.

31. Kelly TR, Zarconi J (1981). Primary hyperparathyroidism: hyperparathyroid crisis. *American Journal of Surgery*, **142**, 539–42.

32. Phitayakorn R, McHenry CR (2008). Hyperparathyroid crisis: use of bisphosphonates as a bridge to parathyroidectomy. *Journal of the American College of Surgery*, **206**, 1106–15.

33. Marcocci C, Chanson P, Shoback D, *et al* (2009). Cinacalcet reduces serum calcium concentrations in patients with intractable primary hyperparathyroidism. *Journal of Clinical Endocrinology and Metabolism*, **94**, 2766–72.

34. Bhattacharyya A, Buckler HM, New JP (2004). Hungry bone syndrome—revisited. *Journal of the Royal College of Physicians of Edinburgh*, **32**, 83–6.

35. Hahner S, Allolio B (2005). Management of adrenal insufficiency in different clinical settings. *Expert Opinion on Pharmacotherapy*, **6**, 2407–17.

36. Bouillon R (2006). Acute adrenal insufficiency. *Endocrinology and Metabolism Clinics of North America*, **35**, 767–75.

37. Mulder AH, Nauta S, Pieters GF, Hermus AR (2008). [Addisonian crisis in patients with known adrenal insufficiency: the importance of early intervention]. *Nederlands Tijdschrift voor Geneeskunde*, **152**, 1497–1500.

38. Allen GC, Rosenberg H (1990). Phaeochromocytoma presenting as acute malignant hyperthermia—a diagnostic challenge. *Canadian Journal of Anaesthesia*, **37**, 593–5.

39. Caputo C, Fishbane S, Shapiro L, *et al* (2002). Pheochromocytoma multisystem crisis in a patient with multiple endocrine neoplasia type IIB and pyelonephritis. *American Journal of Kidney Disease*, **39**, E23.

40. Frankton S, Baithun S, Husain E, Davis K, Grossman AB (2009). Phaeochromocytoma crisis presenting with profound hypoglycaemia and subsequent hypertension. *Hormones*, **8**, 65–70.

41. Kizer JR, Koniaris LS, Edelman JD, St John Sutton MG (2000). Pheochromocytoma crisis, cardiomyopathy, and hemodynamic collapse. *Chest*, **118**, 1221–3.

42. James MF, Cronje L (2004). Pheochromocytoma crisis: the use of magnesium sulfate. *Anesthesia and Analgesia*, **99**, 680–6.

43. Department of Health and Human Services, Centers for Disease Control. Diabetes data & trends. Available online at: http://apps.nccd.cdc.gov/ddtstrs/ (accessed 20 January 2010).

44. Kitabchi AE, Wall BM (1995). Diabetic ketoacidosis. *Medical Clinics of North America*, **79**, 9–37.

45. Munro JF, Campbell IW, McCuish AC, Duncan LJ (1973). Euglycaemic diabetic ketoacidosis. *British Medical Journal*, **ii**, 578–80.

46. Kitabchi AE, Umpierrez GE, Murphy MB (2004). Diabetic ketoacidosis and hyperglycaemic hyperosmolar state. In De Fronzo RA, Ferrannini E, Keen H, Zimmet P (eds), *International Textbook of Diabetes Mellitus*, 3rd edn. John Wiley, Chichester.

47. Edge JA, Roy Y, Bergomi A, *et al* (2006). Conscious level in children with diabetic ketoacidosis is related to severity of acidosis and not to blood glucose concentration. *Pediatric Diabetes*, **7**, 11–15.

48. Kitabchi AE, Umpierrez GE, Murphy MB, *et al.*(2004). Hyperglycemic crises in diabetes. *Diabetes Care*, 27 (Suppl 1), s94–102

49. Nugent B. (2005). Hyperosmolar Hyperglycaemic State. *Emerg Med Clin N Am*, **23**, 629–48.

50. Brown TB (2004). Cerebral oedema in childhood diabetic ketoacidosis. Is treatment a factor? *Emergency Medical Journal*, **21**, 141–4.

51. Glaser N, Barnett P, McCaslin I, *et al* (2001). Risk factors for cerebral edema in children with diabetic ketoacidosis. The Pediatric Emergency Medicine Collaborative Research Committee of the American Academy of Pediatrics. *New England Journal of Medicine*, **344**, 264–9.

52. Handy JM, Soni N (2008). Physiological effects of hyperchloraemia and acidosis. *British Journal of Anaesthesia*, **101**, 141–50.

53. Goyal N, Miller JB, Sankey SS, Mossallam U (2008). Utility of initial bolus insulin in the treatment of diabetic ketoacidosis. *Journal of Emergency Medicine*, e-publication.

54. Trence DL, Hirsch IB (2001). Hyperglycemic crises in diabetes mellitus type 2. *Endocrinology and Metabolism Clinics of North America*, **30**, 817–31.

55. Hillier TA, Abbott RD, Barrett EJ (1999). Hyponatremia: evaluating the correction factor for hyperglycemia. *American Journal of Medicine*, **106**, 399–403.

56. Kitabchi AE, Ayyagari V, Guerra SM (1976). The efficacy of low-dose versus conventional therapy of insulin for treatment of diabetic ketoacidosis. *Annals of Internal Medicine*, **84**, 633–8.

57. Koopmans KP, Brouwers AH, De Hooge MN, *et al.* (2005). Carcinoid crisis after injection of 6-[^{18}F] fluorodihydroxyphenylalanine in a patient with metastatic carcinoid. *Journal of Nuclear Medicine*, **46**, 1240–3.

58. Hughes EW, Hodkinson BP (1989). Carcinoid syndrome: the combined use of ketanserin and octreotide in the management of an acute crisis during anaesthesia. *Anaesthesia and Intensive Care*, **17**, 367–70.

59. Bissonnette RT, Gibney RG, Berry BR, Buckley AR (1990). Fatal carcinoid crisis after percutaneous fine-needle biopsy of hepatic metastasis: case report and literature review. *Radiology*, **174**, 751–2.

60. Castillo JG, Filsoufi F, Adams DH, Raikhelkar J, Zaku B, Fischer GW (2008). Management of patients undergoing multivalvular surgery for carcinoid heart disease: the role of the anaesthetist. *British Journal of Anaesthesia*, **101**, 618–26.

Chapter 10

Hormones as pharmaceutical agents

Focus on steroids and vasopressin

John GT Augoustides, Insung Chung,
and Prakash Patel

Introduction

The hormones, steroids and vasopressin, are established pharmaceutical agents throughout anaesthetic practice, including critical care. There is considerable ongoing clinical
interest in these agents, since they have considerable clinical utility. In this chapter their
established and emerging clinical applications in the care of the cardiac surgical patient,
the non-cardiac surgical patient, and the critically ill patient in the intensive care unit are
reviewed. Future clinical trials will very likely provide further evidence that will lead to
more widespread penetration of these agents throughout peri-operative and intensive
care unit medicine.

The current data already point to the clinical importance of the powerful synergy
between these agents that enhances clinical outcome. This beneficial clinical relationship
between steroids and vasopressin makes sense, since these agents are both intimately
involved in the stress response to surgery and critical illness. Future clinical trials will
undoubtedly include this consideration in their design as they endeavour to optimize
clinical outcomes throughout anaesthetic practice.

The approach taken in this chapter has been evidence based, with a focus on the
highest-quality evidence available and a summary of guidelines for clinical care, wherever
possible. Particular attention has also been paid to rigorous assessment of the evidence
with respect to study design and quality. It is essential to understand what the evidence is,
what its limitations are, and how the evidence should guide clinical care.

Since steroids are common in clinical practice, their comparative potency is summarized in Table 10.1 as a readily available reference for the steroid regimens selected in
clinical trials or recommended by expert panels.

Steroids

Peri-operative steroids in cardiac surgery

Cardiac surgery with cardiopulmonary bypass (CPB) typically triggers a systemic inflammatory response syndrome due to factors such as antigen exposure, ischaemia–reperfusion,

Table 10.1 Comparative potency of clinical steroids (on a per milligram basis)

Steroid	Glucocorticoid effect	Mineralocorticoid effect	Half-life (hours)	Route
Hydrocortisone	1	1	6–8	PO, IV, IM
Prednisone	4	0.1–0.2	18–36	PO
Methylprednisolone	5	0.1–0.2	18–36	IV
Dexamethasone	30	< 0.1	36–54	PO, IV
Fludrocortisone	0	20	18–36	PO

PO, per os (by mouth); IV, intravenous; IM, intramuscular

Adapted from Head DE, Joffe A, Coursin DB (2009). When should peri-operative glucocorticoid replacement be administered? In: Fleisher LA (ed) *Evidence-Based Practice of Anesthesiology* (2nd edition), pp 184–91. Saunders Elsevier, Philadelphia, PA.

and changes in blood flow characteristics.[1] Since this inflammatory response features prominently in the pathophysiology of organ dysfunction after CPB, considerable clinical benefit may be achieved from blockade of this immune response. Since steroids are anti-inflammatory and immunosuppressive, they may offer a pharmacological means of suppressing the inflammatory response to CPB.

Although clinical trials have demonstrated that peri-operative steroid therapy lessens the inflammatory response, this pharmacological intervention has not gained widespread clinical acceptance. This lack of clinical penetrance is most likely due to significant limitations with the scientific evidence such as including surrogate endpoints, limited patient safety data, and limited statistical power.[1–3] To address these clinical concerns with the evidence to date, a systematic review and meta-analysis of the clinical trials tested whether steroids are effective and safe in cardiac surgery with CPB.[4]

The systematic literature review yielded 44 suitable randomized controlled trials (RCTs), performed in the period 1997–2007, for inclusion to yield a cumulative sample size of 3205 subjects.[4] This meta-analysis was performed in a high-quality fashion according to the guidelines of the QUOROM group.[5] The selected trials not only all examined steroids in adult cardiac surgical patients exposed to CPB, but also all had a control group design and a priori specified clinical endpoints.

The quality of each selected RCT was quantified by two independent assessors, utilizing the validated Jadad score for these RCTs.[6,7] The investigators also evaluated for publication bias within the selected trials using funnel plot analysis.

The median sample size across all trials was 51 (range 13–295), with the cardiac surgical procedures being coronary artery bypass grafting and/or valve procedures, all performed with CPB. Steroid protocols across the selected trials varied in duration and drug type. No major adverse clinical outcomes due to steroids were evident in this meta-analysis. Peri-operative steroids appeared to be safe in cardiac surgery with CPB. Steroid exposure significantly reduced the incidence of new atrial fibrillation (relative risk 0.71; 95% CI (CI) 0.59–0.87), post-operative bleeding (weighted mean difference –99.6 mL; 95% CI –149.8 to –49.3), intensive care unit stay (weighted mean difference –0.23 days; 95% CI –0.40 to –0.07), and hospital stay (weighted mean difference –0.59 days; 95% CI –1.17 to –0.02). There was also a trend towards a lower mortality associated with steroid exposure (relative risk 0.73; 95% CI 0.45–1.18).

The authors concluded that, despite the large sample size, adverse effects from steroid therapy are still possible in adult cardiac surgery with CPB, especially since these effects may be dose dependent.[4] Furthermore, the optimal steroid peri-operative protocol with respect to steroid type, dosing regimen, and duration is still unknown. Based on the clinical benefits from steroid therapy in CPB identified in this meta-analysis, the authors suggest that adequately powered RCTs are now justified to validate these clinical outcome advantages and more fully explore the peri-operative safety of this intervention.

A subsequent meta-analysis explored whether the risks and benefits of steroids in adult cardiac surgery with CPB were dose dependent.[8] The literature review identified 50 RCTs (1966–2008; total $N = 3323$) for cumulative analysis according to QUOROM criteria. The main clinical benefits identified in this meta-analysis were that corticosteroids significantly reduced the risk of atrial fibrillation (25.1% vs. 35.1%; relative risk 0.74; 95% CI 0.63–0.86; $P < 0.01$) as well as length of stay in both the intensive care unit (weighted mean difference –0.37 days; 95% CI –0.21 to –0.52; $P < 0.01$) and hospital (weighted mean difference –0.66 days; 95% CI –0.77 to –1.25; $P = 0.03$). Although steroid exposure did not increase infection risk (relative risk 0.93; 95% CI 0.61–1.41; $P = 0.73$), it significantly increased the risk of hyperglycaemia requiring insulin infusion (28.2%; relative risk 1.49; 95% CI 1.11–2.01; $P < 0.01$). A total steroid dose >1000 mg hydrocortisone conferred no additional outcome benefit. Very high dose steroid therapy (defined as a total steroid dose >10 000 mg hydrocortisone) was associated with prolonged mechanical ventilation post-operatively. The authors concluded that low-dose corticosteroid therapy (defined as a total steroid dose <1000 mg hydrocortisone) was clinically effective.

Based on these two recent meta-analyses, low-dose corticosteroid therapy hydrocortisone significantly improves clinical outcome in adult cardiac surgery with CPB. It is important to note that these beneficial effects are not currently supported by adequate evidence in paediatric heart surgery, based on recent meta-analysis of paediatric trials.[9]

The mechanism of these beneficial effects may be related to favourable immunomodulation by peri-operative corticosteroids. An elevated ration of interleukin 6 (IL-6) to interleukin 10 (IL-10) is associated with significantly worse clinical outcome in the systemic inflammatory response syndrome.[10] A recent trial demonstrated that the outcome benefit from corticosteroid therapy in adult cardiac surgery with CPB is associated with a significant reduction in the IL-6/IL-10 ratio.[11] These recent data point to specific immunomodulation by steroids in this clinical setting, an effect that should be further explored in future trials.

There are currently at least two registered steroid RCTs in adult cardiac surgery with CPB. The SIRS (**S**teroids **I**n **CaR**diac **S**urgery Study) trial is evaluating methylprednisolone in adult cardiac surgery with CPB (details available at www.clinicaltrials.gov with study number NCT00427388; accessed 21 January 2010). The second RCT is testing dexamethasone in adult cardiac surgery with CPB (details available at www.clinicaltrials.gov

with study number NCT00293592; accessed 21 January 2010). These two large RCTs are currently in progress with the aim of enrolling over 14 000 subjects. Furthermore, their trial endpoints are meaningful and important clinical outcomes such as mortality and major organ-based complications. The findings of these two trials will most likely determine the future of steroid therapy in adult cardiac surgery with CPB.

In summary, based on recent meta-analysis, low-dose steroids appear to be safe in adult cardiac surgery with cardiopulmonary bypass. Furthermore, they significantly improve clinical outcomes such as atrial fibrillation, bleeding, and length of stay in the intensive care unit and hospital. However, until these favourable results are confirmed in larger RCTs currently in progress, steroid administration cannot be recommended for routine clinical application in adult cardiac surgery with cardiopulmonary bypass.

Peri-operative steroids in non-cardiac surgery

Dexamethasone as an anti-emetic

The corticosteroid, dexamethasone, is established as effective prophylaxis against post-operative nausea and vomiting (PONV), based on multiple systematic reviews that demonstrate its significant efficacy throughout non-cardiac surgery.[12,13] Consequently, it is strongly recommended for prophylaxis in the recent Society of Ambulatory Anaesthesia guidelines for the management of PONV .[14] The recommended dose is 4–5 mg intravenously for patients at increased risk for PONV.[14] This dose of dexamethasone has a similar efficacy for PONV prophylaxis to that of odansetron 4 mg intravenously.[15] The recommended timing for administration of dexamethasone for PONV prophylaxis for maximum effect is at induction of anaesthesia.[16] Based on multiple studies, a single bolus dose of dexamethasone has a very good safety profile.[12–16] However, there is, an increased risk of bleeding after tonsillectomy associated with prophylactic dexamethasone.[17] A recent RCT evaluated whether dexamethasone reduced the risk of PONV after tonsillectomy in a dose dependent fashion ($N = 215$ children; performed between 2005 and 2007 at a major teaching hospital in Switzerland).[17] The dosage regimens of dexamethasone tested against placebo were 0.05 mg/kg, 0.15 mg/kg, and 0.5 mg/kg. Dexamethasone exposure was associated with significantly decreased risk of PONV (in dose-dependent fashion) and additional post-operative analgesia. However, dexamethasone was also associated with significantly increased risk of post-operative tonsillar bleeding ($P = 0.003$), with the 0.5 mg/kg dosage group at highest risk (relative risk 6.80; 95% CI 1.77–16.5). This bleeding risk was so substantial that the trial was terminated early for safety reasons. The authors concluded that although dexamethasone significantly decreased PONV after tonsillectomy in a dose-dependent fashion, it was significantly associated with an increased risk of post-operative bleeding.

Dexamethasone as an analgesic

Lidocaine is very effective for relief of injection pain associated with propofol.[18] An RCT ($N = 70$) demonstrated that dexamethasone 0 15 mg/kg administered prior to propofol injection significantly reduced injection pain (dexamethasone 31% vs. placebo 77%).[19]

A subsequent randomized trial ($N = 140$) demonstrated that dexamethasone 6 mg and lidocaine 20 mg are synergistic for relief of propofol-associated injection pain.[20] The pain relief from this combination was significantly better than with each agent alone or with placebo ($P <0.01$).

The possible peri-operative benefits of dexamethasone for laparoscopic cholecystectomy were recently evaluated in a systematic review and meta-analysis, as outlined by the QUOROM guidelines.[21] The defined clinical endpoints chosen for this trial were PONV and pain after laparoscopic cholecystectomy. The authors included 17 RCTs (1999–2007) with sample sizes ranging from 43 to 5199. As expected, dexamethasone significantly reduced PONV (relative risk 0.55; 95% CI 0.44–0.67). Furthermore, dexamethasone appeared to reduce the severity of post-operative pain (ratio of means 0.87; 95% CI 0.78–0.98), although this conclusion was limited by substantial heterogeneity in the data. The authors concluded that dexamethasone is indicated in laparoscopic cholecystectomy for prophylaxis against PONV and possible analgesia.

The analgesic efficacy of dexamethasone was convincingly demonstrated in a recent randomized placebo-controlled trial in patients undergoing thyroidectomy for benign disease ($N = 72$).[22] In this trial, patients received standardized peri-operative care, but were also randomized to receive dexamethasone 8 mg or normal saline (placebo), given in a blinded fashion by infusion 45 minutes before anaesthetic induction. The selected clinical endpoints were PONV, analgesic requirements, and voice alteration, as reflected by changes in mean frequency on digital voice recordings. The study subjects were followed until 30 days after hospital discharge.

Dexamethasone exposure significantly decreased PONV ($P = 0.001$), post-operative pain ($P = 0.009$), and change in mean vocal frequency ($P = 0.015$). There were no steroid-related complications in this study. Given these clinically significant improvements in PONV, pain, and voice, the investigators strongly advocated routine application of dexamethasone in patients undergoing thyroidectomy. The reduction of post-operative pain by dexamethasone is probably related to modulation of the peri-operative stress response. Steroid administration suppresses inflammatory cytokines that induce hyperalgesia, such as tumour necrosis factor, IL-1 and IL-6.[23]

Steroids in airway management

A recent meta-analysis examined whether, in critically ill adults (including surgical patients), steroids prevent laryngeal oedema after tracheal extubation and reduce the incidence of subsequent repeat tracheal intubation.[24] The systematic literature review identified six RCTs (combined $N = 1923$) that were analysed according to QUOROM criteria. These trials were all of excellent quality, based on their Jadad scores. Compared with placebo, steroid administration prior to planned tracheal extubation significantly reduced laryngeal oedema (odds ratio (OR) 0.38; 95% CI 0.17–0.85; number needed to treat (NNT), 10) and subsequent requirement for repeat tracheal intubation (OR 0.29; 95% CI 0.15–0.58; NNT = 50). Based on subgroup analysis, a multidose steroid protocol significantly improved laryngeal oedema (OR 0.14; 95% CI 0.08–0.23; NNT 5) and requirement for subsequent tracheal reintubation (OR 0.19; 95% CI 0.07–0.50;

NNT 25).[20] This meta-analysis found no adverse clinical effects related to steroid exposure. Based on these favourable results, the authors recommended multidose steroid exposure before planned tracheal extubation for reduction of laryngeal oedema and subsequent rates of repeat tracheal re-intubation. Based on the heterogeneity of steroid regimens, they recommended further trials to determine the optimal steroid dose and optimal time interval between the start of therapy and planned tracheal extubation.

The utility of prophylactic steroids in airway management was further explored in the setting of patients undergoing pulmonary resection requiring selective lung ventilation via a double-lumen endotracheal tube.[25] Since sore throat and hoarseness are common in this clinical setting, steroid therapy may reduce their incidence, given that these peri-operative complications have an inflammatory basis.[26,27] This hypothesis was tested in a randomized placebo-controlled trial ($N = 166$ adults) in three arms: placebo, dexamethasone 0.1 mg/kg, and dexamethasone 0.2 mg/kg (all three medications were administered intravenously in a blinded and randomized fashion just prior to anaesthetic induction). All study subjects were evaluated with a visual analogue scale at 1 and 24 hours after tracheal extubation for sore throat and hoarseness.

The main finding of this study was that dexamethasone 0.2 mg/kg significantly decreased sore throat and hoarseness at both selected time points ($P < 0.002$) after tracheal intubation with a double-lumen endotracheal tube.[21] Furthermore, there was no pre-operative complication associated with dexamethasone exposure, although effects more than 24 hours after tracheal extubation were not assessed.

Airway swelling, trismus, and pain frequently follow major dental surgery such as third molar extraction. The utility of steroids in this setting was recently evaluated by meta-analysis.[28] The systematic literature review identified 12 RCTs (1982–2006) for further analysis, as outlined by the QUOROM criteria.[5] The primary outcomes were early (1–3 days post-operatively) and late (>3 days post-operatively) oedema, trismus, and pain. The main findings of this trial were that steroid exposure significantly decreased oedema (early—mean difference 1.4; 95% CI 0.6–2.2; $P < 0.001$; late—mean difference 1.1; 95% CI 0.1–2.0; $P = 0.03$) and trismus (early—mean difference 4.1 mm; 95% CI 2.8–5.5 mm; $P < 0.001$; late—mean difference 2.7 mm; 95% CI 0.8–4 6 mm; $P = 0.005$), but not pain, after third molar extraction.[28] The authors concluded that peri-operative steroid exposure was associated with mild to moderate reductions in oedema and trismus after third molar surgery.

The utility of peri-operative steroids in airway management for patients with asthma and chronic obstructive pulmonary disease is established in existing guidelines.[29,30]) Although peri-operative steroid exposure decreases the risk of bronchospasm in these patients, their administration is recommended selectively, taking into account disease severity and the planned surgical procedure. Further details are available in the referenced narrative review and recent expert guidelines.[27–31]

Steroid avoidance in the peri-operative period

The toxic effects of steroid therapy, such as poor wound healing, diabetes, immunosuppression, and hypertension, can significantly affect peri-operative outcomes, especially in select populations such as surgical patients with inflammatory bowel disease and solid organ transplant recipients.[32–34] Minimizing peri-operative steroid exposure in these at-risk patient groups has evolved as a management strategy to avoid the steroid-related toxicity.

A meta-analysis of seven observational studies ($N = 1532$) evaluated the relationship between pre-operative steroid exposure and peri-operative complications in patients with inflammatory bowel disease undergoing bowel surgery.[32] The pooled analysis demonstrated that steroid exposure significantly increased all post-operative complications (OR 1.41; 95% CI 1.07–1.87), including infectious complications (OR 1.68; 95% CI 1.24–2.28). Furthermore, peri-operative oral steroid dose >40 mg was associated with a higher risk of total complications (OR 2.04; 95% CI 1.28–3.26). The authors concluded that steroid therapy in patients with inflammatory bowel disease undergoing bowel surgery should be stopped or weaned to a total daily oral dose of <40 mg oral steroid.

Steroid avoidance in immunosuppression regimens immediately after renal transplantation and beyond has evolved as a reasonable management strategy, based on recent trials. Meta-analysis of 30 RCTs ($N = 5949$) explored the extent of outcome benefit from steroid-sparing strategies for immunosuppression in this setting.[33] Steroid avoidance did not significantly affect mortality or graft loss, although the risk of acute rejection was significantly increased (relative risk 1.27; 95% CI 1.00–2.90). Freedom from steroids was significantly associated with reduced clinical severity of hypertension and hyperlipidaemia, as well as a lower incidence of post-transplantation diabetes and cardiovascular events. The authors concluded that steroid avoidance is possible immediately after renal transplantation, especially if antibody induction of immunosuppression is utilized.

Steroid-free immunosuppression after liver transplant has also gained clinical acceptance, given favourable data from recent trials. A recent meta-analysis of 19 RCTs explored the outcome benefits of this strategy.[34] Steroid avoidance had no effect on death, graft loss, or infection. Furthermore, it tended to improve hypertension (relative risk 0.84; $P = 0.08$), and significantly decreased hypercholesterolemia (mean difference –0.41; $P < 0.001$) and cytomegalovirus infection (relative risk 0.52; $P = 0.001$). When steroids were replaced by another immunosuppressive agent, the risks of diabetes (relative risk 0.29; $P < 0.001$), rejection (relative risk 0.68; $P = 0.03$), and severe rejection (relative risk 0.37; $P = 0.001$) were significantly lower. Despite these favourable results, the authors recommended that, because of the significant heterogeneity in the data utilized for the meta-analysis, clinical guidelines should be based on future adequately powered RCTs.[34]

Peri-operative steroid replacement (see also Chapter 7)

Since corticosteroids are commonly prescribed, there are many patients with suppression of the hypothalamic–pituitary–adrenal (HPA) axis secondary to exogenous steroid exposure. These patients are often given supplemental steroids peri-operatively to cover the stress of surgery, even thought the evidence supporting this practice is weak.[35] A recent systematic literature review of this topic included nine studies ($N = 315$; two randomized trials; seven cohort studies).[36] Neither of the randomized trials demonstrated a significant haemodynamic difference between stress steroid exposure and baseline steroid exposure.

In the five cohort studies in which baseline steroid exposure was maintained peri-operatively, there was no adrenal crisis. In the remaining two cohort studies in which baseline steroid exposure was not maintained peri-operatively ($N = 120$), there was a 1.6% incidence (2/120) of unexplained hypotension that responded to hydrocortisone and fluids. Furthermore, a critical literature review confirmed the rarity of peri-operative adrenal crisis in dental patients with exogenous steroid exposure.[37] However, patients who are receiving steroids for primary disease of the HPA axis do require stress steroid therapy peri-operatively.[36–38]

Based on the current evidence, patients on exogenous steroids should have their baseline steroid therapy maintained peri-operatively. In general, stress steroids are not recommended in the peri-operative period, except for patients with primary disease of the HPA axis.[35–37]

Steroids in critical care medicine (see also Chapter 1)

The clinical benefits of steroids in peri-operative and critical care airway management have already been presented based on a recent high-quality meta-analysis.[24] The diagnosis and management of corticosteroid insufficiency in critical care has been an ongoing major research focus with an extensive set of RCTs, meta-analyses, and expert guidelines.[39,40] To summarize these extensive data sets and provide clinical recommendations for patient care, the latest guidelines from the American College of Critical Care Medicine (ACCCM) will be utilized as the clinical framework for this section.[39]

This landmark guideline was complied by consensus by a group of international experts from the Society of Critical Care Medicine and the European Society of Intensive Care Medicine. The process of consensus development followed the modified Delphi method, a validated modus operandi utilizing consecutive rounds of structured expert discussion until group consensus is attained.[41,42] The scientific evidence was further summarized with meta-analysis as part of the preparation for subsequent evidence-based recommendations.[39] The strength of each recommendation was quantified with the modified grades of recommendation assessment, development and evaluation (GRADE) system developed by the American College of Chest Physicians.(43) In the GRADE system there are two classes of recommendations (strong and weak) and three qualities of supporting evidence (high, moderate, and weak). The GRADE system of recommendations and supporting evidence is summarized in Table 10.2.[43] The expert panel developed a set of 12 recommendations which are summarized in Table 10.3. The scientific background to these recommendations will now be reviewed as a framework to understanding the rationale behind their development.

The stress response is mediated mainly by the HPA axis and the sympathoadrenal system.[44] The activation of the sympathoadrenal system results in release of catecholamines such as noradrenaline and epinephrine from the adrenal medulla. Activation of the HPA axis results in release of corticotrophin-releasing hormone (CRH) and arginine vasopressin (AVP). CRH triggers release of adrenocorticotrophic hormone (ACTH) from the anterior pituitary.[39,44] Although vasopressin is vasoactive, it also acts synergistically with

Table 10.2 Recommendation, assessment, development, and evaluation (GRADE) system

What is the grade of recommendation?	What are the benefits and risks?	What is the quality of supporting evidence?	What are the clinical implications?
GRADE 1A Strong recommendation with high-quality evidence	Benefits outweigh risks or vice versa	Randomized trials without major limitations/ overwhelming evidence from observational studies	Strong recommendation applies to most patients in most circumstances
GRADE 1B Strong recommendation with moderate-quality evidence	Benefits outweigh risks or vice versa	Randomized trials without major limitations/ overwhelming evidence from observational studies	Strong recommendation applies to most patients in most circumstances
GRADE 1C Strong recommendation with low-quality evidence	Benefits outweigh risks or vice versa	Observational studies/ case series	Strong recommendation that may change as evidence becomes available
GRADE 2A Weak recommendation with high quality evidence	Benefits closely balanced with risks	Randomized trials without major limitations/ overwhelming evidence from observational studies	Weak recommendation: best action depends on clinical scenario and societal values
GRADE 2B Weak recommendation with moderate quality evidence	Benefits closely balanced with risks	Randomized trials with major limitations/ very strong evidence from observational studies	Weak recommendation: best action depends on clinical scenario and societal values
GRADE 2C Weak recommendation with low-quality evidence	Benefits closely balanced with risks	Observational studies/ case series	Very weak recommendation: alternatives are equally reasonable

Based on data from Guyatt G, Gutterman D, Baumann MH, *et al.* (2006). Grading strength of recommendations and quality of evidence in clinical guidelines: Report from an American College of Chest Physicians Task Force. *Chest*, **129**, 174–81.

CRH to enhance secretion of ACTH which triggers secretion of cortisol from the zona fasciculata of the adrenal cortex.[39,44] The resulting cortisol surge produces widespread metabolic, immune, and cardiovascular effects, all with the general aim of restoring or maintaining homeostasis during stress. It is clear from this physiology that AVP is intimately linked with the cortisol pathway during HPA activation, a link that will be further explored in the section on vasopressin.

This stress response of the HPA and sympathoadrenal axis is frequently dysfunctional in adult critical illness. The first ACCCM recommendation is that this syndrome should be described as critical illness-related corticosteroid insufficiency (CIRCI).[39,44] The syndrome of CIRCI is defined as inadequate cellular corticosteroid activity for the severity of

Table 10.3 American College of Critical Care Medicine recommendations for steroid therapy in adult critical care

	Clinical recommendation	Comments
1.	Dysfunction of HPA axis in adult critical illness is best termed Critical Illness-Related Corticosteroid Insufficiency (CIRCI)	Consensus definition based on expert opinion
2.	The terms absolute or relative adrenal insufficiency have limited application in critical illness	Clinical recommendation based on expert opinion
3.	CIRCI may be diagnosed by a change in the serum cortisol of <9 μg/dL after 250 μg of synthetic ACTH (ACTH stimulation test) or a random total serum cortisol (i.e. bound and free fractions together) <10 μg/dL	Strength of recommendation: GRADE 2B
4.	Free cortisol determination is not recommended for diagnosis of CIRCI because of lack of a defined normal range and a readily available assay	Strength of recommendation: GRADE 2B
5.	The ACTH stimulation test is not recommended for identification of patients with septic shock or ARDS who qualify for steroid therapy	Strength of recommendation: GRADE 2B
6.	Hydrocortisone therapy should be considered in septic shock, especially for poor responders to fluid resuscitation or vasopressor therapy	Strength of recommendation: GRADE 2B
7.	Hydrocortisone therapy (200–300 mg/day) may be indicated in early severe ARDS (P_aO_2/FiO_2 <200) and before day 14 in unresolving ARDS	Strength of recommendation: GRADE 2B
8.	In septic shock, hydrocortisone 50 mg IV should be given 6 hourly (200 mg/day) or as a 100 mg bolus followed by infusion at 10 mg/hour (240 mg/day)	Strength of recommendation: GRADE 1B
	In early ARDS the optimal steroid dose is continuous infusion of methylprednisolone at a total dose of 1 mg/kg/day	
9.	In septic shock, hydrocortisone therapy should last at least 7 days before tapering, assuming no recurrence of sepsis or shock	Strength of recommendation: GRADE 2B
	In early ARDS, hydrocortisone therapy should last at least 14 days before tapering	
10.	Hydrocortisone therapy should not be abruptly terminated, but rather tapered slowly.	Strength of recommendation: GRADE 2B
11.	In addition to hydrocortisone therapy, fludrocortisone therapy (50 μg PO once daily) is optional	Strength of recommendation: GRADE 2B
12.	Dexamethasone is not recommended for treatment of septic shock or ARDS	Strength of recommendation: GRADE 1B

HPA, hypothalamic–pituitary–adrenal; CIRCI, critical illness-related corticosteroid insufficiency; ACTH, adrenocorticotrophic hormone; ARDS, adult respiratory distress syndrome; IV, intravenous; PO, orally.

Data from Marik PE, Pastores SM, Annane D, et al. (2008). Recommendations for the diagnosis and management of corticosteroid insufficiency in critically ill adult patients: consensus statements from an international task force by the American College of Critical Care Medicine. *Critical Care Medicine*, **36**, 1937–49.

the concomitant illness. It is estimated that the incidence of CIRCI is 10–20%, with recent estimates in septic shock as high as 60%.[45–47]

The pathophysiological mechanisms responsible for CIRCI are incompletely understood. Based on the corticosteroid pathway, possible mechanisms include inadequate hormone levels (e.g. CRH, ACTH, vasopressin and/or cortisol) and corticosteroid resistance (e.g. cortisol receptor dysfunction). It is already known that a minority of patients have adrenal failure due to structural damage (haemorrhage, infection, tumour) or functional suppression secondary to exogenous steroid exposure.[44–48] Adrenal haemorrhage may follow blunt trauma, major surgery, sepsis, and burns.[44–49]

However, the majority of patients with CIRCI appear to suffer from reversible dysfunction of the HPA axis.[47] Furthermore, clinical recovery in CIRCI may be delayed due to systemic inflammation-associated glucocorticoid resistance in which there is excessive transcription of inflammatory cytokines, despite high serum cortisol levels.[50] This type of steroid resistance is also described in chronic systemic inflammation as typified by inflammatory bowel disease.[51] Since steroid resistance is a probable mechanism in acute systemic inflammation beyond CIRCI, as typified by cardiac surgery with CPB, it will probably be a focus of future clinical investigation.

Although adrenal insufficiency may be characterized as absolute or relative, these categories in adult critical illness are not only difficult to distinguish but also have limited clinical utility.[52] As a result, the second ACCCM recommendation is that these terms are best avoided in CIRCI.[39] However, the diagnosis of CIRCI is suggested by serum cortisol levels.[53] The third ACCM recommendation is that CIRCI is best diagnosed when the random total cortisol level (protein-bound and serum-free fractions together) is less than 10 µg/dL or when the serum cortisol (δ-cortisol) rises by less than 9 µg/dL in response to 250 µg of synthetic ACTH.[39]

However, these diagnostic endpoints have multiple limitations in practice.[54] The first consideration is that the clinical effects of cortisol depend on the free cortisol level and not the total cortisol level.[55] The determination of a random total cortisol level does not necessarily accurately reflect the free fraction because of fluctuations in binding proteins. Although, consequently, determination of serum-free cortisol is preferable, this test is not readily available and its normal range in critical illness remains undefined. As a result, the fourth ACCM recommendation is that free cortisol determinations are not currently recommended for diagnosis of CIRCI.

The second consideration is that the ACTH stimulation test has limited application in CIRCI. It does not assess the response of the HPA axis to hypotension.[39,47,54] It does not assess the adequacy of stress cortisol serum levels. It is also not adequately reproducible in septic shock.[56] It does not predict response to hydrocortisone therapy in adult respiratory distress syndrome (ARDS) (RCTs)[54–58] or septic shock.(39) The ACCCM panel conducted a meta-analysis of six RCTs in septic shock. In summary, regardless of ACTH response, there was a significant clinical response to hydrocortisone therapy in septic shock (ACTH responders—relative risk 1.37; 95% CI 1.17–1.61; $P < 0.0001$; ACTH non-responders—relative risk 1.38; 95% CI 1.17–1.64; $P = 0.0002$).[39] This lack of predictive power for the ACTH test is probably due to the clinical inability to diagnose steroid tissue resistance. Consequently, the fifth ACCCM recommendation is that glucocorticoid therapy in ARDS and septic shock should not be guided by ACTH testing.

Since diagnostic testing cannot currently guide therapy, significant questions remain. Which criteria can be recommended to guide steroid therapy in septic shock? Which patients with septic shock should receive this intervention? Further results from the ACCCM meta-analysis of six RCTs have helped to answer these important questions from clinicians. This meta-analysis showed that hydrocortisone therapy significantly reversed shock within 7 days of therapy (relative risk 1.39; 95% CI 1.24–1.55; $P < 0.00001$) but did not improve mortality at 28 days (relative risk 0.92; 95% CI 0.79–1.06; $P = 0.25$). The two larger trials in this meta-analysis enrolled patients in septic shock who failed to respond adequately to resuscitation with fluid and vasopressor therapy ($N = 300$ (multi-centre French trial)[58]; $N = 500$ (multicentre European study)[59]). Based on the meta-analysis and the predominant effects of the two larger trials, the sixth ACCCM recommendation is that hydrocortisone therapy should be considered in septic shock, especially in poor responders to fluid and vasopressor therapy.[39]

The results of this important ACCCM meta-analysis are supported by two recent systematic literature reviews.[60,61] The meta-analysis in the second review included eight studies (total $N = 1876$, 1993–2008). Corticosteroid therapy significantly reversed shock within 7 days (64.9% vs. 47.5%; relative risk 1.41; 95% CI 1.22–1.64) regardless of response to ACTH stimulation. Steroid exposure did not significantly improve mortality (42.2% vs. 38.4%; relative risk 1.00; 95% CI 0.84–1.18) or the risk of superinfection (25.3% vs. 22.7%; relative risk 1.11; 95% CI 0.86–1.42).

Corticosteroid therapy in ARDS has been tested in five RCTs (total $N = 518$) with major differences in steroid dose; dosing strategy, and duration of therapy.[39,62] Despite this significant study heterogeneity, they all reported that steroid therapy significantly improved oxygenation, and significantly shortened duration of mechanical ventilation and length of ICU stay (all endpoints had $P < 0.05$). The ACCCM panel demonstrated in a subgroup meta-analysis of patients treated for longer than a week that steroid therapy significantly shortened duration of mechanical ventilation (weighted mean difference 5.59 days; 95% CI 3.49–7.68; $P < 0.001$) and mortality (24% vs. 40%; relative risk 0.62; 95% CI 0.43–0.90; $P = 0.01$).[39]

Based on the heterogeneous data, the seventh ACCM recommendation is that moderate dose glucocorticoid therapy (hydrocortisone 200–300 mg/day) should be considered in early severe ARDS (defined as $Pao_2/Fio_2 < 200$) and before 14 days in the setting of unresolving ARDS. Further trials are required to extend this recommendation to less severe presentations of ARDS.

The remaining five ACCCM recommendations describe the optimal method of administering steroid therapy. The eighth ACCCM recommendation specifies that in septic shock hydrocortisone should be administered as an intermittent regimen (50 mg intravenously every 6 hours) or as a continuous infusion (100 mg bolus, followed by infusion at 10 mg/hour). This recommendation is based on the dosage regimen most commonly utilized in the recent septic shock randomized trials included in the ACCCM meta-analysis.[39] Furthermore, higher steroid doses have been shown in meta-analyses to offer no additional beneficial outcome effects but rather to increase the risks of superinfection, myopathy, and hyperglycaemia.[63–65] This recommendation is further supported by the most recently published meta-analysis of 20 studies from 1966 to 2009 (total $N = 2384$).[66] In this recent analysis, hydrocortisone therapy of 200–300 mg/day increased shock reversal (relative risk 1.12; 95% CI 1.02–1.23; $P = 0.02$), reduced ICU length of stay by 4.49 days (95% CI –7.04 to –1.94; $P < 0.001$), and reduced mortality (relative risk 0.84; 95% CI 0.72–0.97; $P = 0.02$). Furthermore, this lower-dose steroid therapy did not increase adverse events such as gastroduodenal bleeding, superinfection, and/or neuromuscular weakness (all these endpoints had $P \gg 0.05$). Even with this lower steroid dosage, the risk of hyperglycaemia was increased significantly (51.6% vs. 46%; $P < 0.001$). The hyperglycaemia is typically managed easily with insulin infusion.

In early severe ARDS, the eighth ACCCM recommendation suggests that the optimal dosing regimen is methylprednisolone 1 mg/kg/day as a continuous infusion. A further advantage of this infusion technique is the significantly lower severity of the hyperglycaemia that is often associated with bolus steroid therapy.[67]

The ninth ACCCM recommendation has specified the duration of steroid therapy, namely a minimum of 7 days in septic shock and 14 days in ARDS. Thereafter, as per the tenth ACCCM recommendation, steroid therapy should be gradually tapered based on clinical response. This last set of ACCCM recommendations are based on steroid protocols utilized in the recent randomized trials.

The eleventh ACCM recommendation is that supplemental fludrocortisone at a dose of 50 µg/day orally is optional in septic shock. In a recent French multicentre randomized trial, fludrocortisone was utilized in addition to hydrocortisone therapy.[58] At this point, it is considered optional. A randomized trial comparing hydrocortisone alone versus hydrocortisone and fludrocortisone together in septic shock has just been completed (details available at www.clinicaltrial.gov with study number NCT 00320099, accessed 21 January 2010). Its results, when published, might significantly affect this recommendation. The final ACCCM recommendation is that dexamethasone is not recommended in septic shock or ARDS, since it causes prolonged suppression of the HPA axis, further limiting the value of the ACTH stimulation test.[39]

Vasopressin as a vasoactive agent

Vasopressin was described in 1895 when it was discovered that extracts of the posterior pituitary lobe had potent vasopressor effects.[68] Its amino acid sequence was discovered in 1951, and it was synthetically prepared in 1954, a process that earned Du Vigneaud and colleagues the Nobel Prize in 1955.[69,70] Although the benefit of vasopressin in clinical shock was described in 1957,[71] it was not until the 1990s that it was utilized clinically for the vasopressor effects that characterized its discovery more than century earlier.[72] This renewed interest was sparked by the observation that withdrawal of a vasopressin infusion precipitated severe hypotension in a septic patient with bleeding oesophageal varices.[73]

Vasopressin, also known as antidiuretic hormone, is a nonapeptide synthesized in the hypothalamus and secreted from the posterior pituitary. The human hormone is called arginine vasopressin (AVP) as it contains arginine. This descriptive name distinguishes it from its analogues, desmopressin and terlipressin.[74] The triggers for AVP secretion include rising plasma osmolality, as well as decreases in arterial blood pressure and blood volume. Therefore AVP, like corticosteroids, can be considered a stress hormone which acts to maintain homeostasis.

The three types of vasopressin receptors are summarized in Table 10.4 with respect to their locations and functions.[74] It is important to note that there is a direct link between the vasopressin system and the steroid system via the V_3 vasopressin receptors in the anterior pituitary. The release of ACTH is greatly amplified by vasopressin, an interaction that links these two hormonal stress response systems.[75]

The vasopressin agonists used in clinical practice are summarized in Tables 10.5 and 10.6. The focus of this section is to review the roles of vasopressin as a vasoactive agent throughout anaesthetic and critical care practice.

Peri-operative vasopressin in cardiac surgery

Vasodilatory shock after cardiac surgery with cardiopulmonary bypass

Cardiac surgery with CPB is typically associated with serum vasopressin concentration levels >100 pg/mL, which are 20 times higher than the normal levels of 5 ±2 pg/mL.[76] Adult cardiac surgical patients may develop profound vasodilatory shock after CPB as part of the systemic inflammatory response. Independent risk factors for this vasoplegic syndrome include pre-operative heparin exposure, ventricular dysfunction, and chronic angiotensin blockade with angiotensin-converting enzyme (ACE) inhibitors and/or

Table 10.4 Types and functions of vasopressin receptors

Receptor type	Tissue location	Physiological function
V_1	Vascular smooth muscle	Vasoconstriction
V_2	Renal collecting ducts	Osmoregulation via water retention
V_3	Anterior pituitary	Secretion of ACTH

Data from Treschan TA, Peters J (2006). The vasopressin system: physiology and clinical strategies. *Anesthesiology* **105**, 599–612.

Table 10.5 The vasopressin agonists

Agonist	Receptor activity	Clinical utility
Arginine vasopressin	V_1, V_2, V_3	Peri-operative hypotension; septic shock
Desmopressin	V_2	Diabetes insipidus, certain coagulopathies
Terlipressin	V_1	Peri-operative hypotension, septic shock

Data from Treschan TA, Peters J (2006). The vasopressin system: physiology and clinical strategies. *Anesthesiology* **105**, 599–612.

Table 10.6 The vasopressin agonists: typical doses and clinical indications

Agonist	Dose	Clinical comment
Desmopressin	0.3 μg/kg IV	von Willebrand's disease, haemophilia
	5–40 μg nasally	Central diabetes insipidus
Terlipressin	1 mg IV	Refractory intra-operative hypotension
	1–2 mg IV every 6 hours	Septic shock
	1–2 mg IV every 6 hours	Bleeding oesophageal varices
Vasopressin	40 IU bolus intravenously	Cardiopulmonary resuscitation
	0.01–0.04 IU/min	Septic shock (doses >0.1 IU/min avoided to decrease adverse effects)
	10–20 IU bolus followed by infusion up to 0.1 IU/min	Vasoplegic shock after pheochromocytoma resection
	0.04–0.1 IU/min	Vasoplegic shock after cardiopulmonary bypass

IV, intravenous.

Data from Treschan TA, Peters J (2006). The vasopressin system: physiology and clinical strategies. *Anesthesiology* **105**, 599–612.

angiotensin receptor blockers (ARBs).[77,78] This low systemic vascular resistance after CPB is characterized by relative vasopressin deficiency since serum vasopressin levels are <10 pg/mL, 10–20 times lower than expected after exposure to CPB.[79] It follows that exogenous vasopressin would restore systemic vascular tone in this clinical scenario, given its relative deficiency.

Randomized clinical trials have demonstrated that vasopressin infusion at 0.04–0.1 IU/min significantly improves systemic vascular tone in adult vasoplegia after CPB and may allow withdrawal of catecholamine vasopressor support, especially if administered prophylactically in high-risk patients.[79–81] This application of vasopressin is also effective in the management of milrinone-associated vasoplegia after CPB.[82]

Vasodilatory shock after CPB has also increasingly been recognized in the paediatric population, where its prevalence is 3%.[83] The main paediatric risk factor for this syndrome is severe ventricular dysfunction, requiring a ventricular-assist device and/or heart transplant.[83] Clinical trials have already demonstrated the utility of exogenous vasopressin in paediatric vasoplegic shock after CPB with infusions at 0.0001–0.001 IU/kg/min.[84,85]) Given that its efficacy has already been demonstrated in paediatric cardiac surgery, it is likely that vasopressin therapy will have an expanded role in the management of vasoplegia after CPB in this surgical population.

Based on the data from the clinical trials to date, vasopressin deficiency is a major mechanism in vasoplegic shock after CPB, providing the rationale for therapeutic vasopressin infusion within a specified dosage range.[79–86] Although the dosage range utilized in clinical trials appears to be clinically safe, the trials have not been adequately powered or designed to explore adequately the full safety profile of this dosage range.

Potential adverse effects of exogenous vasopressin in the cardiac surgical setting include coronary graft spasm and mesenteric ischaemia. There is strong *in vitro* evidence that vasopressin can cause vasospasm in both the radial artery and internal thoracic artery, with a more pronounced vasospastic effect in the radial artery.[87,88] The clinical significance of these *in vitro* effects has not been fully explored to date.

Furthermore, although vasopressin does cause mesenteric vasoconstriction, current laboratory evidence suggests that, at low doses, it does not precipitate intestinal ischaemia.[89,90] In fact, a low-dose vasopressin infusion was life-saving in an adult cardiac surgical patient with severe post-operative mesenteric ischaemia who developed cardiovascular collapse after successful mesenteric reperfusion.[91] This beneficial cardiovascular profile is further supported by a small observational study ($N = 41$) which demonstrated the cardiac safety and significant benefit of rescue vasopressin infusion in adult cardiac surgical patients with catecholamine-resistant post-cardiotomy shock.[92] In this study, vasopressin therapy was associated with a significant improvement in myocardial performance ($P < 0.05$) and successful cardioversion of tachyarrhythmias to sinus rhythm in 45% of cases.

Right ventricular failure after cardiac surgery with cardiopulmonary bypass

Right ventricular failure after cardiac surgery with CPB is frequently managed with intravenous milrinone infusion. Vasopressin has already demonstrated utility in this setting for the management of milrinone-associated vasoplegia.[82] A second advantage of vasopressin in this clinical scenario is that it does not increase right ventricular afterload, since it is a weak pulmonary vasodilator.[93] Therefore it is a selective systemic vasoconstrictor, which is a major advantage in the management of the pulmonary hypertensive patient with systemic vasoplegia.[94] The clinical efficacy of this pharmacological approach has been demonstrated in both adult and paediatric cardiac surgery.[95,96]

Peri-operative vasopressin in non-cardiac surgery

Vasoplegia associated with angiotensin blockade

Angiotensin II raises systemic blood pressure directly by vasoconstriction and indirectly by stimulation of vasopressin and aldosterone secretion. After renin has formed angiotensin I from angiotensinogen, ACE cleaves angiotensin I to yield angiotensin II. (97) Clinical angiotensin blockade is currently possible with two drug classes, namely the ACE inhibitors (e.g. captopril; ramipril) and the ARBs (e.g. valsartan; losartan).[97] Since these drugs are commonly prescribed for the management of systemic hypertension, heart failure, and/or diabetic nephropathy, they will commonly be encountered in the adult peri-operative setting.[98]

The renin–angiotensin system, the sympathetic system, and the vasopressinergic system are together responsible for vascular tone.[98] Consequently, patients exposed to chronic angiotensin blockade would be expected to be at risk for intra-operative hypotension, since general anaesthesia typically suppresses sympathetic support of vascular tone and chronic angiotensin blockade blunts the rescue role of the renin–angiotensin system. Therefore patients managed chronically with ACE inhibitors and/or angiotensin receptor blockers may be more dependent on the vasopressinergic system for intra-operative vascular tone and avoidance of intra-operative hypotension.[97,98]

Significant hypotension has been demonstrated after induction of general anaesthesia in patients on chronic angiotensin blockade.[99,100] This hypotension may be refractory and require aggressive therapy with ephedrine, noradrenaline, and/or vasopressin agonists such as terlipressin.[101,102] This hypotension associated with angiotensin blockade in the setting of general anaesthesia is most probably the result of lesions in two of the three vasomotor tone systems, namely the sympathetic and renin–angiotensin systems, as described earlier.[97–102] This risk is further exacerbated in the setting of concomitant diuretic therapy, most probably due to the added hypotensive effect of relative hypovolaemia from diuretic exposure.[103] The combination of angiotensin blockade and diuretic therapy is common because it has been strongly recommended in recent guidelines for the management of hypertension.[104]

The risk of hypertension is significantly reduced when angiotensin blockade with ACE inhibitors and/or angiotensin receptor blockers is discontinued at least 10 hours prior to anaesthetic induction.[105,106]. As a consequence, the American College of Physicians recommends that angiotensin blockade is discontinued on the day of surgery, as outlined in their physicians' information and education resource (www.pier.acponline.org, accessed 21 January 2010). Furthermore, this recommendation has been strongly supported in recent anaesthesia guidelines.[107]

While vasopressin therapy is typically very safe in this setting, there are reported risks of coronary and mesenteric ischaemia. There has been at least one reported case of coronary ischaemia and myocardial infarction after administration of terlipressin for intra-operative hypotension.[108] Furthermore, a clinical trial demonstrated that vasopressin therapy for correction of intra-operative hypotension in the setting of angiotensin blockade and general anaesthesia is associated with mesenteric ischaemia. In this trial, mesenteric ischaemia was suggested by reduced gastric mucosal perfusion and an increased serum lactate.[109] As a result of these adverse effects, vasopressin therapy is only recommended for treatment of hypotension refractory to first-line interventions such as fluid administration, reduction of anaesthetic agents, and administration of catecholamines.[97,98]

Vasoplegia associated with phaeochromocytoma resection

The anaesthetic management of phaeochromocytoma is discussed in detail in Chapter 7. The utility of vasopressin in this scenario has been demonstrated in the management of catecholamine-resistant shock after tumour removal.[110–113] The typical bolus dose of vasopressin described has been 5–10 IU, followed by a vasopressin infusion titrated to maintain the mean arterial pressure.

In this setting, vasopressin may offer several advantages. First, it is effective in the presence of residual α-blockade typically utilized in the pre-operative preparation of the patient for surgery.[111–113] Secondly, vasopressin may be required to maintain vascular tone after tumour removal, as vasopressin secretion has been described in phaeochromocytoma.[114,115] Thirdly, the application of vasopressin frequently allows titration of catecholamine support after tumour removal to avoid side-effects such as ventricular arrhythmias.

Vasoplegia in anaphylactic shock

Anaphylactic shock is characterized by profound vasodilatation and the first-line therapy includes epinephrine.[116] However, the vascular response to adrenaline may be inadequate to restore tissue perfusion.[117,118] Vasopressin therapy offers a solution to catecholamine-refractory vasoplegia in anaphylaxis.

Based on a case series, vasopressin therapy has been demonstrated to restore vascular tone and tissue perfusion in severe anaphylaxis in conjunction with first-line measures such epinephrine administration and volume expansion.[118,119] Since anaphylaxis is rare, RCTs to evaluate adrenaline and vasopressin in this disease state do not exist. Clinical recommendations will have to be based on case series and expert opinion. There has been a call to include vasopressin in the early pharmacological response to anaphylactic shock.[119]

Vasoplegia associated with epidural blockade

The sympathectomy associated with epidural blockade triggers endogenous vasopressin secretion to help restore vascular tone.[120,121] In 2004 two case reports demonstrated the utility of vasopressin in maintaining blood pressure during neuraxial anaesthesia.[122,123] A randomized trial ($N =60$) compared vasopressin with noradrenaline or dopamine for management of low vascular tone associated with thoracic epidural anaesthesia.[124] In this trial, vasopressin was significantly faster than dopamine in restoring systemic vascular tone ($P <0.05$), and did not increase serum lactate. However, in contrast with dopamine and noradrenaline, the pH of the gastric mucosa increased significantly in the vasopressin group, indicating splanchnic vasoconstriction.

Vasopressin has also been utilized as a selective systemic vasoconstrictor in patients with severe pulmonary hypertension undergoing procedures requiring anaesthesia.[123] In severe pulmonary hypertension complicated by right ventricular failure, this application of vasopressin maintains right coronary perfusion pressure during neuraxial anaesthesia with no increase in afterload for the right ventricle.[124,125] This pharmacological approach has recently been utilized in parturients with severe primary pulmonary hypertension undergo Caesarean section.[126]

Vasopressin in critical care medicine

Vasopressin in septic shock

Septic shock is typically characterized by advanced systemic vasodilation, relative refractoriness to catecholamines, and a relative deficiency of vasopressin.[127] Recognition of the associated vasopressin deficiency led to the demonstration in multiple clinical trials that vasopressin infusion restored vascular tone in septic shock to improve blood pressure and urine output and to allow significant weaning of concomitant noradrenaline.[128,129] Although these trials established the role of vasopressin in septic shock, they did not demonstrate that vasopressin therapy decreased mortality in septic shock compared with noradrenaline. Therefore a large multicentre study, the Vasopressin and Septic Shock Trial, was undertaken to test for survival benefit due to vasopressin in septic shock.[130]

The hypothesis of this pivotal trial was that low-dose vasopressin rather than noradrenaline would decrease mortality in septic shock. Patients in septic shock managed with a minimum of 5 μg/min of noradrenaline ($N = 778$) were randomized in a double-blind fashion to either low-dose vasopressin (defined as 0.01–0.03 IU/min) or noradrenaline (5–15 μg/min) in addition to open-label vasopressors. Vasopressor management was standardized for all patients enrolled in the trial. The primary endpoint was mortality at 28 days.

There was no significant difference in mortality at 28 days (35.4% vs. 39.3%; $P = 0.11$) or 90 days (43.9% vs. 49.6%; $P = 0.11$). Furthermore, there was no significant difference in serious adverse events (10.3% vs. 10.5%; $P = 1.00$). In the study stratum of less severe septic shock, vasopressin therapy was associated with a lower mortality (26.5% vs. 35.7%; $P = 0.05$). In the severe septic shock subcohort, there was no difference in mortality (44.0% vs. 42.5%; $P = 0.76$). The authors concluded that low-dose vasopressin did not reduce mortality in septic shock, although there may be a survival benefit in patients with less severe septic shock. This study did not take into account the possible confounding effect of corticosteroid therapy, which was not randomized in this trial but rather administered according to clinical judgement at any time in the study period.

To explore the bias of steroid therapy, the authors conducted a post hoc analysis of the study data to test whether low-dose vasopressin in combination with corticosteroid therapy had significant outcome advantage.[131]) The main finding was that, in patients with septic shock who received steroids, vasopressin therapy significantly decreased mortality compared with noradrenaline therapy (35.9% vs. 44.7%; $P = 0.03$). Steroid therapy in septic shock patients exposed to vasopressin significantly increased vasopressin serum levels by 33% at 6 hours ($P = 0.006$) and by 67% at 24 hours ($P = 0.025$). The authors concluded that low-dose vasopressin and steroid therapy significantly decreased mortality in septic shock. It is likely that this therapeutic combination will be tested prospectively in a multicentre randomized trial in the near future.

Adverse effects of vasopressin therapy such as digital ischaemia, hyponatraemia, and mesenteric ischaemia are possible.[132–134] In a single-centre small observational septic shock trial ($N = 63$) ischaemic skin lesions were reported in up to 30% of patients.[135] Although these toxic effects are possible, the latest multicentre trial with the highest power documented no additional significant risk compared with noradrenaline therapy.[130,131] The caveat here is that vasopressin was utilized within a low dosage range.

Vasopressor therapy may remain a major confounder in septic shock trials. The optimal approach is still being defined. While noradrenaline has a central role, recent randomized trials suggest roles for phenylephrine and adrenaline.[136,137] It is essential to interpret future results in septic shock trials in light of the vasopressor regimen and concomitant steroid therapy.

Vasopressin in cardiopulmonary resuscitation

Vasopressin is a core part of the stress response during cardiac arrest.[138] Experimental studies have demonstrated the survival benefit of vasopressin in cardiac arrest.[138] Subsequent randomized clinical trials have demonstrated the utility of bolus vasopressin (20–40 IU per dose) in cardiopulmonary resuscitation.[139,140] Subsequent clinical trials, both individually and in meta-analysis, have demonstrated the clinical equivalency of bolus vasopressin and bolus adrenaline in cardiopulmonary resuscitation for return of spontaneous circulation.[141,142] Current international guidelines recommend vasopressin as an alternative to adrenaline for vasopressor therapy in the management of pulseless cardiac arrest.[138]

Vasopressin therapy in cardiac arrest increases steroid levels because of its stimulation of corticotrophin secretion in the anterior pituitary, as described earlier.[143] Corticosteroid therapy in addition to vasopressin and adrenaline might improve clinical outcome in cardiac arrest. A recent randomized trial demonstrated a significant survival advantage associated with supplemental corticosteroid therapy in guideline-guided cardiopulmonary resuscitation for in-hospital arrest.[144] Further randomized trials are required to confirm this finding before it can recommended for integration into current clinical guidelines.

Conclusions

The clinical utility of steroids and vasopressin is already established in anaesthesia and critical care. Future clinical trials are likely to provide convincing data that will lead to more widespread penetration of these agents throughout peri-operative and ICU medicine. Current data already point to the vital importance of applying the powerful synergy between these agents to enhance clinical outcome. Future clinical trials will undoubtedly include this consideration in their design as they endeavour to optimize clinical outcomes throughout anaesthetic practice.

Key clinical management points

- Based on recent meta-analyses, steroids appear to be safe in adult cardiac surgery with cardiopulmonary bypass. Furthermore, they significantly improve clinical outcomes such as atrial fibrillation and bleeding, as well as length of stay in the intensive care unit and hospital. However, until these favourable results are confirmed in larger randomized controlled trials, steroid administration cannot be recommended for routine clinical application in adult cardiac surgery with cardiopulmonary bypass.

- Dexamethasone is established as an effective prophylaxis against post-operative nausea and vomiting. It is most effective when given at anaesthetic induction. It has been associated with a significantly increased risk of post-operative bleeding in paediatric tonsillectomy.

- Dexamethasone significantly decreases pain associated with propofol injection, as well as post-operative pain in non-cardiac surgery such as laparoscopic cholecystectomy and thyroidectomy.

- Peri-operative steroid therapy decreases laryngeal oedema and enhances extubation success in patients with an endotracheal tube. Furthermore, it significantly decreases sore throat and hoarseness associated with a double-lumen endotracheal tube as well as oedema and trismus after major dental surgery.

- Minimization of peri-operative steroid therapy may improve outcome in selected steroid-dependent surgical populations such as patients with inflammatory bowel disease and patients undergoing solid organ transplantation.

- Patients on exogenous steroids should have their baseline steroid therapy maintained peri-operatively. In general, stress steroids are not recommended in the peri-operative period, except for patients with primary disease of the HPA axis.

- Hydrocortisone therapy should be considered in septic shock, especially poor responders to fluid resuscitation or vasopressor therapy (50 mg every 6 hours (200 mg/day) or a 100 mg bolus followed by infusion at 10 mg/hour (240 mg/day)]. In addition to hydrocortisone therapy, fludrocortisone therapy (50 µg orally once daily) is optional. Hydrocortisone therapy should last at least 7 days and should not be abruptly terminated, but rather tapered slowly

- Hydrocortisone therapy (200–300 mg/day) may be indicated in early severe adult respiratory distress syndrome (ARDS) and before day 14 if it is unresolving. In early ARDS the optimal steroid therapy is continuous infusion of methylprednisolone at a total dose of 1 mg/kg/day and it should last at least 14 days before tapering.

- Vasoplegic shock after cardiac surgery with cardiopulmonary block is characterized by vasopressin deficiency. Vasopressin therapy is able to restore vascular tone in this setting.

Key clinical management points (continued)

- Vasopressin does not cause pulmonary vasoconstriction. As a selective systemic vasoconstrictor, it is particularly useful in vasoplegic shock associated with right ventricular failure and/or severe pulmonary hypertension.

- Vasopressin therapy has demonstrated efficacy in the reversal of vasoplegia associated with angiotensin blockade, phaeochromocytoma resection, anaphylactic shock, and neuraxial blockade.

- Septic shock is associated with vasopressin deficiency. Although vasopressin therapy is effective for the management of the vasoplegia in septic shock, it does not confer a survival advantage, except perhaps in septic shock cases that are of lesser severity or are also managed with steroid therapy.

- Vasopressin is a standard-of-care vasopressor in cardiopulmonary resuscitation.

- As in the case of septic shock, steroid therapy in conjunction with vasopressin therapy may offer a survival advantage in cardiopulmonary resuscitation.

References

1. Chaney MA (2002). Corticosteroids and cardiopulmonary bypass: a review of clinical investigations. *Chest*, **121**, 921–31.
2. Whitlock RP, Rubens FD, Young E, Teoh KH (2005). Pro: steroids should be used for cardiopulmonary bypass. *Journal of Cardiothoracic and Vascular Anesthesia*, **19**, 250–4.
3. Augoustides JG (2007). Use of corticosteroids to prevent atrial fibrillation after cardiac surgery. *Journal of the American Medical Association*, **298**, 283.
4. Whitlock RP, Chan S, Devereaux PJ, *et al.* (2008). Clinical benefit of steroid use in patients undergoing cardiopulmonary bypass: a meta-analysis of randomized trials. *European Heart Journal*, **29**, 2592–600.
5. Moher D, Cook DJ, Eastwood S, Olkin I, Rennie D, Stroup DF (1999). Improving the quality of reports of meta-analyses of randomized controlled trials: the QUOROM statement. Quality of Reporting of Meta-analyses. *Lancet*, **354**, 1896–1900.
6. Jadad AR, Moore RA, Carroll D, *et al.* (1996). Assessing the quality of reports of randomized clinical trials: is blinding necessary? *Controlled Clinical Trials*, **17**, 1–12
7. Downs SH, Black N (1998). The feasibility of creating a checklist for the assessment of the methodological quality both of randomized and nonrandomized studies of health care interventions. *Journal of Epidemiology and Community Health*, **52**, 377–84.
8. Ho KM, Tan JA (2009). Benefits and risks of corticosteroid prophylaxis in adult cardiac surgery: a dose–response meta-analysis. *Circulation*, **119**, 1853–66.
9. Robertson-Malt S, Afrane B, Elbarbary M (2007). Prophylactic steroids for paediatric open heart surgery. *Cochrane Database of Systematic Reviews*, **4**, CD005550
10. Taniguchi T, Koido Y, Aiboshi J, Yamashita T, Suzaki S, Kurokawa A (1999). Change in the ratio of interleukin-6 to interleukin-10 predicts a poor response in patients with the systemic inflammatory response syndrome. *Critical Care Medicine*, **27**, 1262–4.
11. Weis F, Beiras-Fernandez A, Schelling G, *et al.* (2009). Stress doses of hydrocortisone in high-risk patients undergoing cardiac surgery: effects on interleukin-6 to interleukin-10 ratio and early outcome. *Critical Care Medicine* **37**, 1685–90

12. Henzi I, Walder B, Tramer MR (2000). Dexamethasone for the prevention of postoperative nausea and vomiting: a quantitative systematic review. *Anesthesia and Analgesia*, **90**, 186–94.

13. Carlisle J, Stevenson CA (2006). Drugs for preventing postoperative nausea and vomiting. *Cochrane Database of Systematic Reviews*, **3**, CD004125

14. Gan TJ, Meyer TA, Apfel CC, *et al.* (2007). Society for Ambulatory Anesthesia guidelines for the management of postoperative nausea and vomiting. *Anesthesia and Analgesia*, **105**, 1615–28.

15. Apfel CC, Kortila K, Abdalla M, *et al.* (2004). A factorial trial of six interventions for the prevention of postoperative nausea and vomiting. *New England Journal of Medicine*, **350**, 2441–51.

16. Wang JJ, Ho ST, Tzeng JI, Tang CS (2000). The effect of timing of dexamethasone administration on its efficacy as a prophylactic antiemetic for postoperative nausea and vomiting. *Anesthesia and Analgesia*, **91**, 136–9.

17. Czarnetzki C, Elia N, Lysakowski C, *et al.* (2008). Dexamethasone and risk of nausea and vomiting and postoperative bleeding after tonsillectomy in children: a randomized trial. *Journal of the American Medical Association*, **300**, 2621–30.

18. Picard P, Tramer MR (2000). Prevention of pain on injection with propofol: a quantitative systematic review. *Anesthesia and Analgesia*, **90**, 963–9.

19. Singh M, Mohta M, Sethi AK, Tyaqi A (2005). Efficacy of dexamethasone pretreatment for alleviation of propofol injection pain. *European Journal of Anaesthesiology*, **22**, 888–90.

20. Kwak KH, Ha J, Kim Y, Jeon Y (2008). Efficacy of combination intravenous lidocaine and dexamethasone on propofol injection pain: a randomized double-blind, prospective study in adult Korean surgical patients. *Clinical Therapeutics* **30**, 1113–19.

21. Karanicolas PJ, Smith SE, Kanbur B, Davies E, Guyatt GH (2008). The impact of prophylactic dexamethasone on nausea and vomiting after laparoscopic cholecystectomy: a systematic review and meta-analysis. *Annals of Surgery*, **248**, 751–62.

22. Worni M, Schudel HH, Seifert E, *et al.* (2008). Randomized controlled trial on single dose steroid before thyroidectomy for benign disease to improve postoperative nausea, pain and vocal function. *Annals of Surgery*, **248**, 1060–6.

23. Sapolsky RM, Romero LM, Munck AU (2000). How do glucocorticoids influence the stress response? Integrating permissive, suppressive, stimulatory, and preparatory actions. *Endocrine Reviews*, **21**, 55–89.

24. Fan T, Wang G, Mao B, *et al.* (2008). Prophylactic administration of parenteral steroids for preventing airway complications after extubation in adults: meta-analysis of randomized placebo controlled trials. *British Medical Journal*, **337**, a1841.

25. Park SH, Han SH, Do SH, Kim JW, Rhee KY, Kim JH (2008). Prophylactic dexamethasone decreases the incidence of sore throat and hoarseness after tracheal extubation with a double-lumen endobronchial tube. *Anesthesia and Analgesia*, **107**, 1814–18.

26. Christensen AM, Willemoes-Larsen H, Lundby L, Jakobsen KB (1994). Postoperative throat complaints after tracheal intubation. *British Journal of Anaesthesia*, **73**, 786–7.

27. Knoll H, Ziegeler S, Schreiber JU, *et al.* (2006). Airway injuries after one-lung ventilation: a comparison between double-lumen tube and endobronchial blocker. A randomized, prospective, controlled trial. *Anesthesiology* **105**, 471–7

28. Markiewicz M, Brady MF, Ding EL, Dodson TB (2008). Corticosteroids reduce postoperative morbidity after third molar surgery: a systematic review and meta-analysis. *Journal of Oral and Maxillofacial Surgery*, **66**, 1881–94.

29. Yamakage M, Iwasaki S, Namiki A (2008). Guideline-oriented perioperative management of patients with bronchial asthma and chronic obstructive pulmonary disease. *Journal of Anesthesia*, **22**, 412–28.

30. Bousquet J, Clark TJH, Hurd S, *et al.* (2007). GINA guidelines on asthma and beyond. *Allergy*, **62**, 102–12.

31. Rabe KF, Hurd S, Anzueto A, *et al.* (2007). Global strategy for the diagnosis, management, and prevention of chronic obstructive pulmonary disease. GOLD executive summary. *American Journal of Respiratory and Critical Care Medicine*, **176**, 532–55.

32. Subramanian V, Saxena S, Kang JY, Pollok RCG (2008). Preoperative steroid use and risk of postoperative complications in patients with inflammatory bowel disease undergoing abdominal surgery. *American Journal of Gastroenterology*, **103**, 2373–81.

33. Pascual J, Zamora J, Galeano C, Royuela A, Quereda C (2009). Steroid avoidance or withdrawal for kidney transplant recipients. *Cochrane Database of Systematic Reviews*, **1**, CD005632.

34. Segev DL, Sozlo SM, Shin EJ, *et al.* (2008). Steroid avoidance in liver transplantation: meta-analysis and meta-regression of randomized trials. *Liver Transplantation*, **14**, 512–25.

35. de Lange DW, Kars M (2008). Perioperative glucocorticosteroid supplementation is not supported by evidence. *European Journal of Internal Medicine*, **19**, 461–7.

36. Marik PE, Varon J (2008). Requirements of perioperative stress doses of corticosteroids: systematic review of the literature. *Archives of Surgery*, **143**, 1222–6.

37. Gibson N, Ferguson JW (2004). Steroid cover for dental patients on long-term steroid medication: proposed clinical guidelines based upon a critical review of the literature. *British Dental Journal*, **197**, 681–5.

38. Jung C, Inder WJ (2008). Management of adrenal insufficiency during the stress of medical illness and surgery. *Medical Journal of Australia*, **188**, 409–13.

39. Marik PE, Pastores SM, Annane D, *et al.* (2008). Recommendations for the diagnosis and management of corticosteroid insufficiency in critically ill adult patients: Consensus statements from an international task force by the American College of Critical Care Medicine. *Critical Care Medicine*, **36**, 1937–49.

40. Richardson L, Hunter S (2008). Is steroid therapy ever of benefit to patients in the intensive care unit going into septic shock? *Interactive Cardiovascular and Thoracic Surgery*, **7**, 898–905.

41. Fink A, Kosecoff J, Chassin M, Brook RH (1984). Consensus methods: characteristics and guidelines for use. *American Journal of Public Health*, **74**, 979–83.

42. Williams PL, Webb C (1994). The Delphi technique: a methodological discussion. *Journal of Advanced Nursing*, **19**, 180–6.

43. Guyatt G, Gutterman D, Baumann MH, *et al.* (2006). Grading strength of recommendations and quality of evidence in clinical guidelines: Report from an American College of Chest Physicians Task Force. *Chest*, **129**, 174–81.

44. Carrasco GA, Van de Kar LD, Carrasco GA, *et al.* (2003). Neuroendocrine pharmacology of stress. *European Journal of Pharmacology*, **463**, 235–72.

45. Widmer IE, Puder JJ, Konig C, *et al.* (2005). Cortisol response in relation to the severity of stress and illness. *Journal of Clinical Endocrinology and Metabolism*, **90**, 4579–86.

46. Annane D, Maxime V, Ibrahim F, Alvarez JC, Abe E, Boudou P (2006). Diagnosis of adrenal insufficiency in severe sepsis and septic shock. *American Journal of Respiratory and Critical Care Medicine*, **174**, 1319–26.

47. Marik PE, Zaloga GP (2002). Adrenal insufficiency in the critically ill: a new look at an old problem. *Chest*, **122**, 1784–96.

48. Arlt W, Allolio B (2003). Adrenal insufficiency. *Lancet*, **361**, 1881–93.

49. Vella A, Nippoldt TB, Morris JC, III (2001). Adrenal haemorrhage: a 25-year experience at the Mayo Clinic. *Mayo Clinic Proceedings*, **76**, 161–8.

50. Meduri GU, Yates CR (2004). Systemic inflammation-associated glucocorticoid resistance and outcome of ARDS. *Annals of the New York Academy of Sciences*, **1024**, 24–53.

51. Creed TJ, Probert CS (2007). Steroid resistance in inflammatory bowel disease: mechanisms and therapeutic strategies. *Alimentary Pharmacology and Therapeutics*, **25**, 111–22.

52. Meyer NJ, Hall JB. Relative adrenal insufficiency in the ICU: can we at least make the diagnosis? *American Journal of Respiratory and Critical Care Medicine*, **174**, 1282–3.

53. Annane D, Sebille V, Troche G, Raphael JC, Gajdos P, Bellisant E (2000). A 3-level prognostic classification in septic shock based on cortisol levels and cortisol response to corticotropin. *Journal of the American Medical Association*, **283**, 1038–45.

54. Arafah BM (2006). Hypothalamic–pituitary–adrenal function during critical illness: limitations of current assessment methods. *Journal of Clinical Endocrinology and Metabolism*, **91**, 3725–45.

55. Cooper MD, Stewart PM (2003). Corticosteroid insufficiency in acutely ill patients. *New England Journal of Medicine*, **348**, 727–34.

56. Loisa P, Uusaro A, Ruokonen E (2005). A single adrenocorticotropic hormone stimulation test does not reveal adrenal insufficiency in septic shock. *Anesthesia and Analgesia*, **101**, 1792–8.

57. Meduri GU, Golden E, Freire AX, *et al.* Methylprednisolone infusion in patients with early severe ARDS: results of a randomized trial. *Chest*, **131**, 954–63.

58. The Acute Respiratory Distress Syndrome Network (2006). Efficacy and safety of corticosteroids for persistent acute respiratory distress syndrome. *New England Journal of Medicine*, **354**, 1671–84.

59. Annane D, Sebille V, Charpentier C, *et al.* (2002). Effect of treatment with low doses of hydrocortisone and fludrocortisone on mortality in patients with septic shock. *Journal of the American Medical Association*, **288**, 62–71.

60. Sprung CL, Annane D, Keh D, *et al.* (2008). Hydrocortisone therapy for patients with septic shock. *New England Journal of Medicine*, **358**, 111–24.

61. Sligl WI, Milner DA, Sundar S, Mphatswe W, Majundar SR (2009). Safety and efficacy of corticosteroids for the treatment of septic shock: a systematic review and meta-analysis. *Clinical Infectious Diseases*, **49**, 93–101.

62. Meduri GU, Golden E, Freire AX, *et al.* (2007). Methylprednisolone infusion in patients with early severe ARDS: results of a randomized trial. *Chest*, **131**, 954–63.

63. Keh D, Sprung CL (2004). Use of corticosteroid therapy in patients with sepsis and septic shock: an evidence-based review. *Critical Care Medicine*, **32**, S527–33.

64. Minneci PC, Deans KJ, Banks SM, Eichacker PQ, Natanson C (2004). Meta-analysis: the effect of steroids on survival and shock during sepsis depends on the dose. *Annals of Internal Medicine*, **141**, 47–56.

65. Minnecci PC, Deans KJ, Eichacker PQ, Natanson C (2009). The effects of steroids during sepsis depend on dose and severity of illness: an updated meta-analysis. *Clinical Microbiology and Infection*, **15**, 308–18.

66. Annane D, Bellisant E, Bollaert PE, *et al.* (2009). Corticosteroids in the treatment of severe sepsis and septic shock in adults: a systematic review. *Journal of the American Medical Association*, **301**, 2362–75.

67. Weber-Carstens S, Deja M, Bercker S, *et al.* (2007). Impact of bolus application of low-dose hydrocortisone administration on glycemic control in septic shock patients. *Intensive Care Medicine*, **33**, 730–3.

68. Oliver GS, Schafer EA (1895). On the physiological action of extracts of pituitary body and certain other glandular organs. *Journal of Physiology*, **18**, 277–9.

69. Turner RA, Pierce JG, Du Vigneaud V (1951). The purification and the amino acid content of vasopressin preparation. *Journal of Biological Chemistry*, **191**, 21–8.

70. Du Vigneaud V, Gash DT, Katsoyannis PG (1954). A synthetic preparation possessing biological properties associated with arginine-vasopressin. *Journal of the American Chemical Society*, **76**, 4751–2.

71. Wislicki L (1957). Hypotension after neo-synephrine infusion treated by pitressin. *Acta Medica Orientalia*, **16**, 174–7.

72. Landry DW, Levin HR, Gallant EM, *et al.* (1997). Vasopressin deficiency contributes to the vasodilation of septic shock. *Circulation*, **95**, 1122–5.

73. Oliver JA, Landry DW (2007). Endogenous and exogenous vasopressin in shock. *Current Opinion in Critical Care*, **13**, 376–82.

74. Treschan TA, Peters J (2006). The vasopressin system: physiology and clinical strategies. *Anesthesiology*, **105**, 599–612.

75. Tanoue A, Ito S, Honda K, *et al.* (2004). The vasopressin V1b receptor critically regulates hypothalamic-pituitary-adrenal axis activity under both stress and resting conditions. *Journal of Clinical Investigation*, **113**, 302–9.

76. Levine FH, Philbin DM, Kono K, *et al.* (1981). Plasma vasopressin levels and urinary sodium excretion during cardiopulmonary bypass with and without pulsatile flow. *Annals of Thoracic Surgery*, **32**, 63–7.

77. Argenziano M, Chen JM, Choudri AF, *et al.* (1998). Management of vasodilatory shock after cardiac surgery: identification of predisposing factors and use of a novel pressor agent. *Journal of Thoracic and Cardiovascular Surgery*, **116**, 973–80.

78. Mekontso-Dessap A, Houel R, Souselle C, Kirsch M, Thebert D, Loisance DY (2001). Risk factors for post-cardiopulmonary bypass vasoplegia in patients with preserved left ventricular function. *Annals of Thoracic Surgery*, **71**, 1428–32.

79. Argenziano M, Choudri AF, Oz MC, Rose EA, Smith CR, Landry DW (1997). A prospective randomized trial of arginine vasopressin in the treatment of vasodilatory shock after left ventricular assist device placement. *Circulation*, **96** (Suppl), II-286–90.

80. Argenziano M, Chen JM, Cullinane S, *et al.* (1999). Arginine vasopressin in the management of vasodilatory hypotension after cardiac transplantation. *Journal of Heart and Lung Transplantation*, **18**, 814–17.

81. Morales DL, Garrido MJ, Madigan JD, *et al.* (2003). A double-blind randomized trial: prophylactic vasopressin reduces hypotension after cardiopulmonary bypass. *Annals of Thoracic Surgery*, **75**, 926–30.

82. Gold JA, Cullinane S, Chen J, Oz MC, Oliver JA, Landry DW (2000). Vasopressin as an alternative to noradrenaline in the treatment of milrinone-induced hypotension. *Critical Care Medicine*, **28**, 249–52.

83. Killinger JS, Hsu DT, Schleien CL, Mosca RS, Hardart GE (2009). Children undergoing heart transplant are at increased risk for postoperative vasodilatory shock. *Pediatric Critical Care Medicine*, **10**, 335–40.

84. Lechner E, Hofer A, Mair R, Moosbauer W, Sames-Dolzer E, Tulzer G. Arginine-vasopressin in neonates with vasodilatory shock after cardiopulmonary bypass. *European Journal of Pediatrics*, **166**, 1221–7.

85. Lechner E, Dickerson HA, Fraser CD, Jr, Chang AC. Vasodilatory shock after surgery for aortic valve endocarditis: use of low-dose vasopressin. *Pediatric Cardiology*, **25**, 558–61.

86. Jochberger S, Velik-Salcher C, Mayr VD, *et al.* (2009). The vasopressin and copeptin response in patients with vasodilatory shock after cardiac surgery: a prospective, controlled study. *Intensive Care Medicine*, **35**, 489–97.

87. Novella S, Martinez AC, Pagan RM, *et al.* (2007). Plasma levels and vascular effects of vasopressin in patients undergoing coronary artery bypass grafting. *European Journal of Cardiothoracic Surgery*, **32**, 69–76.

88. Wei W, Yang CQ, Furnary A, He GW (2005). Greater vasopressin-induced vasoconstriction and inferior effects of nitrovasodilators and milrinone in the radial artery than in the internal thoracic artery. *Journal of Thoracic and Cardiovascular Surgery*, **129**, 33–40.

89. Khan TA, Bianchi C, Ruel M, Feng J, Selke FW. Differential effects of the mesenteric microcirculatory response to vasopressin and phenylephrine after cardiopulmonary bypass. *Journal of Thoracic and Cardiovascular Surgery*, **133**, 682–8.

90. Asfar P, Bracht H, Radermacher P (2008). Impact of vasopressin analogues on the gut mucosal microcirculation. *Best Practice and Research. Clinical Anaesthesiology*, **22**, 351–8.

91. Luckner G, Jochberger S, Mayr VD, *et al*. (2006). Vasopressin as adjunct vasopressor for vasodilatory shock due to non-occlusive mesenteric ischaemia. *Anaesthetist*, **55**, 283–6.

92. Dunser MW, Mayr AJ, Stallinger A, *et al*. (2002). Cardiac performance during vasopressin infusion in postcardiotomy shock. *Intensive Care Medicine*, **28**, 746–51.

93. Evora PR, Pearson PH, Schaff HV (1993). Arginine vasopressin induces endothelium- dependent vasodilatation of the pulmonary artery: V_1-receptor mediated production of nitric oxide. *Chest*, **103**, 1241–5.

94. Augoustides JG, Ochroch EA (2005). Inhaled selective pulmonary vasodilators. *International Anesthesiology Clinics*, **43**, 101–14.

95. Tayama E, Ueda T, Shojima T, *et al*. (2007). Arginine vasopressin is an ideal drug after cardiac surgery for the management of low systemic vascular resistance hypotension concomitant with pulmonary hypertension. *Interactive Cardiovascular and Thoracic Surgery*, **6**, 715–19.

96. Scheurer MA, Bradley SM, Atz AM (2005). Vasopressin to attenuate pulmonary hypertension and improve systemic blood pressure after correction of obstructed total pulmonary venous return. *Journal of Thoracic and Cardiovascular Surgery*, **129**, 464–6.

97. Augoustides JG (2008). Angiotensin blockade and general anesthesia: so little known, so far to go. *Journal of Cardiothoracic and Vascular Anesthesia*, **22**, 177–9.

98. Lange M, Van Aken H, Westphal M, Morelli A (2008). Role of vasopressinergic V_1 receptor agonists in the treatment of perioperative catecholamine-refractory arterial hypotension. *Best Practice and Research. Clinical Anaesthesiology*, **22**, 369–81.

99. Coriat P, Richer C, Douraki T, *et al*. (1994). Influence of chronic angiotensin-converting enzyme inhibition on anesthetic induction. *Anethesiology*, **81**, 299–307.

100. Brabant SM, Bertrand M, Eyraud D, Darmon PL, Coriat P (1999). The hemodynamic effects of anesthetic induction in vascular surgical patients chronically treated with angiotensin II receptor antagonists. *Anesthesia and Analgesia*, **89**, 1388–92.

101. Meersschaert K, Brun L, Gourdin M, *et al*. (2002). Terlipressin–ephedrine versus ephedrine to treat hypotension at the induction of anesthesia in patients chronically treated with angiotensin converting-enzyme inhibitors: a prospective randomized, double-blinded, crossover study. *Anesthesia and Analgesia*, **94**, 835–40.

102. Boccara G, Ouattara A, Godet G, *et al*. (2003). Terlipressin versus noradrenaline to correct arterial hypotension after general anesthesia in patients chronically treated with renin–angiotensin system inhibitors. *Anesthesiology*, **98**, 1338–42.

103. Kheterpal S, Khodaparast O, Shanks A, O'Reilly M, Tremper KK (2008). Chronic angiotensin-converting enzyme inhibitor or angiotensin receptor blocker therapy combined with diuretic therapy is associated with increased episodes of hypotension in noncardiac surgery. *Journal of Cardiothoracic and Vascular Anesthesia*, **22**, 177–9.

104. Chobanian AV, Bakris GL, Black HR, *et al*. (2003). The seventh report of the Joint National Committee on Prevention, Detection, Evaluation and Treatment of High Blood Pressure. *Journal of the American Medical Association*, **289**, 2560–72.

105. Bertrand M, Godet G, Meersschaert K, Brun L, Salcedo E, Coriat P (2001). Should the angiotensin II antagonists be discontinued before surgery? *Anesthesia and Analgesia*, **92**, 26–30.

106. Comfere T, Sprung J, Kumar MM, *et al*. (2005). Angiotensin system inhibitors in a general surgical population. *Anesthesia and Analgesia*, **100**, 636–44.

107. Augoustides JGT (2009) Should all antihypertensives be discontinued before surgery? In: Fleisher LA (ed) *Evidence-Based Practice of Anesthesiology* (2nd edn), pp 49–54. Saunders Elsevier, Philadelphia, PA.

108. Medel J, Boccara G, van de Steen E, *et al*. (2001). Terlipressin for treating intraoperative hypotension: can it unmask myocardial ischemia? *Anesthesia and Analgesia*, **93**, 53–5.

109. Morelli A, Tritapepe L, Rocco M, *et al.* (2005). Terlipressin versus noradrenaline to counteract anesthesia-induced hypotension in patients treated with renin-angiotensin system inhibitors: effects on systemic and regional hemodynamics. *Anesthesiology*, **102**, 12–19.

110. Tan SG, Koay CK, Chan ST (2002). The use of vasopressin to treat catecholamine-resistant hypotension after phaechromocytoma resection. *Anaesthesia and Intensive Care*, **30**, 477–80.

111. Augoustides JG, Abrams M, Berkowitz D, Fraker D (2004). Vasopressin for hemodynamic rescue in catecholamine resistant vasoplegic shock after resection of massive pheochromocytoma. *Anesthesiology*, **101**, 1022–4.

112. Deutsch E, Tobias JD (2006). Vasopressin to treat hypotension after pheochromocytoma resection in an eleven-year-old boy. *Journal of Cardiothoracic and Vascular Anesthesia*, **20**, 394–6.

113. Roth JV (2007). Use of vasopressin bolus and infusion to treat catecholamine-resistant hypotension during pheochromocytoma resection. *Anesthesiology*, **106**, 883–4.

114. Boccara G, Mann C, Guillon G (1998). Secretion of vasopressin from a human pheochromocytoma. *Annals of Internal Medicine*, **128**, 1049.

115. Grazzini E, Breton C, Derick S, *et al.* (1999). Vasopressin receptors in human adrenal medulla and pheochromocytoma. *Journal of Clinical Endocrinology and Metabolism*, **84**, 2195–203.

116. Levy JH, Adkinson NF (2008). Anaphylaxis during cardiac surgery: implications for clinicians. *Anesthesia and Analgesia*, **106**, 392–403.

117. Laxenaire MC, Mertes PM (2001). Anaphylaxis during anaesthesia: results of a two-year survey in France. *British Journal of Anaesthesia*, **87**, 549–58.

118. Schummer W, Schummer C, Wipperman J, Fuchs J (2004). Anaphylactic shock: is vasopressin the drug of choice? *Anesthesiology*, **101**, 1025–7.

119. Schummer C, Wirsing M, Schummer W (2008). The pivotal role of vasopressin in refractory anaphylactic shock. *Anesthesia and Analgesia*, **107**, 620–4.

120. Carp H, Vadhera R, Jayaram A, *et al.* (1994). Endogenous vasopressin and renin-angiotensin systems support blood pressure after epidural block in humans. *Anesthesiology*, **80**, 1000–7.

121. Ecoffey C, Edouard A, Pruszczynski W, *et al.* (1985). Effects of epidural anaesthesia on catecholamines, renin activity, and vasopressin changes induced by tilt in elderly men. *Anesthesiology*, **62**, 294–7.

122. Vaquero Roncero LM, Julian Gonzalez R, and Muriel Villoria C (2004). Refractory hypotension during anaesthesia in a patient treated with angiotensin receptor blockers. *Revista Española de Anestesiología y Reanimación*, **51**, 338–41.

123. Braun EB, Palin CA, Hogue CW (2004). Vasopressin during spinal anaesthesia in a patient with primary pulmonary hypertension treated with intravenous epoprostenol. *Anesthesia and Analgesia*, **99**, 36–7.

124. De Kock M, Laterre PF, Andruetto P, *et al.* (2000). Ornipressin (Por 8): an efficient alternative to counteract hypotension during combined general/epidural anaesthesia. *Anesthesia and Analgesia*, **90**, 1301–7.

125. Jochberger S, Dunser MW (2008). Arginine vasopressin as a rescue vasopressor to treat epidural anaesthesia-induced arterial hypotension. *Best Practice and Research. Clinical Anaesthesiology*, **22**, 383–91.

126. Price LC, Forrest P, Sodhi V, Adamason DL, Nelson-Piercy C (2007). Use of vasopressin after Caesarean section in idiopathic pulmonary arterial hypertension. *British Journal of Anaesthesia*, **99**, 552–5.

127. Holmes CH, Walley KR (2008). Arginine vasopressin in the treatment of vasodilatory septic shock. *Best Practice and Research. Clinical Anaesthesiology*, **22**, 275–86.

128. Olivier JA, Landry DW (2007). Endogenous and exogenous vasopressin in shock. *Current Opinion in Critical Care*, **13**, 376–82.

129. Russell JA (2007). Vaspressin in vasodilatory and septic shock. *Current Opinion in Critical Care* **13**, 383–91.

130. Russell JA, Walley KR, Singer J, *et al.* (2008). Vasopressin versus noradrenaline infusion in patients with septic shock. *New England Journal of Medicine*, **358**, 877–87.

131. Russell JA, Walley KR, Gordon AC, *et al.* (2009). Interaction of vasopressin infusion, corticosteroid treatment and mortality of septic shock. *Critical Care Medicine*, **37**, 811–18.

132. Ertmer C, Rehberg S, Westphal M (2008). Vasopressin analogues in the treatment of shock states: potential pitfalls. *Best Practice and Research. Clinical Anaesthesiology*, **22**, 393–406.

133. Asfar P, Bracht H, Radermacher P (2008). Imapct of vasopressin analogues on the gut mucosal microcirculation. *Best Practice and Research. Clinical Anaesthesiology*, **22**, 351–8.

134. Sharshar T, Annane D (2008). Endocrine effects of vasopressin in critically ill patients. *Best Practice and Research. Clinical Anaesthesiology*, **22**, 265–73.

135. Dunser MW, Mayr AJ, Tur A, *et al.* (2003). Ischemic skin lesions as a complication of continuous vasopressin infusion in catecholamine-resistant vasodilatory shock: incidence and risk factors. *Critical Care Medicine*, **31**, 1394–8.

136. Morelli A, Ertmer C, Rehberg S, *et al.* (2008). Phenylephrine versus noradrenaline for initial hemodynamic support of patients with septic shock: a randomized, controlled trial. *Critical Care*, **12**, R143.

137. Myburgh JA, Higgins A, Jovanovska A, *et al.* (2008). A comparison of epinephrine and noradrenaline in critically ill patients. *Intensive Care Medicine*, **34**, 2226–34.

138. Wenzel V, Raab H, Dunser MW (2008). Role of arginine vasopressin in the setting of cardiopulmonary resuscitation. *Best Practice and Research. Clinical Anaesthesiology*, **22**, 287–97.

139. Wenzel V, Krismer AC, Arntz HR, *et al.* (2004). A comparison of vasopressin and epinephrine for out-of-hospital cardiopulmonary resuscitation. *New England Journal of Medicine*, **350**, 105–13.

140. Gueugniaud PY, David JS, Chanzy E, *et al.* (2008). Vasopressin and epinephrine vs epinephrine alone in cardiopulmonary resuscitation. *New England Journal of Medicine*, **359**, 21–30.

141. Mukoyama T, Kinoshita K, Nagao K, Tanjoh K (2009). Reduced effectiveness of vasopressin in repeated doses for patients undergoing prolonged cardiopulmonary resuscitation. *Resuscitation*, **80**, 755–61.

142. Sillberg VA, Perry JJ, Stiell JG, Wells GA (2008). Is the combination of vasopressin and epinephrine superior to repeated doses of epinephrine alone in the treatment of cardiac arrest? A systematic review. *Resuscitation*, **79**, 380–6.

143. Kornberger E, Prengel AW, Krismer A, *et al.* (2000). Vasopressin-mediated adrenocorticotrophin release increases plasma cortisol concentrations during cardiopulmonary resuscitation. *Critical Care Medicine*, **28**, 3517–21.

144. Mentzelopoulos SD, Zakynthinos SG, Tzoufi M, *et al.* (2009). Vasopressin, epinephrine and corticosteroids for in-hospital cardiac arrest. *Archives of Internal Medicine*, **169**, 15–24.

Chapter 11

Endocrine surgery: a personal view

Tom R Kurzawinski

Endocrinology and endocrine surgery have emerged as distinctive specialties following a series of discoveries made in the last century. The word 'hormone' was only coined just over 100 years ago by Ernest Starling, Professor of Physiology at University College London. Although the first successful operations on endocrine organs were reported at the turn of the nineteenth century, it was the discovery of hormones and their receptors which helped to define several endocrine disorders caused by excessive or deficient production of particular hormones. This launched endocrinology as a scientific discipline.

Since then, the developments in both disciplines have been closely entwined and mutually beneficial. The ability to measure hormone concentrations accurately refined the indications for surgical interventions, and blocking or replacing their actions made surgery much safer. Advances in anaesthetics, surgical techniques, transplantation, and pharmacology offered new treatments and a chance to cure some of the debilitating endocrine conditions. Rapid progress in radiological and isotope imaging, and more recently genetics, has further strengthened our ability to establish accurate diagnosis and plan appropriate treatment.

The revolution in endoscopic technology and the arrival of minimally invasive surgery has been an important development in surgical techniques and has had a great impact on endocrine surgery. Consequently, endocrine surgery has become one of the most precise and refined of surgical interventions. Success is, in part, due to a close cooperation between the endocrinologist, radiologist, anaesthetist, and surgeon, working together to establish the correct diagnosis, localize the lesion, and prepare the patient for operation. Technological progress has allowed surgeons to introduce new operating strategies and replace explorative 'open' operations with a more targeted and less traumatic approach. Endocrine surgery is ideally suited for the minimally invasive approach, otherwise known as 'keyhole' surgery. In most cases, removal of a small, often benign, tumour will result in a cure without the need for complex reconstruction. Less trauma, smaller incisions, and limited manipulation inside the human body result in less pain, shorter hospital stays, and better scars.

Over time, close partnerships have developed between the anaesthetist and the surgeon—not a 'marriage of convenience', but a real example of teamwork, on which the successful outcome of the operation depends. This particularly applies to endocrine surgery, where mutual understanding and good communication between anaesthetist and surgeon before, during, and after the operation is vital for achieving the best results and avoiding complications. It has been my experience over the years that the best part-nerships take a long time to build, and operating in stable teams should be encouraged and insisted upon. As doctors responsible for the well-being of our patients we should endeavour to preserve best practice and resist ad hoc arrangements of the 'one size fits all' variety.

The terms 'endocrine surgery', as a specialty, and 'endocrine surgeon' are difficult to define, because endocrine organs are found in many different anatomical locations and therefore can be of interest to surgeons from a variety of specialties. Although neurosur-geons seems to have exclusive claim on pituitary surgery, other endocrine organs such as the thyroid, parathyroids, adrenals, and pancreas are operated on by surgeons with a background in general, ear, nose, and throat, head and neck, urological, and hepatopan-creatobiliary surgery. Thyroid operations are by far the most common, and therefore are performed in the majority of hospitals. Parathyroid, pancreatic, and adrenal operations are less common, and are usually performed in larger academic centres by surgeons with more specific expertise and skills. It is in these centres, which attract a large volume of work, that endocrine surgeons operating on endocrine organs are based. Whatever the training background of surgeons operating on endocrine organs, they should never work alone but in cooperation with a team of experts consisting of endocrinologists, radiolo-gists, nuclear physicians, pathologists, geneticists, oncologists, and obviously anaesthet-ists who have special interest in this field. Many well-functioning units have developed this multidisciplinary approach and this model of shared care should be encouraged.

This book is written primarily for anaesthetists who want to develop expertise in the endocrine field, and contains several chapters covering anatomy, physiology, clinical, biochemical and radiological diagnosis and peri-operative management of the specific diseases of endocrine organs. Because of constraints of space, not all aspects of endocrine surgery are discussed in this chapter, and it should be read in association with other chap-ters in this book. In writing it, I have tried to avoid unnecessary repetitions or, even more embarrassing, contradictions, which are common in textbooks with many contributors. My intention was to give the reader a broad but personal surgical perspective of the subject.

Parathyroid surgery (see Chapter 5)

Surgery is the cornerstone of managing patients with hyperparathyroidism and remains the only simple and effective treatment for patients with this condition. The surgical approach to hyperparathyroidism has recently become a focus of intense debate, touch-ing on many relevant issues relating to epidemiology, health economics, clinical and biochemical diagnosis, imaging, and medical and surgical treatment of this condition. Traditional classification of hyperparathyroidism as primary, secondary, and tertiary reflects aetiology of the disease, but other distinctive characteristics such as sporadic or familial, benign or malignant, and recurrent disease also highlight important features of parathyroid pathology relevant to the surgeon. Although clinical issues involved in the decision-making in primary and tertiary hyperparathyroidism are not the same, surgical considerations overlap to some extent, and in this chapter surgery for both conditions will be discussed together.

Incidence, presentation, and indications for surgery

Since the first successful parathyroid surgery performed by Felix Mandl in 1925 in Vienna, primary hyperparathyroidism (PHPT) has changed from a rare to a common clinical condition. At first, all patients diagnosed with primary hyperparathyroidism had symptoms and were found to have either severe bone disease (osteitis fibrosa cystica), which caused pathological, frequently multiple, fractures, or kidney stones. The *aide memoire* of the time, helping to remember symptoms of this disease, was 'painful bones, kidney stones, abdominal groans, psychic moans, and fatigue overtones'. Introduction of routine automated calcium blood tests and better, more sensitive, and more specific parathyroid hormone (PTH) assays have significantly increased the number of patients diagnosed with this condition, many of them being diagnosed in the pre-symptomatic stage. Currently, the annual incidence of PHPT is estimated to be approximately 20 per 100 000, with a prevalence in post-menopausal women of 21 in 1000, which is equivalent to 3 in 1000 patients in the general population.[1,2] Most of these patients have no obvious symptoms and only mildly elevated calcium, and only 20% of them meet indications for surgical intervention.[3] Although most patients diagnosed with hyperprathyroidism are either treated conservatively or merely observed, the number of operations on parathyroid glands is steadily rising.

Diagnosis and localization studies

Diagnosis of hyperparathyroidism is based on plasma biochemistry. Hypercalcaemia with inappropriately elevated PTH levels is a strong indicator of this condition. Additional tests such as renal function tests, vitamin D_3 levels, and urine calcium help to determine the aetiology of hyperparathyroidism and exclude other conditions, such as familial benign hypercalcaemia or vitamin D_3 deficiency, which do not require surgery. With the diagnosis firmly established, the next step is to decide whether the patient should undergo surgery. Localization studies of abnormal parathyroid should only be requested if parathyroidectomy is indicated. Localization studies play no part in establishing diagnosis of hyperparathyroidism but are essential for planning surgery. In the past, with patients undergoing full exploration of the neck and assessment of all parathyroids, the usefulness of these studies was limited, as experienced surgeons were able to find enlarged glands and cure the majority of patients. The introduction of minimally invasive parathyroidectomy and a targeted approach changed all that and the statement that 'the only thing you have to localize before parathyroid surgery is an experienced surgeon' is a witty commentary of the past but not applicable to the present day. Neck ultrasound and sestamibi scan are the best tools for assessing the number, position, and size of enlarged parathyroids. In patients with primary hyperparathyroidism single parathyroid adenoma can be detected with either technique in about 80% of cases, but if both investigations are used to predict the position of an enlarged gland concordantly, sensitivity of localization rises to 90–95%.[4] CT and MRI scans of the neck and chest, angiography, and venous sampling are reserved for difficult cases such as familial or recurrent hyperparathyroidism.[4]

Operating technique and outcomes

The classical approach to parathyroid surgery has been bilateral neck exploration through a large collar incision, identification of all parathyroids, and excision of the enlarged glands. Although this approach has proved very successful in terms of curing hypercalcaemia in about 85–95% of patients with PHPT, it has been challenged by the introduction of unilateral neck exploration, which yielded a similar cure rate and was made possible by improved localization studies.[5] The concept of limited exploration was taken forward by the introduction of minimally invasive parathyroidectomy, which targets only one of the glands, carefully located with the help of ultrasound and sestamibi scanning. Minimally invasive operations are performed through neck incisions less than 3 cm, using either a direct open approach or an endoscope.[6–8] It is estimated that about three-quarters of patients with PHPT are suitable for the minimally invasive approach. Many surgeons use intra-operative PTH monitoring to confirm that biochemical cure has been achieved after removing the pre-operatively localized enlarged gland. The criterion for cure is at least a 50% decrease in PTH plasma concentration measured at 5, 10, and 15 minutes after the removal of an adenoma. Persistently high levels of PTH indicate the presence of a second parathyroid adenoma or multiple-gland hyperplasia and necessitate further exploration.[9,10] Minimally invasive parathyroidectomies can also be performed using local anaesthetic. Surgical treatment of hyperparathyroidism is very successful, and the cure rate for patients with concordant ultrasound and sestamibi findings, even without intra-operative PTH monitoring, is 97%. In patients with discordant pre-operative imaging, when only ultrasound or sestamibi finds the lesion or the tests disagree on its location, intra-operative PTH measurements are essential to maintain this high cure rate.[9]

Standard neck exploration and identification of all parathyroid glands remains the procedure of choice in patients with more than one enlarged gland or with tertiary, recurrent, or familial hyperparathyroidism. It is in these situations that removal of four parathyroid glands might be necessary to achieve a cure and patients require long-term supplementation with oral calcium and vitamin D_3. Surgery for tertiary and familial hyperparathyroidism is more demanding than for single adenomas, and cure rate by first-time surgery is lower (around 85%). Autografting some of the parathyroid tissue into the forearm is acceptable practice in patients with renal hyperparathyroidism, but in the author's opinion is not advisable in genetically determined syndromes such as multiple endocrine neoplasia type 1 (MEN 1), hyperparathyroidism–jaw tumour syndrome, or neonatal severe hyperparathyroidism. Some of the parathyroids can be located in an ectopic position, such as the mediastinum, and may require either sternotomy or minimally invasive endoscopic access.[11] Parathyroid carcinoma is a rare cause of PHPT and its treatment, apart from parathyroidectomy, often involves ipsilateral thyroid lobectomy and lymphadenectomy.[12]

Thyroid surgery (see Chapter 4)

Thyroid surgery has been performed for well over 100 years, but early operations were marred by frequent serious complications and high mortality rate. Continuous improvement in anaesthetic and surgical techniques, as well as in pre- and post-operative care, reduced the risk of adverse outcomes. The incidence of complications is a sensitive measure of the quality of surgery; serious complications are now uncommon (<1%) and mortality from thyroid surgery is close to zero.[13] There is an association between volume of thyroid surgery and outcomes; lower complication rates and shorter hospital stays are achieved by surgeons performing this type of surgery more frequently.[13,14]

Incidence, presentation, and indications for surgery

In a world where 5% of the population have goitres, it is perhaps not surprising that thyroid surgery is the most frequently performed endocrine operation.[15] The most common indication for thyroidectomy is colloid goitre. Many patients with enlarged thyroids are asymptomatic and conservative treatment can be recommended for most of them. About a quarter will have progression of symptoms and will require surgery within 10 years of diagnosis.[16] Classical indications for surgery in multinodular goitres are compression symptoms such as dysphagia, stridor, and venous obstruction. Emergence of autonomous nodules causing thyrotoxicosis and nodules suspected of malignancy are also straightforward indications for surgery. However, many thyroidectomies are performed for less clear indications such as neck discomfort or cosmetic reasons (patient's preference). Endocrinologists and surgeons differ in their approach to managing multinodular goitre, with the former frequently advocating conservative management treatment with either thyroxine or radio-active iodine and the latter favouring surgery.[17]

One of the greatest concerns before surgery for very large goitres is tracheal stenosis and deviation, which can result in difficult intubation. Plain X-ray can help, but a CT scan gives a better view of tracheal distortion and aids planning intubation strategy. The author and many of his peers have never encountered a case of tracheomalacia, and therefore it is assumed that this must be an extremely rare condition. Most of the retrosternal goitre can be resected using the neck approach and sternotomy is rarely indicated.

Surgery for thyroid cancer and potentially malignant solitary nodules constitutes about 20–30% of all thyroidectomies. Although thyroid nodules are found in 5% of middle-aged women and 1% of adult men in the UK,[18] only about 5% of them are thyroid carcinomas. Most thyroid cancers present as solitary nodules and are frequently asymptomatic. Changes of voice or symptoms caused by metastasis to bones or lungs are clearly indicators of advanced disease. About 90% of thyroid cancers are well-differentiated tumours, with papillary more common than follicular; the remaining 10% are medullary and rare anaplastic cancers.[19] Papillary and follicular cancers have very good prognosis with a 10-year survival of 80–90%. Medullary thyroid cancers may be either sporadic or familial and, together with phaeochromocytoma and parathyroid hyperplasia, present as MEN 2. Ninety-eight per cent of patients with MEN 2 syndrome have a mutation of the RET oncogene and can be diagnosed by genetic screening. Children and young adults found to be positive for the RET mutation should be considered for prophylactic thyroidectomy to prevent development of medullary cancer.[20]

Thyrotoxicosis, caused by either autoimmune Graves' disease or an autonomous nodule, is the third indication for thyroid surgery. Surgery for thyrotoxicosis is performed less frequently because of the increasing popularity of treatment with radio-active iodine. All patients undergoing surgery should have thyrotoxicosis and its symptoms controlled pharmacologically with carbimazole, propylthiouracyl, or, less frequently, pre-treatment with Lugol's iodine solution. Some of the patients with thyrotoxicosis are very difficult to control and because of this are considered for surgery. Patients who are clinically asymptomatic, but still have suppressed thyroid-stimulating hormone (TSH) and marginally elevated tri-iodothyronine (T_3) or thyroxine (T_4), should not have their operation cancelled automatically as this result could be the best achievable for them. Peri-operative treatment with β-blockers should be considered for patients who have tachycardia despite normal thyroid function tests.

Diagnosis and assessment of thyroid function and solitary nodules

Thyroid assessment should include clinical, biochemical, radiological, and cytological evaluation. Clinical assessment, consisting of careful history-taking and neck palpation, can be extremely effective in establishing diagnosis and should always be performed first and guide the need for further tests.

Thyroid function is assessed by measurement of T_4, T_3, and TSH levels; thyroid antibodies can be also useful. Evaluation of patients being treated for thyroid malignancy includes measurement of thyroglobulin in patients with well-differentiated thyroid cancers or calcitonin in medullary cancer.[21,22]

Ultrasound is the most useful method of imaging thyroid and an ideal tool for identifying the number and size of nodules and enlarged lymph nodes. It is frequently used to guide biopsy of suspicious non-palpable nodules and for sampling metastatic lymph nodes. CT and MRI scans are both very good at estimating thyroid mass, its retrosternal extension, its tracheal stenosis, and its relation to other neck structures. Radio-active iodine scanning has a role in assessing function of the thyroid nodules, and is essential as a diagnostic and treatment modality for patients who have undergone surgery for papillary or follicular thyroid cancer.[23]

The pre-operative pathological diagnosis of thyroid nodules is usually obtained using fine-needle aspiration cytology; core biopsies are indicated only in rare situations.[19,23,24]

Operating technique

Thyroid surgery remains predominantly an open operation and minimally invasive thyroidectomies are performed infrequently. The possible reasons behind slow uptake of 'keyhole' thyroid surgery by endocrine surgeons is that it offers no significant advantage over standard thyroidectomy through a small collar incision. Minimally invasive surgery is also limited to small thyroid nodules and lymphadenectomy can be very difficult.

Both open and minimally invasive techniques can achieve excellent cosmetic results, minimal pain, and short hospital stay.[8,25] Choice of surgical technique and extent of thyroid surgery depends on the type of pathology and both the short- and long-term aims of the operation. The main principles of thyroid surgery should always be careful dissection, visualization of laryngeal nerves, and preservation of parathyroid glands.

The most common thyroid operations are as follows.

- Lobectomy or hemithyroidectomy—removal of one of the thyroid lobes (left or right hemithyroidectomy) performed mainly for solitary thyroid nodules.
- Near total thyroidectomy, which removes almost all thyroid tissue—performed for large colloid goitres and thyrotoxicosis due to Graves' disease.
- Total thyroidectomy removes all functioning thyroid tissue and is the most common operation for both well-differentiated thyroid cancer and medullary cancer.
- Lymphadenectomy is frequently performed during surgery for malignancy. Central lymphadenectomy involves removal of lymphatic tissue from around the thyroid. Lateral modified neck dissection is indicated for proven or suspected metastases in the carotid lymphatic chain.

Post-operative care and complications after thyroid and parathyroid surgery

Bleeding

The incidence of bleeding after neck surgery is uncommon at about 1%, but is potentially a serious problem. Blood loss during surgery is minimal nowadays in the great majority of cases, but severe intra-operative haemorrhage can still occur when operating on very large vascular goitres with retrosternal extension. However, post-operative bleeding remains a challenge and can be life-threatening. Bleeding into a tight cervical space raises the pressure within the neck and impairs lymphatic and venous drainage, which in turn causes laryngeal oedema and stridor. Patients who develop swelling of the neck after neck surgery and respiratory difficulties should be treated immediately by opening the wound and evacuating the haematoma, but this may not resolve the respiratory problem. Endotracheal intubation will be necessary if symptoms persist and should be performed by the most experienced anaesthetist available, as it could be very difficult. Patients should return to theatre to control bleeding and close the wound.

Infection

Infection after thyroid and parathyroid surgery is rare and therefore routine prophylactic antibiotics are not indicated but should be considered for immunocompromised patients and re-operations. Wound infection rate is less than 2%, and the majority of infections are minor and can be treated conservatively with antibiotics. Severe post-operative staphylococcal and streptococcal wound infection is extremely rare but can be fatal.

Voice impairment

Injury of the recurrent laryngeal nerve(RLN) or the external branch of the superior laryngeal nerve causes voice impairment and diminishes quality of life. Voice changes may be permanent or transient, and the length and severity of dysphonia depends on the type of nerve injury. Transection of the nerve (neurotmesis) leads to permanent vocal cord paralysis, but bruising of the nerve (neuropraxia) without interrupting its continuity can result in a temporal vocal cord paresis. Eventual recovery of function can take as little as a few hours or as long as several months (average 6–8 weeks). The incidence of nerve injury varies from 1% to 20% and depends not only on the surgeon's experience but also on the technical difficulty of the operation determined by the size of the goitre, extensive malignant spread, re-operation, or type of surgery.[26] Unilateral RLN injury causes a hoarse voice, but bilateral injury is much more debilitating and can result in total loss of voice and difficulty in breathing and swallowing, which sometimes requires tracheostomy and feeding gastrostomy. Injury to the external branch of the laryngeal nerve is less noticeable, but can cause some hoarseness with difficulty in singing high notes.

As the effects of damage to the laryngeal nerves can be devastating, avoiding injury to the laryngeal nerves has become one of the top priorities in thyroid and parathyroid surgery. In 1938, Lahey[27] reported a significantly lower incidence of RLN injury following clear visualization of the nerves during surgery compared with operating without nerve identification. Many studies have confirmed this observation and routine identification of the nerves became the 'gold standard' in thyroid surgery, resulting in significant reduction of this complication to about 1%. Recently, intra-operative neuromonitoring has been proposed as a way of aiding nerve identification and predicting their post-operative function. Improved functional outcomes have been reported by some groups,[28,29] but routine use of this technique is still considered controversial and it is not widely implemented.[30]

Hypoparathyroidism

Parathyroid glands, usually four in number, secrete PTH and are responsible for maintaining stable serum calcium levels. They are located very close to the thyroid, often share its blood supply, and are sometimes attached firmly to the thyroid capsule. It is normally possible for the surgeon to identify and preserve some, if not all, of these glands, but during thyroid operation they can be inadvertently removed, bruised, or devascularized, and therefore, even after skilful surgery, they may not function straight away. Hypocalcaemia after hemi-thyroidectomy is very rare, but following near-total or total thyroidectomy 1 in 3 patients have temporary hypocalcaemia, and 1 in 50 have permanent hypocalcaemia, caused by the injury to the parathyroid glands. Dissection of central neck lymph nodes increases this risk. Removal of a single parathyroid adenoma rarely causes hypocalcaemia, but after resection of multiple parathyroid glands a drop in calcium concentration is expected. Patients with low calcium may experience a tingling sensation in their hands, fingers and toes, lips, or around the nose. Very low serum calcium can produce painful muscle cramps and spasms, or even shortness of breath due to spasm of respiratory muscles.

Calcium levels should be measured either within 12 hours of the operation or immediately if symptoms of hypocalcaemia occur. Measurement of PTH levels 3–4 hours after surgery accurately predicts hypocalcaemia and can facilitate a safe early discharge.[31] Symptomatic patients with calcium levels less than 2 mmol/L should be given intravenous infusion of calcium (1.7 mL/kg calcium gluconate 10% diluted with 500 mL of 5% glucose) over 4–6 hours. If calcium remains low, oral supplementation should be commenced with oral alfacalcidol (1–2 µg/day) and Sandocal (1 g four times daily) Plasma calcium concentrations should be checked regularly and medications adjusted accordingly. Detectable levels of PTH in the blood after discharge from the hospital usually indicate parathyroid recovery, and oral calcium and vitamin D_3 can be gradually reduced and withdrawn. In the great majority of patients hypocalcaemia is a transient phenomenon lasting for few days. However, in some patients the parathyroid function might take several months to recover. If permanent hypocalcaemia occurs, this should be treated with the lifelong alfacalcidol.

Hypothyroidism

Thyroid surgery often results in hypothyroidism. Common symptoms are fatigue and weight gain, but quite often patients develop subclinical hypothyroidism detected only by measuring serum TSH levels. Removal of half the thyroid gland causes hypothyroidism in about 10–30% of patients. Maintaining thyroid function after lobectomy depends on the volume of remaining thyroid tissue and its functional capacity, which could be affected by pre-existing thyroiditis or the patient's age.

Near-total and total thyroidectomy always requires post-operative T_4 replacement. If thyroidectomy was performed for a benign condition, the initial dose depends on the patient's weight and age, and is about 50–100 µg or 1.3 µg/kg body weight. This dose is gradually titrated according to clinical symptoms and the results of thyroid function tests. The usual dose is between 1 and 2.2 µg/kg and the tablets are taken once daily. The aim is to achieve clinical euthyroidism and maintain thyroid function tests within normal limits.

After total thyroidectomy for cancer the initial replacement is with T_3 at a dose of 40–60 µg daily. T_3 is a short-acting hormone with shorter half-life than T_4 and therefore has to be taken two or three times daily. Using T_3 rather than T_4 reduces the time of thyroid replacement withdrawal necessary to render the patient hypothyroid before treatment with radio-active iodine is given. Once treatment with radio-active iodine is completed, T_3 is replaced with lifelong T_4. The aim of the treatment with T_4 after thyroidectomy for cancer is not only to maintain euthyroid status but also to suppress the pituitary-released TSH to undetectable levels. High or even normal serum TSH levels can stimulate tumour growth and result in recurrence of thyroid cancer. Doses of T_4 are relatively higher after cancer surgery than after benign disease, and accordingly thyroid function tests might suggest mild hyperthyroidism. However, suppression of serum TSH is one of the most important parts of the treatment of patients with thyroid cancer and any changes to the dose of T_4 should be discussed with members of the thyroid multidisciplinary team.

Surgery for gastroenteropancreatic neuroendocrine tumours

Neuroendocrine tumours form a heterogeneous group of rare neoplasms originating from neuroendocrine cells of pancreatic islets and the gastroenteric and respiratory tract, and from parafollicular C-cells of the thyroid, pituitary gland, and adrenal medulla. The term neuroendocrine tumour is preferred to carcinoid, which is still commonly used to describe serotonin-secreting tumours of the gastroenteric tract. The term apudoma is of historical value.

Incidence, presentation, and genetics

Neuroendocrine tumours of gut and pancreas constitute 2% of all malignant gastrointestinal neoplasms. The incidence of these tumours per 100 000 in the general population is about 1% for carcinoid and 0.4% for pancreatic neuroendocrine tumours (PNETs), but their prevalence is relatively high because of their slow growth and prolonged survival.[32] The incidence of PNETs has increased by a factor of 2–3 in the last two decades, possibly because of the increased radiological detection of asymptomatic tumours.[33]

Non-functional tumours, which form the largest group of PNETs (30–40%), are diagnosed when there is no biochemical or clinical evidence of hormonal imbalance.[34] Non functional PNETs are either asymptomatic, and are detected on imaging for non-specific abdominal complaints, or cause symptoms by either obstructing the lumen of the gastrointestinal tract, pancreatic duct, and bile duct or producing abdominal distension or organ failure due to the shear mass of the primary tumour and metastases.

PNETs are called functional if oversecretion of the particular hormone can be detected by blood tests and also causes a well-defined clinical syndrome:

- **Carcinoid syndrome (see Chapter 6)** occurs in 10% of patients with carcinoid tumour who usually develop liver metastases which release serotonin and other vasoactive compounds into the systemic circulation. The carcinoid syndrome is characterized by flushing, diarrhoea, and less commonly wheezing, carcinoid heart disease, and pellagra. Carcinoid crisis, usually precipitated by anaesthetic induction, surgery or embolization, or radiofrequency treatment, is the extreme clinical manifestation of the carcinoid syndrome, presenting with profound flushing, bronchospasm, tachycardia, and fluctuating blood pressure.[35]

- **Zollinger–Ellison syndrome (gastrinoma)** is caused by oversecretion of gastrin by duodenal (50%) and pancreatic tumours (50%), which in turn stimulates parietal cells in the stomach, causing hyperacidity. Gastrinomas are most common between the ages of 30 and 50. Clinical symptoms include dyspepsia, severe upper gastrointestinal ulcerations frequently complicated by perforation and bleeding, vomiting, and diarrhoea. Gastrinomas are frequently malignant (60–90%) and metastasize to the liver and lymph nodes. They are frequently (25–40%) associated with MEN 1 syndrome, when they tend to be small, multiple, and extra-pancreatic and have better survival that of sporadic gastrinomas.[36]

- **Insulinoma** is the most common type of functional islet cell neoplasm, accounting for about three-quarters of all functioning islet tumours. It presents with hypoglycaemia, caused by overproduction of insulin, associated with fits, sweating, weakness, dizziness, and personality changes.[37] Most insulinomas (90%) are solitary, sporadic, and benign, and only 5–10% of them are multiple tumours associated with MEN 1. Insulinomas are mainly pancreatic tumours with only 1% of them in an extrapancreatic location. They occur most frequently between the ages of 30 and 60 years and are usually about 2 cm in size at detection.[37]

- **VIPoma**, also known as WDHA syndrome (watery diarrhoea, hypochlorhydria, and hypokalaemia), is an islet cell tumour secreting vasoactive intestinal peptide. The average age at diagnosis is 50 years, and the main presenting features are watery diarrhoea, dehydration, and weight loss. About 80–90% are derived from the pancreas and more than 50% of them are malignant.[38]

- **Glucagonoma** is caused by overproduction of glucagons and its defining symptoms are skin rashes, weight loss, and deep vein thrombosis. Laboratory testing reveals high glucagon levels and hyperglycaemia. The average age at presentation is 55 years, and 80% of glucagonomas are malignant. They are mostly sporadic, but 13% are associated with MEN 1.[38]

- **Somatostatinoma**, **GRHoma** (secreting growth hormone releasing factor or hormone), **ACTHoma** (secreting adrenocorticothropin), and **PTHrPoma** (secreting PTH-related protein) are very rare syndromes with incidences of less than 0.1 per 100 000. Clinical presentation is determined by hypersecretion of the particular hormone, and includes diabetes and gallstones (somatostatinoma), acromegaly (GRHoma), Cushing's syndrome (ACTHoma), and hypercalcaemia (PTHrPoma). These tumours are located mainly in the pancreas and ampullary region, and most of them behave in a malignant fashion.[38]

The great majority of neuroendocrine tumours (NETs) are sporadic, but around 10% of them are associated with MEN 1, MEN 2, neurofibromatosis type 1, von Hippel–Lindau disease, and tuberous sclerosis. PNETs most commonly associated with hereditary syndromes are gastrinoma (25–40%) and somatostatinoma (45%). Careful family history, clinical examination, and biochemical as well as radiological tests can give rise to clinical suspicion of familial disease. All patients with a family history of NETs should be referred to a geneticist for counselling and gene testing as diagnosis of familial syndrome has implications for both the patient and their family.[39]

Diagnosis and pre-operative staging

Precise diagnosis and staging of NETs is a challenging and complex task influenced by the plethora of hormones they may produce, variable locations, widely different tumour sizes, which may vary from undetectable to huge, and the relative unpredictability of their biological behaviour. To assess so many variables, a combination of clinical, hormonal, radiological and nuclear imaging, and histological information is necessary.

Thorough clinical evaluation, including both history and examination, is essential and should always form the basis of the assessment. It is usually lack of a good medical history or an unnoticed 'tell-tale sign' which leads to delays in diagnosis which are sometimes measured in years. Formulation of a hypothetical diagnosis based on clinical symptoms and signs should guide further investigations.

Symptomatic patients with a clinical presentation suggesting a hormone-secreting tumour should undergo comprehensive hormonal assessment which may assist in making the initial diagnosis, help with assessing response to treatment, and have some prognostic value. General peptides indicating the presence of a NET are plasma chromogranin A and B, which are produced by neuroendocrine tumours regardless of their secretory status, serum pancreatic polypeptide, calcitonin, and human chorionic gonadotrophin α and β. To assess the secretory status of pancreatic tumours, fasting levels of gastrin, insulin, glucagon, vasoactive intestinal peptide, pancreatic polypeptide, somatostatin, and on rare occasions GHRH, ACTH, or PTHrP should be measured.[38] Diagnosis of insulinoma is confirmed biochemically by a fasting glucose test performed over 12–72 hours during which hypoglycaemia (glucose levels <2.48 mmol/L with insulin levels >5 IU/mL) and high C peptide levels are observed.[40,41]

Radiological and nuclear imaging plays an important role in the assessment and staging of patients with PNETs. Choice of the investigation depends on the clinical situation and type of information asked for. Symptomatic patients with elevated hormone levels require localization of the oversecreting tumour. This could be difficult as some of the insulinomas or gastrinomas may be very small and difficult to detect. Accuracy of abdominal ultrasound, CT scan, or MRI in detecting a small primary tumour depends on the experience of the centre, but generally the quoted sensitivity is <50%. Endoscopic ultrasound is the best test for localizing small pancreatic tumours, with a sensitivity around 90%, and it has largely replaced more invasive intra-arterial calcium stimulation with hepatic venous sampling.[42–44]

NETs express somatostatin receptors (SSTRs), and radiolabelled somatostatin analogues are widely used for detecting primary and metastatic tumours. With the exception of insulinoma, which has a low expression of SSTRs, somatostatin receptor scintigraphy plays a central role in the imaging of NETs with sensitivity of 61–96% for detecting primary or metastatic lesions.[42,45] Newly developed glucagon-like peptide 1 and [18F]fluoro-dihydroxyphenylalanine (DOPA) scintigraphy could be very helpful in improving detection rates for small insulinomas and staging other NETs.[46,47]

Surgery, management, and outcomes

Surgery is the only curative treatment for NETs. Primary carcinoid tumours smaller then 2 cm rarely metastasize, but nodal and liver metastases are present at the time of diagnosis in 40–70% of patients with larger tumours.[38] Carcinoid tumours of the gastrointestinal tract commonly present as surgical emergencies, such as appendicitis, intestinal obstruction, or bleeding, and are usually resected in admitting hospitals. Once definitive histology confirms diagnosis of carcinoid, further radical resection (e.g. right hemicolectomy with regional lymph node clearance for carcinoid of the appendix) should be considered.[38]

Many patients with NETs develop liver metastases, and curative liver resection, sometimes combined with radiofrequency ablation (RFA), is possible in about 10% of cases. Bilobar distribution of metastases precludes curative resection, but in selected patients debulking resection, embolization of the hepatic artery, and RFA can be carried out for palliation, with the intention of reducing tumour size and hormone output.[38] The 5-year survival after liver resection for neuroendocrine metastases is 74–87%.[48,49]

Surgery on functioning carcinoids and some PNETs, especially large ones, can cause a crisis because of the release of excessive amount of hormones. The prophylactic measure to prevent carcinoid crisis is intravenous administration of 50 mg of octetride for 12 hours before and 48 hours after surgery.[50] Similar precautions, such as administration of glucose for insulinoma and proton pump inhibitors for gastrinoma, should be undertaken when operating on PNETs.

Pancreatic surgery for PNETs can be classified into formal resections such as distal pancreatectomy and pancreatoduodenectomy (Whipple's procedure) or enucleation of the tumour from the parenchyma.[33,51] Pancreatic surgery is technically difficult, and until recently most of these operations were performed at the time of laparotomy. Laparoscopic pancreatic surgery for NETs is relatively new, but increasingly some of the enucleations and distal pancreatectomies for small functioning tumours are performed laparoscopically.[52–54] The success rate of surgery for insulinoma is 92–98% and 5-year survival is up to 94%.[38,55] The formation of a post-operative pancreatic fistula is more frequent after enucleation than after resection (15% vs. 4%) and seems to be similar for open and laparoscopic surgery.[41,53] If insulinoma cannot be found during surgery, blind pancreatic resection is not recommended.[40,55] Patients with Zollinger–Ellison syndrome due to sporadic gastrinoma should have the tumour resected as the disease-free survival at 5 years is 40%, but MEN 1 patients with gastrinoma are less likely to benefit from surgery (disease-free 5-year survival 4%).[56]

Non-secreting PNETs are usually large at the time of the diagnosis and require open rather then laparoscopic surgery. Because of their indolent biology, they are more amenable to resection and have better long-term survival than pancreatic cancer. Factors predicting survival are age, grade, distant metastases, tumour functionality, and type of resection.[33] The overall 5- and 10-year survivals for PNETs are 50–80% and 38%, respectively.[33,38]

Adrenal surgery (see Chapters 7 and 8)

Adrenal surgery is performed relatively infrequently, and even the largest tertiary referral centres in the UK, Europe, and the USA rarely carry out more than 30–50 adrenelectomies a year. Recently, however, increased numbers of patients with adrenal pathology have been referred to our service. The reason for this increase in adrenal surgery is probably a combination of a larger number of high-resolution abdominal scans detecting adrenal pathology, more detailed assessment of hormonal function, and concentration of adrenal surgery in centres offering laparoscopic rather than open adrenelectomies. In adrenal surgery, close cooperation between anaesthetist and surgeon is essential.

Adrenal pathology, diagnosis, and indications for surgery

Adrenal incidentaloma

Adrenal masses are common and are frequently discovered incidentally. An adrenal incidentaloma is an adrenal mass discovered by chance during a radiological examination performed for indications other than evaluation of adrenal disease.[57] The frequency of adrenal nodules in 25 studies reporting on 87 065 autopsy studies was 6%, and the prevalence of adrenal incidentalomas detected radiologically is around 4%.[58,59] The frequency of incidentalomas increases with age.[57] The risk of an incidentaloma being a metastasis in patients with previous history of cancer could be as high as 45–73%.[60] The majority of incidentalomas are non-hypersecreting adenomas (70%), but careful assessment can detect subclinical hyperfunction in 16% of patients.[60] The most common hormonal abnormalities caused by incidentalomas are cortisol- or aldosterone-secreting adenomas (5–8% and 1–4%, respectively) and phaeochromocytomas (5–8%).[57,60] Incidentalomas showing hormonal hyperfunction, which can be either subclinical or clinically obvious, should be treated surgically. The size of most incidentalomas at discovery is 1–3 cm. Adrenal masses measuring 4–6 cm, enlarging in size on sequential scans, ones with attenuation of more than 10 Hounsfield units, and delayed washout of contrast are highly suspicious of being malignant (adrenocortical carcinoma or metastasis) and should be resected.[57,60,61]

Cushing's disease/syndrome

Cushing's disease (pituitary-dependent hypercorticolism, see Chapter 7) is the most common form of cortisol oversecretion pathology. ACTH-secreting tumours are located in the pituitary and therefore trans-sphenoidal surgery is the obvious initial treatment (see Chapter 2).[62] However, as the initial remission rate after pituitary surgery for Cushing's disease is only 60–80% and the late relapse rate is up to 25%, some patients still require bilateral adrenelectomy to cure this condition.[62,63]

Cushing's syndrome is commonly caused by either cortisol-secreting adrenal adenomas or rarely adrenocortical carcinomas, but can also be caused by ectopic secretion of ACTH by tumours of mostly neuroendocrine origin (see Chapter 7).[63] An adrenal mass secreting cortisol is an indication for unilateral adrenelectomy. Bilateral adrenelectomy is required to treat Cushing's syndrome due to ectopic ACTH secretion.[63]

The screening test for detecting patients with hypercorticolism is an overnight dexamethasone suppression test. If it is found to be positive, further confirmatory tests should include measurements of serum corticotrophin and blood and 24-hour urine cortisol levels (see Chapter 7).

The typical patient with Cushing's syndrome presents a significant challenge to both anaesthetist and surgeon because of central obesity, short fat neck (buffalo hump), easy bruising, poor wound healing, proximal muscle weakness, and cognitive changes. Frequent comorbidities, such as hypertension, impaired immunity, diabetes mellitus, and osteoporosis, must be also appropriately managed during the peri-operative period.[57] Pharmacological control of hypercorticolism, which can be achieved with ketaconazole, metyrapone, or somatostatin analogues, is not routinely indicated before surgery but can be used if patients have to wait for their operation for a long time or if they are considered unfit for surgery.[62]

Adrenocortical carcinoma

Adrenocortical carcinoma (ACC) is a very rare malignancy with an incidence of 1–2 per million population. It is more common in women and the peak incidence is in the fourth and fifth decades.[64] Clinical presentation depends on whether or not the tumour is hormonally active, which is the case in about 60% of cases. Excess cortisol causes rapidly progressing Cushing's syndrome, androgen-secreting tumours in women cause hirsutism and virilization, and aldosterone hypersecretion leads to hypertension and hypokalaemia. Hormonally inactive adrenocortical cancers often present with abdominal discomfort, pain, and weight loss. Increasingly often they are discovered as incidentalomas during abdominal imaging.[64] Pre-operative staging should include CT or an MRI scan which could be particularly helpful for assessing extension of ACC into the inferior vena cava. The role of positron emission tomography (PET) scans in staging and follow-up of patients with ACC is not certain. Most adrenocortical carcinomas are large at diagnosis and the operation of choice is open adrenelectomy with lymphadenectomy, not a laparoscopic approach. Surgery often needs to be extensive, as neighbouring organs can be invaded and must be removed *en bloc*. Tumour spillage should be avoided at all costs to prevent local recurrence. The prognosis is poor and reported 5-year survival is 16–38%.[64]

Primary aldosteronism

Primary aldosteronism (PA) can be caused by several different adrenal pathologies of which aldosterone-producing adenoma (Conn's syndrome) and bilateral idiopathic adrenal hyperplasia are the most common (35% and 60%, repectively).[65,66] Other, less common, forms of PA include primary (unilateral) adrenal hyperplasia, aldosterone-producing adrenocortical carcinoma, and familial hyperaldosteronism. Primary aldosteronism is the most common form of secondary hypertension, and its estimated prevalence in patients with hypertension is 5–13% which is much higher than 1–2% quoted until recently.[65,66] This sudden increase in the number of patients diagnosed with PA is due to recognition of the fact that many patients with this condition do not have low potassium, and therefore screening for PA by measuring potassium underestimates its prevalence. The recommended test for determining whether hypertensive patients have PA is to measure the ratio of plasma aldosterone concentration (PAC) to plasma rennin activity (PRA). An increased PAC-to-PRA ratio in itself is not diagnostic of primary aldosteronism, and further tests demonstrating inappropriate aldosterone secretion are required to confirm this diagnosis.[65] Adrenal venous sampling is sometimes necessary to differentiate unilateral from bilateral disease, although the procedure is technically difficult and it takes a long time to become expert in performing it.[67] Treatment of PA depends on the type of the disease. The aim is to normalize aldosterone levels and, by achieving this, to prevent morbidity and mortality caused by hypertension, hypokalaemia, and cardiovascular and renal damage.[65,68] Unilateral adenoma or hyperplasia should be treated with unilateral laparoscopic adrenelectomy. Adrenelectomy corrects hypoka-laemia in 98% of patients and improves control of blood pressure in 90%, although only 35% have complete resolution of hypertension with no need for further medications. The best predictors of curing PA are two or less antihypertensive medications, body mass index below 25 kg/m², duration of hypertension of less than 6 years, and female sex.[69] Patients with bilateral adrenal hyperplasia or familial aldosteronism should be treated medically with a mineralocorticoid receptor antagonist (spironolactone or eplerenone) in combination with other antihypertensive medications if required.

Phaeochromocytoma

Phaeochromocytomas of the adrenal medulla (85%) and paragangliomas arising from extra-adrenal chromaffin tissues (15%) are unusual but fascinating tumours secreting catecholamines such as adrenaline, noradrenaline, and dopamine (see Chapter 8).[70] It is notoriously difficult to predict their biological behaviour from histological features, but the majority of them are benign and only 10% are malignant.[57] Biochemical diagnosis is established by measurement of catecholamine and metanephrine levels in the urine and plasma. All patients at presentation should be carefully assessed with either a CT or MRI scan to find out whether they have localized or metastatic disease. Nuclear scanning with MIBG ([^{123}I]meta-iodobenzylguanidine) should be considered before surgery to confirm the diagnosis and exclude multifocal disease.[57] Patients with phaeochromocytoma must be carefully prepared for surgery appropriately to minimize the risk of hypertensive crisis. If biopsy of a large retroperitoneal tumour is considered, the possibility of the mass being a paraganglioma should be excluded biochemically, and in uncertain cases α-blockade (and possibly β-blockade) should be initiated before biopsy.[71] Diagnosis of phaeochro-mocytoma during pregnancy is unusual and difficult to make. Treatment depends on the time of diagnosis in relation to pregnancy. Women in the first and second trimesters should be managed pharmacologically, but surgical resection during the second trimester is recommended.[72] During surgery for phaeochromocytoma extensive manipulation of the tumour should be avoided to prevent a sudden rise of blood pressure. It is of great importance to work with an experienced anaesthetist who is able to control surges of hypertension during the dissection and hypotension after the removal of tumour.

Laparoscopic and open adrenelectomy

Arrival of laparoscopic surgery had a great impact on adrenal surgery. Since the first description of laparoscopic adrenelectomy (LA) in 1992, most adrenelectomies are now performed using a minimally invasive approach.[73] Many case series have demonstrated the advantages of LA versus open adrenelectomy, including less analgesia and trauma, a shorter hospital stay, and better cosmetic results.[74] Despite the lack of prospective rand-omized trials comparing these two techniques, the laparoscopic approach is now the preferred option for most adrenal pathologies. Even large tumours up to 10 cm can be successfully removed using this technique.[75] Partial cortical-sparing LA, a procedure of particular interest for patients with hereditary syndromes, can be performed for selected patients with well-defined lesions. However, open adrenelectomy should be considered for patients with high cardiopulmonary risk or previous extensive abdominal surgery, and patients who have adrenal masses larger than 10–12 cm. Open adrenelectomy is preferred for patients with suspicion of malignant adrenal mass. The overall morbidity associated with LA is 9.5%, with bleeding and injury to surrounding organs being the most common reported complications. Severe hypercarbia and acidosis are rare.[74] The reoperation rate is 1.2% and overall mortality is low at 0.2%.[74] LA can be performed trans- or retroperitoneally. The former is more popular, but both procedures are equally safe and effective.[74,76] LA for phaeochromocytoma is associated with a higher conversion rate, longer operating time, and more blood loss compared with LA for other indications. Haemodynamic changes during LA and open adrenelectomy for phaeochromocytoma have been said to be similar (see Chapter 8).[74] Low intra-abdominal pressures (8–10 mmHg) have been recommended as resulting in fewer haemodynamic disturbances.[77] Dissection of the adrenal gland should be very careful, as fragmentation of the gland can result in local recurrence.[74] LA for Conn's and Cushing's syndromes, both unilateral and bilateral, are very successful in curing these diseases and have almost completely replaced need for open surgery for these indications.

References

1. Melton LJ, III (1991). Epidemiology of primary hyperparathyroidism. *Journal of Bone and Mineral Research*, **6** (Suppl 2), S25—30.

2. Adami S, Marcocci C, Gatti D (2002). Epidemiology of primary hyperparathyroidism in Europe. *Journal of Bone and Mineral Research*, **17** (Suppl 2), N18–23.

3. Bilezikian JP, Potts JT, Jr., Fuleihan G, *et al.* (2002). Summary statement from a workshop on asymptomatic primary hyperparathyroidism: a perspective for the 21st century. *Journal of Bone and Mineral Research*, **17** (Suppl 2), N2–11.

4. Bartsch DK, Rothmund M (2009). Reoperative surgery for primary hyperparathyroidism. *British Journal of Surgery*, **96**, 699–701.

5. Russell CF, Dolan SJ, Laird JD (2006). Randomized clinical trial comparing scan-directed unilateral versus bilateral cervical exploration for primary hyperparathyroidism due to solitary adenoma. *British Journal of Surgery*, **93**, 418–21.

6. Pang T, Stalberg P, Sidhu S, *et al.* (2007). Minimally invasive parathyroidectomy using the lateral focused mini-incision technique without intraoperative parathyroid hormone monitoring. *British Journal of Surgery*, **94**, 315–19.

7. Miccoli P, Berti P, Materazzi G, Massi M, Picone A, Minuto MN (2004). Results of video-assisted parathyroidectomy: single institution's six-year experience. *World Journal of Surgery*, **28**, 1216–18.

8. Henry JF (2006). Minimally invasive surgery of the thyroid and parathyroid glands. *British Journal of Surgery*, **93**, 1–2.

9. Lew JI, Solorzano CC, Montano RE, Carneiro-Pla DM, Irvin GL, III (2008). Role of intraoperative parathormone monitoring during parathyroidectomy in patients with discordant localization studies. *Surgery*, **144**, 299–306.

10. Barczynski M, Konturek A, Cichon S, Hubalewska-Dydejczyk A, Golkowski F, Huszno B (2007). Intraoperative parathyroid hormone assay improves outcomes of minimally invasive parathyroidectomy mainly in patients with a presumed solitary parathyroid adenoma and missing concordance of preoperative imaging. *Clinical Endocrinology*, **66**, 878–85.

11. National Institute for Health and Clinical Excellence (2009). *NICE Guideline IPG247. Thoracoscopic Excision of Mediastinal Parathyroid Tumours.* Available online at: http://www.nice.org.uk/guidance/IPG247 (accessed 24 January 2010).

12. Rawat N, Khetan N, Williams DW, Baxter JN (2005). Parathyroid carcinoma. *British Journal of Surgery*, **92**, 1345–53.

13. McHenry CR (2002). Patient volumes and complications in thyroid surgery. *British Journal of Surgery*, **89**, 821–3.

14. Sosa JA, Bowman HM, Tielsch JM, Powe NR, Gordon TA, Udelsman R (1998). The importance of surgeon experience for clinical and economic outcomes from thyroidectomy. *Annals of Surgery*, **228**, 320–30.

15. Gaitan E, Nelson NC, Poole GV (1991). Endemic goiter and endemic thyroid disorders. *World Journal of Surgery*, **15**, 205–15.

16. Winbladh A, Jarhult J (2008). Fate of the non-operated, non-toxic goitre in a defined population. *British Journal of Surgery*, **95**, 338–43.

17. Bhagat MC, Dhaliwal SS, Bonnema SJ, Hegedus L, Walsh JP (2003). Differences between endocrine surgeons and endocrinologists in the management of non-toxic multinodular goitre. *British Journal of Surgery*, **90**, 1103–12.

18. Tunbridge WM, Evered DC, Hall R, *et al.* (1977). The spectrum of thyroid disease in a community: the Whickham survey. *Clinical Endocrinology*, **7**, 481–93.

19. Mazzaferri EL (1993). Management of a solitary thyroid nodule. *New England Journal of Medicine*, **328**, 553–9.

20. Machens A, Niccoli-Sire P, Hoegel J, *et al.* (2003). Early malignant progression of hereditary medullary thyroid cancer. *New England Journal of Medicine*, **349**, 1517–25.

21. Spencer CA, Fatemi S (2006). Thyroglobulin. In: Mazzaferri EL, Harmer C, Mallick UK, Kendall-Taylor P (eds) *Practical Management of Thyroid Cancer: A Multidisciplinary Approach.* Springer-Verlag, London.

22. Pinchera A, Elisei R (2006). Medullary thyroid cancer: diagnosis and mangement. In: Mazzaferri EL, Harmer C, Mallick UK, Kendall-Taylor P (eds) *Practical Management of Thyroid Cancer: A Multidisciplinary Approach.* Springer-Verlag, London

23. Hegedus L (2004). Clinical practice. The thyroid nodule. *New England Journal of Medicine*, **351**, 1764–71.

24. Schlumberger MJ (1998). Papillary and follicular thyroid carcinoma. *New England Journal of Medicine*, **338**, 297–306.

25. Stalberg P, Delbridge L, van Heerden J, Barraclough B (2007). Minimally invasive parathyroidectomy and thyroidectomy—current concepts. *Surgeon*, **5**, 301–8.

26. Hermann M, Alk G, Roka R, Glaser K, Freissmuth M (2002). Laryngeal recurrent nerve injury in surgery for benign thyroid diseases: effect of nerve dissection and impact of individual surgeon in more than 27,000 nerves at risk. *Annals of Surgery*, **235**, 261–8.

27. Lahey FH (1938). Routine dissection and demonstration of recurrent laryngeal nerves in subtotal thyroidectomy. *Surgery, Gynecology and Obstetrics*, **66**, 775–7.

28. Dralle H, Sekulla C, Haerting J, *et al.* (2004). Risk factors of paralysis and functional outcome after recurrent laryngeal nerve monitoring in thyroid surgery. *Surgery*, **136**, 1310–22.

29. Barczynski M, Konturek A, Cichon S (2009). Randomized clinical trial of visualization versus neuromonitoring of recurrent laryngeal nerves during thyroidectomy. *British Journal of Surgery*, **96**, 240–6.

30. National Institute for Health and Clinical Excellence (2009). NICE Guideline IPG 255. Intraoperative nerve monitoring during thyroid surgery. Available online at: http://www.nice.org.uk/guidance/IPG255 (accessed 24 January 2010).

31. Grodski S, Lundgren CI, Sidhu S, Sywak M, Delbridge L (2009). Postoperative PTH measurement facilitates day 1 discharge after total thyroidectomy. *Clinical Endocrinology*, **70**, 322–5.

32. Watson RG, Johnston CF, O'Hare MM, *et al.* (1989). The frequency of gastrointestinal endocrine tumours in a well-defined population—Northern Ireland 1970–1985. *Quarterly Journal of Medicine*, **72**, 647–57.

33. Bilimoria KY, Talamonti MS, Tomlinson JS, *et al.* (2008). Prognostic score predicting survival after resection of pancreatic neuroendocrine tumors: analysis of 3851 patients. *Annals of Surgery*, **247**, 490–500.

34. Eriksson B, Oberg K (2000). Neuroendocrine tumours of the pancreas. *British Journal of Surgery*, **87**, 129–31.

35. Soga J, Yakuwa Y, Osaka M (1999). Carcinoid syndrome: a statistical evaluation of 748 reported cases. *Journal of Experimental and Clinical Cancer Research*, **18**, 133–41.

36. Soga J, Yakuwa Y (1998). The gastrinoma/Zollinger–Ellison syndrome: statistical evaluation of a Japanese series of 359 cases. *Journal of Hepatobiliary–Pancreatic Surgery*, **5**, 77–85.

37. Soga J, Yakuwa Y, Osaka M (1998). Insulinoma/hypoglycemic syndrome: a statistical evaluation of 1085 reported cases of a Japanese series. *Journal of Experimental and Clinical Cancer Research*, **17**, 379–88.

38. Ramage JK, Davies AH, Ardill J, *et al.* (2005). Guidelines for the management of gastroenteropancreatic neuroendocrine (including carcinoid) tumours. *Gut*, **54** (Suppl 4), iv1–16.

39. Toumpanakis CG, Caplin ME (2008). Molecular genetics of gastroenteropancreatic neuroendocrine tumors. *American Journal of Gastroenterology*, **103**, 729–32.

40. Dolan JP, Norton JA (2000). Occult insulinoma. *British Journal of Surgery*, **87**, 385–7.

41. Tucker ON, Crotty PL, Conlon KC (2006). The management of insulinoma. *British Journal of Surgery*, **93**, 264–75.

42. Chiti A, Fanti S, Savelli G, *et al.* (1998). Comparison of somatostatin receptor imaging, computed tomography and ultrasound in the clinical management of neuroendocrine gastro-entero-pancreatic tumours. *European Journal of Nuclear Medicine*, **25**, 1396–1403.

43. Slooter GD, Mearadji A, Breeman WA, *et al.* (2001). Somatostatin receptor imaging, therapy and new strategies in patients with neuroendocrine tumours. *British Journal of Surgery*, **88**, 31–40.

44. Anderson MA, Carpenter S, Thompson NW, Nostrant TT, Elta GH, Scheiman JM (2000). Endoscopic ultrasound is highly accurate and directs management in patients with neuroendocrine tumors of the pancreas. *American Journal of Gastroenterology*, **95**, 2271–7.

45. Schillaci O, Spanu A, Scopinaro F, *et al.* (2003). Somatostatin receptor scintigraphy in liver metastasis detection from gastroenteropancreatic neuroendocrine tumors. *Journal of Nuclear Medicine*, **44**, 359–68.

46. Wild D, Macke H, Christ E, Gloor B, Reubi JC (2008). Glucagon-like peptide 1-receptor scans to localize occult insulinomas. *New England Journal of Medicine*, **359**, 766–8.

47. Kauhanen S, Seppanen M, Ovaska J, *et al.* (2009). The clinical value of [^{18}F]fluoro-dihydroxyphenylalanine positron emission tomography in primary diagnosis, staging, and restaging of neuroendocrine tumors. *Endocrine-Related Cancer*, **16**, 255–65.

48. Que FG, Nagorney DM, Batts KP, Linz LJ, Kvols LK (1995). Hepatic resection for metastatic neuroendocrine carcinomas. *American Journal of Surgery*, **169**, 36–42.

49. Iwao M, Nakamuta M, Enjoji M, *et al.* (2001). Primary hepatic carcinoid tumor: case report and review of 53 cases. *Medical Science Monitor*, **7**, 746–50.

50. Roy RC, Carter RF, Wright PD (1987). Somatostatin, anaesthesia, and the carcinoid syndrome. Peri-operative administration of a somatostatin analogue to suppress carcinoid tumour activity. *Anaesthesia*, **42**, 627–32.

51. Crippa S, Bassi C, Salvia R, Falconi M, Butturini G, Pederzoli P (2007). Enucleation of pancreatic neoplasms. *British Journal of Surgery*, **94**, 1254–9.

52. Gagner M, Pomp A, Herrera MF (1996). Early experience with laparoscopic resections of islet cell tumors. *Surgery*, **120**, 1051–4.

53. Fendrich V, Langer P (2007). Minimally invasive surgery for pancreatic endocrine tumours. *British Journal of Surgery*, **94**, 1187–18.

54. Isla A, Arbuckle JD, Kekis PB, *et al.* (2009). Laparoscopic management of insulinomas. *British Journal of Surgery*, **96**, 185–90.

55. Rostambeigi N, Thompson GB (2009). What should be done in an operating room when an insulinoma cannot be found? *Clinical Endocrinology*, **70**, 512–15.

56. Norton JA, Fraker DL, Alexander HR, *et al.* (1999). Surgery to cure the Zollinger–Ellison syndrome. *New England Journal of Medicine*, **341**, 635–44.

57. Young WF, Jr. (2007). Clinical practice. The incidentally discovered adrenal mass. *New England Journal of Medicine*, **356**, 601–10.

58. Kloos RT, Gross MD, Francis IR, Korobkin M, Shapiro B (1995). Incidentally discovered adrenal masses. *Endocrine Reviews*, **16**, 460–84.

59. Bovio S, Cataldi A, Reimondo G, *et al.* (2006). Prevalence of adrenal incidentaloma in a contemporary computerized tomography series. *Journal of Endocrinological Investigation*, **29**, 298–302.

60. Barzon L, Sonino N, Fallo F, Palu G, Boscaro M (2003). Prevalence and natural history of adrenal incidentalomas. *European Journal of Endocrinology*, **149**, 273–85.

61. Miller JC, Blake MA, Boland GW (2009). Definitive characterisation of adrenal lesions. *British Medical Journal*, **338**, a3092.

62. Mullan KR, Atkinson AB (2008). Endocrine clinical update. Where are we in the therapeutic management of pituitary-dependent hypercortisolism? *Clinical Endocrinology*, **68**, 327–37.

63. Chow JT, Thompson GB, Grant CS, Farley DR, Richards ML, Young WF, Jr. (2008). Bilateral laparoscopic adrenalectomy for corticotrophin-dependent Cushing's syndrome: a review of the Mayo Clinic experience. *Clinical Endocrinology*, **68**, 513–19.

64. Allolio B, Fassnacht M (2006). Clinical review. Adrenocortical carcinoma: clinical update. *Journal of Clinical Endocrinology and Metabolism*, **91**, 2027–37.

65. Young WF (2007). Primary aldosteronism: renaissance of a syndrome. *Clinical Endocrinology*, **66**, 607–18.

66. Ganguly A (1998). Primary aldosteronism. *New England Journal of Medicine*, **339**, 1828–34.

67. Young WF, Stanson AW (2009). What are the keys to successful adrenal venous sampling (AVS) in patients with primary aldosteronism? *Clinical Endocrinology*, **70**, 14–17.

68. Rossi GP, Bernini G, Desideri G, *et al.* (2006). Renal damage in primary aldosteronism: results of the PAPY study. *Hypertension*, **48**, 232–8.

69. Zarnegar R, Young WF, Jr., Lee J, *et al.* (2008). The aldosteronoma resolution score: predicting complete resolution of hypertension after adrenalectomy for aldosteronoma. *Annals of Surgery*, **247**, 511–18.

70. Lenders JW, Eisenhofer G, Mannelli M, Pacak K (2005). Phaeochromocytoma. *Lancet*, **366**, 665–75.

71. Sood SK, Balasubramanian SP, Harrison BJ (2007). Percutaneous biopsy of adrenal and extra-adrenal retroperitoneal lesions: beware of catecholamine secreting tumours! *Surgeon*, **5**, 279–81.

72. Brunt LM (2001). Phaeochromocytoma in pregnancy. *British Journal of Surgery*, **88**, 481–3.

73. Gagner M, Lacroix A, Bolte E (1992). Laparoscopic adrenalectomy in Cushing's syndrome and pheochromocytoma. *New England Journal of Medicine*, **327**, 1033.

74. Assalia A, Gagner M (2004). Laparoscopic adrenalectomy. *British Journal of Surgery*, **91**, 1259–74.

75. Walz MK, Petersenn S, Koch JA, Mann K, Neumann HP, Schmid KW (2005). Endoscopic treatment of large primary adrenal tumours. *British Journal of Surgery*, **92**, 719–23.

76. Hanssen WE, Kuhry E, Casseres YA, de Herder WW, Steyerberg EW, Bonjer HJ (2006). Safety and efficacy of endoscopic retroperitoneal adrenalectomy. *British Journal of Surgery*, **93**, 715–19.

77. Sood J, Jayaraman L, Kumra VP, Chowbey PK (2006). Laparoscopic approach to pheochromocytoma: is a lower intraabdominal pressure helpful? *Anesthesia and Analgesia*, **102**, 637–41.

Index